T0325260

Advance Praise for *Revolutionary Surgeons*

"Readers will be surprised and edified by learning about the professional and personal lives of notable Revolutionary era surgeons on both sides of the Atlantic, as well as the reality of what wounded and ill soldiers encountered during eight long years of the American Revolutionary War. Patriot American surgeons and physicians were operating out of the same Anglo-British and Euro-centric tradition as their politically Loyalist professional colleagues. In *Revolutionary Surgeons* we learn about those shared bases in Enlightenment medicine and the gritty real work of military and community surgical practice during the Revolutionary era. Based on close readings of notable physicians' biographies, Dr. Hasselgren seamlessly interweaves their personal lives, occasional rivalries, innovative procedures, and both famous and obscure patients' experiences.

"Those wanting to immerse themselves in the formative years of the United States will find much to be educated and edified by Per-Olof Hasselgren's book, which brings an authoritative and compassionate approach to the subject that only a distinguished Harvard Medical faculty member could."
—Samuel A. Forman, author of *Dr. Joseph Warren: The Boston Tea Party, Bunker Hill, and the Birth of American Liberty* and *Ill-Fated Frontier: Peril and Possibilities in the Early American West*

"Intriguing in scope, and deftly written, *Revolutionary Surgeons* is a spirited tale of driven personalities, magnificent ideas, and tragic shortcomings. It is a fascinating and timely survey of America's surgical beginnings; an essential source for those interested in understanding the role that surgeons played during the Revolutionary War, militarily, politically, and socioeconomically."

—Ira Rutkow, author of *A History of Medicine in America; Bleeding Blue and Gray; Civil War Surgery and the Evolution of American Medicine; Surgery: An Illustrated History*, named a *New York Times* Notable Book of the Year; Dr. Rutkow is a recipient of the American Medical Writers Association Medical Book Award, and the Fletcher Pratt Literary Award of the Civil War Round Table of New York. She has been inducted into The Johns Hopkins University's Society of Scholars, and awarded Union College's Founders' Medal.

Revolutionary Surgeons

PATRIOTS *and* LOYALISTS *on the* CUTTING EDGE

Per-Olof Hasselgren

A KNOX PRESS BOOK
An Imprint of Permuted Press
ISBN: 978-1-64293-888-3
ISBN (eBook): 978-1-64293-889-0

Revolutionary Surgeons:
Patriots and Loyalists on the Cutting Edge
© 2021 by Per-Olof Hasselgren
All Rights Reserved

Cover Image: From "The Death of General Warren at the Battle of Bunker's Hill, June 17, 1775" by John Trumbull, c1831, Museum of Fine Arts, Boston. MA

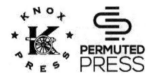

Permuted Press, LLC
New York • Nashville
permutedpress.com

Published in the United States of America
1 2 3 4 5 6 7 8 9 10

CONTENTS

INTRODUCTION

Although most aspects of the American Revolution have been well researched and documented, the medical and surgical treatment in the army during the Revolutionary War, as well as the surgeons' political and military engagements, have often been overlooked.

Surgeons played important roles in the American Revolution. Many were actively involved in politics as well as on the battlefields. Surgeries performed at the time were heroic, both from the surgeons' standpoint and, in particular, from the perspective of patients who agreed to undergo major, utterly painful procedures, performed without anesthesia.

The young nation in the process of being born had to grapple with several important organizational issues related to military and civilian medical care, the establishment of hospitals, and the equipment and supplies of the surgeons. In addition, the training and licensing of physicians were not well regulated—or regulated at all.

Before the establishment of medical schools in America, students striving toward careers in medicine and surgery could either apply for an apprenticeship with an established physician in the colonies, or travel to Europe for training. Going to Europe for studies (commonly to London and Edinburgh) was expensive and typically required the support of wealthy parents. The payoff, however, was training under prestigious surgeons, and exposure to modern ways to treat patients. Physicians returning from training abroad were held in high esteem and looked upon as the most educated and expert doctors in their communities, especially if they came back with an MD degree.

Even though a local apprenticeship required a fee paid to the master, the cost was only a fraction of two or three years of training in London, or elsewhere in Europe. The duration of a surgical apprenticeship in the colonies was about two years (but sometimes longer), and the cost was around one hundred pounds, paid upfront to the master. For this fee, the apprentice would live in the master's home and become part of the household. For the medical training, the master allowed the apprentice to participate in all aspects of his medical and surgical practice, including seeing patients in his office and participating in-home visits. The apprentice would also assist during surgical and obstetric procedures. In addition, the master provided theoretical education and guided reading in anatomy, physiology, and pharmacology. The apprenticeship was typically secured with a contract signed by the practitioner and by somebody (often the trainee's father) promising to pay the master, stating that the master would provide instructions "in the…Mysterys of Physick and Surgery." At the end of the apprenticeship, the master would issue a certificate, confirming both the training and that the physician student was qualified to start his own practice.

At the outbreak of the revolution, there were about 3,000 "doctors" in the colonies serving a population of approximately 2.5 million. Only about 350 physicians were fully trained and licensed, and even fewer had additional training in Europe.

Most "hospitals" at the time of the American Revolution were temporary, and consisted of private homes, barns, meetinghouses, churches, and other public buildings. During the 1700s, only two major hospitals—in today's sense of the word—were in use. A hospital was established in Philadelphia in 1755 with the support of Benjamin Franklin. In 1771, King George III granted a charter to establish the New York Hospital. Construction of the hospital began in 1773. Tragically, the building was destroyed in a major fire before its completion and had to be rebuilt. The reconstruction was delayed because of the Revolutionary War, and the hospital could not be fully opened until 1791.

The same cities saw the first medical schools in America founded in Philadelphia in 1765, and New York City in 1768. Boston had to wait until 1782 to see the establishment of Harvard Medical School.

There are many reasons why it is of interest to learn about surgeons and surgery at the time of the American Revolution. There were surgeons who participated in the deliberations of the Continental Congresses. Four of the fifty-six signers of the Declaration of Independence were physicians, including the renowned Philadelphia surgeon Benjamin Rush. Among the members of the Massachusetts Provincial Congresses in 1774 and 1775, twenty-two were surgeons, most of whom came to be actively involved in bloody engagements during various Revolutionary War military campaigns. Indeed, historians have commented that if it hadn't been for the fatal injury sustained by a certain surgeon at Bunker Hill, it is possible that the first commander-in-chief of the United States would have been a surgeon.

Although it may be easy to forget, many colonists were opposed to the idea of breaking away from Britain, and there were also members of the medical profession who were Loyalists and wanted to remain faithful to the king. One prominent surgeon, who was probably a "closet" Loyalist, was accused by George Washington of being a traitor, and was found guilty of spying for the British enemy. One of the busiest surgeons in Massachusetts had to send his family away for safety reasons when the locals in Salem, just north of Boston, discovered that their surgeon was a Loyalist.

This book tells the stories of surgeons who played important political, military, and medical roles at the time of the American Revolution. It also provides insight into the medical care and surgical procedures during this era. Much innovation in medicine during the 1700s took place in Europe, in particular in England and France. Young, aspiring American surgeons voyaged across the ocean for training with famous colleagues at world-renowned institutions, mainly in London and Edinburgh.

Surgeries during the 1700s were hurried (to reduce the patients' suffering), performed with unclean instruments, risky, and often resulted in death of the patients. The procedures were, to a great extent, surgeries for injuries—both civilian, caused by accidents, and war-related, incurred on the battlefields. In the civilian life, there were many opportunities to get injured—people fell off horses and carriages and fractured their legs and skulls, and they sustained injuries when working on the farms, ships, and in the harbors. Several conditions unrelated to trauma were also managed by surgeons, including bladder stones, hernias, breast tumors, and tumors of the abdomen.

During wartime, surgeons had ample opportunities to practice their skills in treating gruesome injuries caused by swords, bayonets, guns, and cannons—and the eighteenth century saw its share of wars. Multiple conflicts between England and France, as well as between other European countries, resulted in numerous bloody battles. In 1754, tensions between France and Britain escalated into the French and Indian War on the American continent. The war spread and developed into a worldwide conflict known in Europe as the Seven Years' War (1756–1763). The Revolutionary War (1775–1783) added to the need for surgeons on the American continent, with surgeons participating on both sides of the conflict. Surgeries performed for injuries suffered on the battlefields, such as amputations, disarticulations, and treatment of fractures and wounds, were great in number.

There are many circumstances related to surgeries during the 1700s that are worthy of reflection. First, surgeries were remarkably performed without anesthesia. Today, it is almost impossible to comprehend that people would agree to have surgery while being awake and undergoing indescribable suffering. The pain and risks were staggering, and many people chose to continue to suffer from their conditions and ultimately die rather than submit themselves to the horrendous pain inflicted by the surgery.

Second, bacteria were unknown, and the role of antiseptic techniques was not understood. Infectious complications were common—if not the rule. Formation of pus in the wound was actually considered laudable and a sign of proper healing. In other, less happy situations, the infections caused the death of patients who had survived the surgery itself.

Third, many American surgeons traveled to Europe for training and brought new insight and ideas with them when returning to the colonies. The propagation of cutting-edge knowledge, however, was slow. Awareness of novel surgical techniques first had to travel across the Atlantic for weeks or months before hitting the American shore. Once these techniques finally arrived on the American continent, establishing know-how throughout the colonies was also a slow process.

Additionally, although many surgeons were involved in the American Revolution and became important freedom fighters, other surgeons were Loyalists and opposed the idea of separation from the motherland. One such surgeon was Dr. James Lloyd, who trained Joseph Warren during his apprenticeship. Dr. Edward Holyoke in Salem started out as a Loyalist, but became a Patriot when he recognized where the wind was blowing. Another surgeon, Dr. Benjamin Church, was a Patriot by name but probably a Loyalist in his heart. He was found guilty of spying for the British. Although he claimed that the reason he provided secret information to the enemy was to ultimately prevent a bloody military conflict on the American continent, he was found guilty of treason and was expelled from America, only to be lost at sea under unclear circumstances.

Finally, recognizing the role of surgeons and surgery during the 1700s requires an understanding of the society and its view on healthcare. The eighteenth century was the age of enlightenment. Philanthropy and humanitarianism emphasized that society had a responsibility to care for its dependents, including the mentally ill, poor, women, children, soldiers, and sailors. Many hospitals were established with the purpose of caring for the indigent, particularly in London, where a number of such hospitals were opened. The clinical experience surgeons from America acquired in these hospitals was an important part of their training.

Although important advances in surgery took place in many European countries during the eighteenth century, England and France were the two hotbeds. Because many American surgeons journeying to Europe for training went to England, the British and Scottish surgeons had the greatest influence on surgery in the colonies. Surgeons in London and Edinburgh were particularly important for the training of surgeons from the colonies.

Even though this is not a surgical textbook, some technical aspects of procedures are discussed. In general, though, most of the surgeries are described in layman's terms and from patients' perspectives, to give a better understanding of the human and emotional aspects surrounding the surgeries.

The surgeons described in the book were not only skillful and courageous in the execution of their craft, but they also displayed many less favorable traits, including betrayal, jealousy, backstabbing, adultery, and selfish ambitions. Many of these characteristics, of course, make them stand out as mere mortals, despite their revered places in history.

The American Revolutionary War ended only eight years after its start in 1775, but the events leading up to the rebellion and its aftermath left a stamp on most of the century. Therefore, the history of surgeons and surgery at the time of the American Revolution is, to a great extent, the history of surgery during the eighteenth century.

It is astonishing that any surgery could be performed during the 1700s—or, for that matter, at any time before 1846, the year of the first surgery performed under ether anesthesia. It is also amazing that many patients actually survived their surgeries. Because knowledge about bacteria had not yet entered the stage, antisepsis was not practiced. This was made even worse by a general lack of cleanliness. Because of poor or nonexistent sanitary conditions in military camps and in society as a whole, the spread of infectious diseases was unbridled, resulting in epidemics killing large numbers of people. It has been estimated that more soldiers died from causes other than injuries sustained on the battlefield during the Revolutionary War, and it was a widespread understanding that it was more dangerous to be admitted to a hospital than to participate in a battle.

Bleeding after surgery was often profuse and sometimes stopped in the most gruesome way. An iron spatula that was heated on burning coal till it was glowing was applied to the wound—almost like branding cattle. The method cauterized not only blood vessels, but surrounding muscles, fat, and other tissues as well, filling the room with fumes and the smell of burning flesh, in addition to screams from the suffering patients.

Because of the pain inflicted on the patient during surgery, speed was of essence. This decreased the precision of the surgical procedures. There were stories of amputations being performed in seconds that resulted in the amputation of not only the patient's leg, but also of fingers belonging to the assistants holding it down.

The eighteenth century saw important advancements in medicine in general, and surgery in particular. It was a time when scientific observations began to influence medicine, and surgery started to emerge as a specialty of its own. Despite the fact that anesthesia would not arrive on the scene until the following century, surgeons were able to perform remarkable and heroic procedures. The patients, of course, were the true heroes, allowing surgeons to cut and slice into them while experiencing unimaginable pain. It was also a time when knowledge about the human anatomy expanded rapidly, which explains why the 1700s have been called "the age of the surgeon-anatomist."

In addition to disorders requiring the knife, there were a large number of nonsurgical conditions that needed physicians' attention, including diarrhea, malnutrition, and epidemics such as smallpox, tuberculosis (consumption), yellow fever, cholera, typhus, and venereal diseases. In the 1700s, surgeons were often involved in the management of such conditions as well.

Even though this is not a book about the American Revolution per se, a short list of important events related to the revolution will allow readers to put them in the context of the surgeons who were active at the time.

Important Dates Related to the American Revolution

1764. The British Parliament passes the Sugar and Currency Acts.

1765. The Stamp Acts imposed by the Parliament
The Stamp Act riots in Albany, New York, and Boston
The founding of the Sons of Liberty

1767. The Townshend Acts

1768. Samuel Adams organizes protests against continued creation of repressive laws by Parliament.
Four thousand British troops deployed in Boston

1770. The Boston Massacre (March 5)

1773. The Destruction of the Tea, later called the "Boston Tea Party" (December 16)

1774. The Intolerable Acts imposed by Parliament
The First Continental Congress meets in Philadelphia.

1775. The midnight rides of Paul Revere and William Dawes
The Battles at Lexington and Concord (April 19), spawning the Revolutionary War
The Siege of Boston
The Battle of Bunker Hill (June 14)
The Second Continental Congress in Philadelphia

George Washington appointed commander in chief

1776. Henry Knox brings cannons from Fort Ticonderoga to Boston.

The British army evacuates Boston (March 17)

The Declaration of Independence (July 4)

The Battle of Long Island

British troops capture New York

Washington's crossing of the Delaware River on night of Christmas Dayday

1777. The Continental Army suffers many defeats and is close to being disbanded.

The British army is defeated at Saratoga.

The Continental Army enters winter camp at Valley Forge.

Baron von Steuben arrives from Germany and begins training Washington's troops.

1778. France enters the war on the Rebels' side.

British troops leave Philadelphia.

1780. Benedict Arnold's betrayal

1781. The Articles of Confederation

The British army is defeated at Yorktown.

1783. The peace treaty of Paris brings the American Revolution to conclusion.

1787. The Constitutional Convention meets in Philadelphia and creates the American Constitution.

1788. The Constitution is ratified.

1789. George Washington is elected the first American president, and John Adams vice president.

CHAPTER 1

JOSEPH WARREN—
Surgeon, Patriot, Hero

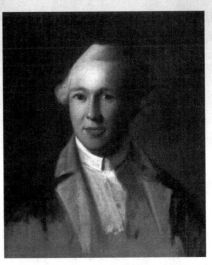

Joseph Warren (1741–1775). Portrait by John Singleton Copley, circa 1772. At the time the portrait was painted, Warren was only three years away from being killed at the Battle of Bunker Hill. (World History Archive)

The British hated him. At Bunker Hill, the Redcoats not only killed him; they also trampled and mutilated his dead body, decapitated him, and threw him into an unmarked grave. It would take almost a year before the burial pit was found and the body could be identified. Had Bunker Hill not happened, it is possible that the first president of the United States would have been a surgeon.[1]

The Early Years

Joseph Warren (1741–1775) was born in Roxbury, a town of only 500 that was just southwest of Boston. His father, also named Joseph, was a farmer and an apple grower. Joseph was the firstborn child, with three more sons added to the family over the next twelve years. He was two months shy of turning thirty-four when the Revolutionary War broke out.

When Joseph was fourteen, his father fell down from an apple tree, broke his neck, and died "in a few moments."[2] At the time of the accident, Joseph had just started his studies at Harvard University. Thanks to efforts by his mother, Mary, and financial support from neighbors, Joseph was able to complete his studies and graduate in 1759. In those days, when a young boy was sponsored by a town or village to go to college, it was common practice for him to return the favor by teaching at a local school. Adhering to that tradition, Joseph served as a teacher at Roxbury Latin Grammar School for two years after graduating from Harvard. Today, a statue of Warren stands outside the Roxbury Latin School to memorialize his service to the community, commemorating the ties between Roxbury and Warren.

Not many details are known from Warren's college years. It has been reported that he enjoyed and was successful at chemistry. Studies in the Greek and Latin languages were obligatory for all students. It is possible that Warren was a member of the debating club. He was interested in theater, and produced and directed plays in his own dormitory room.

Although it is not known if Warren participated in many extracurricular activities, there would certainly have been opportunities. Harvard students could frequent taverns in Cambridge that were described as "marts of luxury, intemperance, and ruin." There were ample opportunities to find places for drinking, gambling, and "the company of loose women." Students could easily find drinking holes and other venues where prostitutes were available. It was also no secret that "women of ill fame" provided services in the dorm rooms at Harvard.[3]

What is known about Joseph's lifestyle during his Harvard years would suggest that he did not often pursue "illicit pleasures." Being ranked low on the social scale, he probably conducted a life that was simpler and less expensive than that of his wealthier classmates. His dorm room was frugally furnished with "a lone shelf, a wooden bench, and a bed. He had partially furnished his room with a 'great' chair and small mirror from his Roxbury home."[4] These were much simpler accommodations than what many of his fellow students enjoyed. Likely, Warren spent much of his free time at his home in Roxbury, helping his mother with the farm and orchard and looking after his younger brothers.

During his college years, it became clear to Warren that he wanted to pursue a career in medicine and surgery. Warren was a driving force behind the Anatomical Club, also called the Spunkers.[5] Members of the Spunkers were Harvard undergraduates who were planning to go into medicine. The main focus of the club was to foster interest and knowledge in anatomy. In order to make that possible, the members (including Joseph and, later, his brother John) resorted to, or were at least aware of, grave robbery and procurement of bodies from freshly executed criminals to provide corpses for dissection. The Anatomical Club is usually considered a forerunner to Harvard Medical School.

While teaching at Roxbury Latin Grammar School after graduating from Harvard, Warren pursued self-studies to qualify for a Master of Arts degree. His thesis, delivered as an oral dissertation in Latin, was approved and he was granted his degree in 1762. By then, he was already well into his apprenticeship with Dr. James Lloyd, a renowned local physician, surgeon, and obstetrician.

Apprenticeship with Dr. James Lloyd

Warren started his apprenticeship with Dr. Lloyd in 1761. Lloyd had received surgical training in England and had been taught by William Cheselden and Samuel Sharp. He was esteemed by Bostonians. During the French and Indian War, he had served as a young surgeon in the British army.

Lloyd's practice included many patients from the higher society of colonial Boston. He was reported to have "a more respectable circle of professional business than any other physician of his day."[6] It was no wonder that the apprenticeships offered by Lloyd were considered excellent and prestigious, and therefore highly competitive.

Lloyd must have seen Warren as a promising future student because he was allowed to start his training with the fee of one hundred pounds on credit. Half of the amount was in his mother's name, and half in his own. Warren could look forward to an outstanding experience when he arrived for his apprenticeship. His training with Lloyd not only prepared him for his medical practice, but it also resulted in a lifelong friendship between the two doctors.

Although medicine, and surgery in particular, underwent dramatic developments during the 1700s, many old theories about the origin of diseases and their treatments remained popular. The ancient theory that diseases reflected imbalances between the four humors of the body (blood, yellow bile, black bile, and phlegm) was still prevalent, explaining why bleeding, purging, and cupping continued to be part of the treatment of many conditions throughout the eighteenth century. In addition to the surgical training, which was the main focus of the apprenticeship, Warren also learnt about bloodletting and cupping, and received instructions in herbal and chemical medications. Physicians at that time prepared medicines themselves and dispensed many prescriptions in their offices, a practice that often became an important source of extra income.

Another area of training during the apprenticeship was that of dentistry, mainly extraction of diseased teeth or implantation of prosthetic ones. Transplantation of teeth from dead or living donors was a peculiar practice during the 1700s. The practice originated in Europe, but also caught on in the colonies.

Because anesthesia had not yet made its debut, other methods were used to diminish the pain and agony associated with surgical procedures. Large amounts of wine and laudanum (a mixture of opium and alcohol) were given to the patients, but despite this, they had to be held down by strong assistants to make the procedures possible. Although the patients suffered the most, it must have also been hard on the surgeons to recognize the pain and suffering they inflicted, and to listen to the screams of horror during the surgeries. It took unimaginable courage for patients to consent to surgery, knowing what awaited them. Only patients with life-threatening conditions or diseases that resulted in severe pain and suffering would consider surgery.

In order to reduce the agonizing pain, speed was of essence. Surgeries were frequently associated with complications, including severe infections, significant blood loss, and high death rates. Surgical operations during the 1700s have been described as "brutal, fast, dirty, and all too often deadly."[7]

Amputation was a common procedure during the 1700s. It was most often performed because of severe infections, gangrene caused by poor blood supply to the extremity, or compound (open) fractures. During the Revolutionary War, injuries sustained on the battlefield became a common indication for amputations.

"Cutting for the stone" (removal of bladder stones or lithotomy) was another procedure performed by surgeons in those days. Lloyd had been exposed to the latest techniques in lithotomy when training in London, and brought that knowledge back to Massachusetts. It is likely that, in London, William Cheselden's innovative work in this field had influenced Lloyd, and that he performed "lateral lithotomy" for bladder stones, although the suprapubic approach was being used as well.[8] Warren was probably exposed to both techniques during his apprenticeship and could apply both. Most likely, Warren treated many patients with bladder stones, since it was a common condition in the 1700s.

The Smallpox Epidemic of 1764

After completing two years of apprenticeship, Warren was ready to start his own practice. Warren began seeing patients in Roxbury in June of 1763, but moved his practice into Boston after only a couple of months. Surgery was not yet accepted as a separate specialty, and physicians preferentially practicing surgery also took care of patients with nonsurgical problems, such as infections, diarrheas, and even toothache.

Within a year after opening his practice, Warren became engaged in an event that was not new to Boston, but disastrous every time it hit—an outbreak of smallpox. Although mainly trained as a surgeon, Warren became involved in the treatment of smallpox victims and efforts to try to stop the epidemic.

Smallpox epidemics were recurrent events in colonial America, with previous outbreaks occurring in Boston in 1721, 1730, and 1752. One method by which protection against the dreaded disease could be obtained was inoculation. The inoculation was performed by introducing pus (containing smallpox virus) from ripe pustules of a smallpox patient into a superficial skin incision made on the person who was being inoculated. This typically resulted in a "mild," controlled case of smallpox, still severe enough to make the person suffer from significant illness with fevers, malaise, back and headaches, nausea, vomiting, and eruption of skin lesions. These signs and symptoms could last for several weeks or even months. Although most individuals survived, inoculation could also result in death. Inoculation rendered the individual more or less immune to the disease in the future. Even if the inoculated individual was affected by smallpox later in life, the risk of death from the disease was substantially reduced.[9]

During the 1721 epidemic, inoculation was introduced in Boston by Reverend Cotton Mather and Dr. Zabdiel Boylston. The procedure was initially met with outrage and anger by the community, mainly because it was considered dangerous and potentially deadly. The clergy was strong in their opposition (Reverend Mather was an exception); they thought smallpox was God's way of punishing sinful people, and trying to prevent the malady would interfere with God's plans and create "distrust of God's overruling care."[10] The local populace became polarized, and angry words and threats were flying. Indeed, so strong was the opposition to the inoculation that Boylston had to go into hiding. Despite that, he was arrested for his actions and his wife and children were threatened by a hand grenade thrown into their home. On another occasion, Mather's home was firebombed with a message attached to the missile reading, "Cotton Mather, You Dog, Dam you, I'll inoculate you with this, with a Pox to you."[11]

The first cases of the 1764 epidemic occurred in January in the North End of Boston. The epidemic spread rapidly, with new people getting sick and dying on a daily basis. Governor Francis Bernard arranged for a group of physicians headed by Dr. Nathaniel Perkins, and including doctors Benjamin Church, Elisha Lord, James Lloyd, and Joseph Warren, to provide inoculations to the general population. The place for the inoculations was Castle William, a military fort on the strategic Castle Island, just outside Boston. According to an announcement in the *Boston Gazette* on March 5, 1764, inoculations were available from that day until the middle of May.[12] The work performed by the physicians at Castle William was an act of charity, provided without cost. Performing the inoculations exposed the physicians to the deadly disease, and the doctors were hailed as heroes by the populace of Boston.

Interestingly, John Adams, the future president, was one of the individuals inoculated at Castle William in April of 1764. Adams was twenty-nine at the time. After the inoculation, Adams was kept for observation in a room of the temporary "smallpox hospital," together with other people who had been inoculated. No inoculated person was released until the last pustule had healed. In a letter to his then fiancée Abigail, Adams described his encounter with Joseph Warren at Castle William and wrote of Warren as a "pretty, tall, genteel, fair faced young Gentleman."[13]

The smallpox epidemic of 1764 kept Warren busy. Although the inoculations subjected him to great dangers, they also provided an opportunity to establish important contacts and build a reputation in the city—factors that became important in the effort to establish a medical practice. After the outbreak Warren and his colleagues were celebrated as heroes by the Bostonians.

Building a Medical and Surgical Practice

The reputation Warren earned from his involvement in the inoculations helped boost his practice. Accepting apprentices also helped Warren gain a reputation and provided increased income, as well as the manpower to sustain an expanding practice. During his surgical career, Warren trained five apprentices, all of whom would play important roles not only in the medical and surgical fields, but in the American Revolution as well. They were all Harvard graduates and had been members of the Spunkers at Harvard. The list of trainees included names such as Samuel Adams

Jr. (son of the prominent patriot Samuel Adams), John Warren (Joseph's younger brother and the future founder of Harvard Medical School), and William Eustis (who later switched from medicine to politics and ended up secretary of war under John Madison during the 1812 conflict, then ambassador to Holland, and ultimately governor of Massachusetts).

After almost a decade of continuous growth, Warren felt that he needed—and could afford—more space for his practice and private residency. In 1770, Warren rented a house on Hanover Street in the North End, and used the house both for patient care and living quarters for his family. Based on the typical layout of houses in Boston during the 1700s, the home occupied by Warren probably had two floors, and perhaps an attic loft for the accommodation of servants (often slaves from Africa) and apprentices. The bedrooms were on the second floor. On the first floor, there was a centered front entryway flanked by a room on each side. One of those rooms served as the doctor's office (the "chirurgery"), containing a writing desk, bookshelves, and a chair and table for examination of the patients. The surgeon also kept instruments in the consultation room, such as lancets for bloodletting, cupping glasses, tools for tooth extractions, tourniquets, scalpels, a saw and a big knife for amputations, and forceps used during difficult deliveries. Large syringes were used for rectal or vaginal enemas. The room opposite the office was commonly used as a dining room for the family, or as an informal waiting room for patients on busy days.

Warren's practice was a solo practice, and even if his apprentices relieved some of the burden of being constantly on call, Warren had to be available to his patients all days of the week. In addition, Warren was increasingly involved in politics, and was becoming a well-known Patriot opposing the British. He was an active member of various committees and organizations (including the Sons of Liberty), and he was a prolific writer.

The exact nature of Warren's practice is not well known. It is clear, however, that although Warren had received surgical training, his practice (like that of most other surgeons of the time) was not only surgical, but also included the treatment of conditions not requiring the knife (similar to the services provided by today's general practitioners).

Not only was Warren's practice diverse from a medical standpoint, but his patient population was varied as well. His patients represented people from all layers of society, ranging from the poor and uneducated to the wealthy and intellectual. Many patients would become important players in American politics and governing, including future Patriots, governors, and even a future United States president. Patients' positions in society, race, wealth or lack thereof, and political orientation did not play a role in who Warren agreed to see. Surgeons who had trained with Warren or who had been influenced by his thinking and moral values in other ways often referred to his motto: "When in distress every man becomes our neighbor."

Thomas Hutchinson was an example of a patient with a prominent position in society and a political affiliation opposite that of Warren. Hutchinson was a Loyalist and the lieutenant governor of Massachusetts when, in May 1767, Warren treated him for what may have been a mild stroke (symptoms described by Hutchinson himself as a "paralytic illness of 6–7 weeks' duration").[14] Hutchinson recovered from his illness, and although his recovery may have occurred thanks to Warren's care, Hutchinson in his own writing also gave credit to "country air and horseback riding."

Several other individuals for whom Warren provided medical care were prominent in the American Revolution, and in other aspects of American politics. We have already seen that Warren participated in the inoculation of John Adams against smallpox in 1764. Warren also took care of John Adams and his family for other medical reasons, and functioned as a family doctor for the Adams family. John Quincy Adams—John and Abigail Adams's son, who would become the sixth president of the United States—was treated in his boyhood by Warren for a finger fracture. Josiah Quincy Jr., who together with John Adams served as a defense lawyer for British soldiers involved in the Boston Massacre, suffered from pulmonary tuberculosis and died from the disease at a young age. He was cared for in his final days by his friend Warren. Additional prominent Patriots who were Warren's patients included Samuel Adams, John Hancock, and James Otis Jr.

Warren also provided medical care to less influential persons. For example, in 1769–1722, he held an appointment as physician at the Almshouse and Manufactory.[15] The occupant of this position was appointed by the Governor's Council to provide care for the poor. Although Warren billed patients in his private practice, the collection rate was low.

The appointment at the Almshouse and Manufactory was reimbursed by the Province of Massachusetts and became an important supplementary income for Warren. Dr. Benjamin Church had held the same post before Warren. The position at the Almshouse and Manufactory reflected the government's involvement in those days to provide health care for the poor and elderly, and this type of "socialized medicine" was well accepted by the general population. In fact, both Whigs and Tories agreed that society should help the poor get appropriate health care; the question that generated debate was, instead, who would be appointed to positions like Warren's.

In September 1774, William Dawes, another important Patriot, became a patient of Warren. Dawes was a tanner working with Paul Revere in the North End. The circumstances that resulted in Dawes becoming Warren's patient are interesting. Dawes and some of his friends had broken into a British army guardhouse and stolen two cannons. When Dawes helped lift the cannons, one of his sleeve buttons penetrated the skin at the wrist and had to be removed surgically by Warren. A year earlier, Dawes had participated in the Tea Party. Later, Dawes played an additional important role in the American Revolution when he, along with Revere, was dispatched by Warren for the "midnight ride."

The Business Aspects of Warren's Practice: 1763–1775

Important information about Warren's practice has been generated from account books and daybooks. These sources of information provide statistics regarding the number of patients being seen, charges, payments, and, in some instances, diagnoses and treatments. Several of these documents are preserved at the Massachusetts Historical Society. The business and other aspects of Warren's practice were described recently by Samuel A. Forman in his excellent book, *Dr. Joseph Warren: The Boston Tea Party, Bunker Hill, and the Birth of American Liberty.*

Warren's practice was a private practice with fee for service. The practice grew steadily during his twelve-year medical career. During the first couple of years, Warren saw between five hundred and one thousand patients annually. At the end of his career, the corresponding figure became about three thousand. When calculated as the average number of patients seen per day, the figure was about three during the period 1763–1768, and grew to about eight patients per day during the last two years of the practice. Although these may not sound like impressive numbers, since home visits were common and time consuming (Warren had to get to most of those visits on horseback), he had enough patients to keep him busy. Warren's practice was actually one of the busiest medical enterprises in New England at the time, with only one practice exceeding it: Dr. Holyoke of Salem saw on average ten patients per day during the same period.

Although Warren was reimbursed by the province of Massachusetts for services provided at the Almshouse and Manufactory, the remainder of his practice revenue was generated from billing his private patients. The total billing for Warren's private patients was about seventy Massachusetts pounds during the first couple of years, and grew to more than £400 in 1774. Based on statistics in Warren's account books, the collection rate for his private patients was about 30 percent. During the three years of his appointment at the almshouse, the income from the service at the almshouse accounted for almost seventy percent of Warren's total revenue.

The Women in Warren's Life

Warren had a close and loving relationship with his mother, Mary; a relationship that became even closer after she was widowed. Their close relationship was exemplified by the financial support Mary gave to her son's education, making it possible for him to finish his studies at Harvard and complete the apprenticeship with Dr. Lloyd. From letters that have been preserved, it is clear that Warren dearly loved and respected his mother.

Warren married Elizabeth Hooton on September 6, 1764. He was twenty-three, and she was still a teenager, only seventeen years old. Elizabeth's mother had died earlier, and her father passed away at a relatively young age, only a couple of months before her marriage to Warren, leaving Elizabeth with a substantial inheritance. It is possible that the courtship between Joseph and Elizabeth was kindled by visits to Elizabeth's father's sickbed that Joseph made, along with his master, Dr. Lloyd. Elizabeth's and Joseph's marriage was mentioned in Boston newspapers and described as a union between "Doct. Joseph Warren, one of the physicians in this Town" and Ms. Hooton, "an accomplished young lady with a handsome Fortune."[16] Although not many details are known about the courtship leading to their marriage, or about their lives and feelings as a young married couple, some historians have speculated that the marriage, at least in the beginning, was a marriage of convenience rather than a marriage of passionate love. Elizabeth caught a young and handsome physician with looks described as "pleasing to the ladies," and Joseph got a wealthy wife. Rumors had it that Warren did not hesitate to spend some of his wife's money, not always in her company.

The marriage produced four children. Although the last children's dates of birth were well documented, the birthdate of their first-born child was not registered. This has given rise to the assumption that Elizabeth was pregnant with their first child at the time of the wedding.

The marriage between Elizabeth and Joseph lasted only about nine years. Elizabeth died on May 23, 1773, at the young age of twenty-six. It is possible that the cause of death was an infectious disease spreading in Boston during that time, which may explain why Paul Revere's first wife also died at a young age, only a few days before Elizabeth.

There were other women in Warren's life, several of them surrounded by interesting circumstances. Although Warren's involvement with some of those women is speculative, some of the stories are intriguing. For example, it has been suggested that Warren was romantically involved with Margaret Kemble Gage, the wife of the Massachusetts Governor General Thomas Gage.[17] It is possible that she was the person who supplied Warren with intelligence about troop movements just before the Battles of Lexington and Concord (her husband was convinced that she was guilty of passing the secrets along, something that pained him deeply as she was the love of his life). Other historical sources suggest that it was Paul Revere, not Warren, who was the recipient of Margaret Gage's secrets.

Another relationship surrounded by some secrecy is that between Warren and Sally Edwards.[18] Sally was still just a teenager when she became pregnant. Some historians suspect that Warren was the father, due to the circumstances around Sally's pregnancy and her delivery of a baby girl on June 29, 1775 (only twelve days after the Battle of Bunker Hill), as well as the economic support of Sally provided by some of Warren's friends.

When Warren's wife, Elizabeth, died, he was left a widower with four children to care for. He managed to get the children out of Boston just before the siege of the city began. The children were sheltered in the home of his friend, Dr. Dix, in Worcester, a town approximately twenty miles west of Boston. Most of the responsibility to support and care for the children was given to Mercy Scollay.[19] Warren had met Mercy when she was a patient of his in 1774. She was about the same age as Warren, and according to daybooks carried by Warren, he had seen her as a patient several times in May of 1774, and given her prescriptions for various medicines and purging agents. At some point, they seem to have become personal friends, and she developed a keen interest in the welfare of the children, but she was also not uninterested in Warren. From information in Warren's daybooks, it has been deduced that she came to see Warren in his practice, not exclusively for medical reasons.

Mercy's devotion to Warren and his children is illustrated by her continued care for the siblings after Warren's death. The orphaned children were ultimately adopted by Joseph's brother John, but Mercy continued to be instrumental in securing the safe placement of the children, their financial support, and education. Later in life, Mercy explained that she was "religiously bound to the promise I made my friend that in case he fell a victim to the rage of power I would be the protectress of his offspring."

Not surprisingly, it has been speculated that Mercy was both governess to Warren's children and his mistress. One historian has suggested that Warren and Mercy were engaged and planning to be married. According to this narrative, the custody of the four children became a source of conflict between Mercy and the Warren family after Warren's death. Interestingly, the economic burden of providing for the children was eased by support from Benedict Arnold, who at this point was still an influential Patriot. Mercy never married after Warren's death, and she died childless at the age of eighty-four in 1826.

Efforts to Regulate the Training and Practice of Physicians

During the 1700s, particularly before the Revolution, medicine and surgery in the colonies were not strictly regulated (or regulated at all). This resulted in many unqualified "physicians" practicing medicine and surgery, especially in the countryside. Warren saw this as a great problem and wanted to get the profession on a more respectable footing by suppressing the "Heard of Empiricks who have bro't such intolerable contempt on the Epithet Country Practitioner." To improve the quality and accountability of medical practitioners, Warren became a driving force behind the formation of the Medical Society in Boston. It held its first meeting at Gardner's Tavern in March of 1765. The Boston Society was a forerunner to the Massachusetts Medical Society that was founded in 1781, and is still an active organization today.

Warren the Writer

Like today, people in the 1700s who wanted to express their views publicly and sway the public opinion turned to the press (of course, nowadays, social media fills more and more of the press's function). In the mid-1700s, there were two major newspapers read by Bostonians. The *Boston Gazette,* published by Benjamin Edes and John Gill, commonly expressed views reflecting those of the Whigs. The other paper, the *Boston Evening Post,* represented the ideas of the Tories, and was the voice of the local governing officials and the British government. Between the two newspapers, there was a fierce competition for readers. Debate articles expressing sharp and sometimes insulting language engaged the citizens of Boston. The custom in the 1700s was for the authors to use pseudonyms, although it was often obvious and understood by the readership exactly who the writer was.

Warren was a prolific author, penning many articles under different pseudonyms. Most of his writing was published in the *Boston Gazette,* and many articles used a sharp tongue, offending people with an opposite view. His pieces were widely read and discussed, and often created powerful personal enemies, sometimes even resulting in lawsuits.

Warren wrote articles addressing both medical and political issues. As time went on, his writing became more political and opinionated. The progression of his authorship reflected his increasing opposition to the British, and made him an important spokesman for the Patriots.

In the medical arena, Warren used the pseudonym "Graph Iatoos" when in 1765, he argued for the creation of a medical society in Boston, improved medical education, and the discouragement of unqualified practitioners. He also wanted to increase collegiality in the medical profession, "that they may avoid condemning & calumniating each other before the Plebians." In addition, he stressed the importance of coordinated care of individual patients when multiple physicians needed to be involved.

In October 1765, Warren wrote an editorial in the *Boston Gazette* under the pseudonym "B.W." In this essay, Warren expressed concerns about the taxation of the colonies and the threat to the civil liberties that the different British Acts posed. In particular, Warren was troubled by the Stamp Act riots that resulted in the destruction of private property in his own North End neighborhood. He warned that if the Stamp Tax was allowed to stand, "you may next expect a Tax on your Lands; and after that one Burden on the back of another, till you are reduced to a State of the most abject Poverty." Warren had thus started to express ideas that that would put him solidly among the Whigs and the Sons of Liberty.

Warren's next series of political articles was published in the *Boston Gazette,* 1766–1767. This time, Warren used the pseudonym "Paskalos." The main subject of these pieces was the dispute between the local Whigs and Tories about Governor Bernard's reports to London that discredited the Boston Patriots. The Whigs were upset about this misrepresentation of the Patriots, and Paskalos was quite sharp in his critique of Governor Bernard. Warren's articles provoked equally angry essays written by Tories and published in the *Boston Evening Post.* This war of words kept escalating—probably to the delight of the publishers, who saw their newspapers selling in large numbers.

After an interlude of writing medical articles, Warren returned to the political arena under the pseudonym "A True Patriot" in early 1768. In a series of discourses, A True Patriot was again critical of Governor Bernard.[20] The pieces were also a response to the Townshend Acts, which soon became another thorn in Bostonians' flesh.

The Townshend Acts were passed by the Parliament in 1767 and 1768, and were designed to raise additional revenue in the American colonies. The income generated by the Townshend Acts was used to pay salaries to governors and judges. The Acts were named after Charles Townshend, the chancellor of the exchequer. They included the Revenue Act (1767), the Indemnity Act (1767), the Commissioners of Customs Act (1767), the New York Restraining Act (1767), and the Vice Admiralty Act (1768).

Although most of the Townshend Acts were ultimately repealed by Parliament, the strong opposition against them among the colonists was a major reason why British troops occupied Boston in 1768. The presence of British soldiers would boil over in the Boston Massacre of 1770. Thus, the introduction of the various Townshend Acts had significant consequences, and would play an important role in the American Revolution.

In one of the articles published in the *Boston Gazette,* Warren (writing as "A True Patriot") was particularly harsh against Governor Bernard and wrote, "If such Men are by God appointed / The Devil may be the Lord's anointed."[21] To openly compare the royal governor with the devil was one insult too many. The governor and his council decided to take legal actions and sue for libel. The Massachusetts House of Representatives, however, rejected their recommendation to prosecute the editors of the *Boston Gazette*—a victory of sort for the freedom of the press.

The "True Patriot" did not only write angry and defaming pieces but also authored articles that were more statesmanlike. Part of that writing explains why some historians believe Joseph Warren may have become the leader of the Revolution—and subsequently even president of the United States—had he not met a premature death at Bunker Hill. In one of those pieces, Warren wrote, "The beneficent Lord of the universe delights in viewing the happiness of all men: And so far as civil government is of divine institution, it was calculated for the greatest good of the whole community: And whenever it ceases to be of general advantage, it ceases to be of divine appointment...."

A new journal, *Massachusetts Spy,* was established in July 1770. In November 1771, Warren contributed an article under the pseudonym "Mucius Scaevola." In the article, Warren argued that Thomas Hutchinson, who had replaced Bernard as governor, was not a constitutional governor but an intruder and a "pretended Governor." This writing was seen by Hutchinson and the Governor's Council as unacceptable, and a direct challenge of British authority. Hutchinson and his Council threatened the *Massachusetts Spy* with libel, but when the lawsuit was dropped, it was viewed as yet another victory for the freedom of the press. The previously friendly relationship between Warren and Hutchinson, who had been one of Warren's patients, had drastically deteriorated when Warren became one of the leading Patriots, and more and more aggressive in opposing British rule.

Warren the Politician

Warren joined the Sons of Liberty in 1767. Samuel Adams, one of the most influential leaders of the British resistance, was one of the founders of the Sons of Liberty, and he became an important political mentor for Warren. Warren joined a group of individuals who were counseled by Samuel Adams, which included John Hancock, Paul Revere, Benjamin Church, and Thomas Young. Warren and Samuel Adams did not only interact in politics and the Patriots' movement, but they also had medical interactions. Samuel Adams's family consulted Warren for various health issues starting in 1768. Adams was suffering from tremor of his hands, raising concerns for a degenerative neurological condition. Adams's wife, Elizabeth, had lost three of her five pregnancies. Other members of the extended Adams family were also among Warren's patients, including Samuel Adams's younger cousin John Adams, his wife, Abigail, and their children. These and other doctor–patient relationships provided ample opportunities for Warren to build relationships with politically important and active individuals, who also wanted to increase the independence and home rule in the colonies, and to repeal the multitude of taxes and other regulations that the London Parliament imposed on the American colonies.

The Townshend Acts made it clear to Warren that he needed to become even more involved with the local Patriots. New taxes made it obvious that although the Stamp Act had been repealed, the Parliament continued to have the power (and desire) to "impose taxes in all cases whatsoever." The taxes were applied to a number of products that were essential for the colonists, including paper, lead, glass, and tea. The duties were immensely unpopular among the Bostonians, and the British had to send a warship, *The HMS Romney*, to Boston to enforce collection of the import taxes. This further worsened the tense relationships between the inhabitants of Boston and the British officials.

In the summer of 1768, one of John Hancock's merchant ships, *Liberty*, arrived in Boston with a cargo of wine.[22] Customs agents tried to board the ship but were stopped and forced back to land. The government filed a lawsuit claiming that Hancock had violated the law by bringing the imported wine ashore without paying the import tax. Warren became a mediator in the legal fight, using his favorable standing with both Hancock (a Patriot and fellow Freemason) and the customs commissioner Benjamin Hallowell (who was a patient of Warren and had been seen by Warren for medical care more than ninety times between 1764 and 1768). Warren managed to work out a compromise that avoided a permanent seizure of Hancock's ship, and saved face for the customs officials. The government's prosecutors dropped the case against Hancock a couple of months later.

Warren later became a driving force in the opposition against the Townshend taxes. He was a leading proponent for boycotts of British products, a strategy that had also been used against the Stamp Act. The three essential components of the boycott were the nonimportation, requesting American merchants not to order taxable British products; the nonconsumption, convincing American consumers not to use British products; and the subsequent replacement of British products with homegrown alternatives. The boycott became a double-edged sword. It not only had a negative impact on the British who wanted to sell their products to the colonists, but it also harmed the business of American merchants. However, even if the enthusiasm among merchants and colonists who could not get their hands on necessary products was not great, the Patriots, particularly Warren, continued to forcefully push for the boycott.

The earlier riots against the Stamp Act and the strong opposition against the Townshend Duties, made Tories and the British government nervous about potential violence. To counter that risk, the British decided to send troops to the American continent. This, however, inflamed the situation even more.

On October 1, 1768, four thousand British troops disembarked at the Long Wharf in Boston. The situation in the city had become tense as British soldiers were often despised and sometimes even harassed by segments of the local population. In a 1769 letter written to officials in London, Warren warned that "the People here, they will never think their grievances redressed till every Revenue Act is repealed, the Board of

Commissioner dissolved and the Troops removed...."[23] At the same time, Warren expressed optimism that if these things were accomplished, "we doubt not that the harmony which heretofore subsisted between Great Britain and the Colonies will be happily restored—an event ardently wished for by every friend to the British Empire." Although the British gave into many of the colonists' demands, they did not repeal the import tax on tea or recall the military. Their presence in Boston continued to increase the city's anxiety, and ultimately resulted in the eruption of violence. This included the British tax collector John Robinson beating James Otis Jr. in September 1769, the killing of the young apprentice Christopher Seider in February 1770, and the Boston Massacre on March 5, 1770.

Warren was involved in all of these events. He was James Otis's physician and attended to the head injury Robinson had given him. Warren also became involved in events during 1770. That year saw further unrest and violence in Boston. Angry colonists continued to express their outrage against British taxes, regulations imposed on the colonies, and the presence of a large military force in Boston.

The Killing of Christopher Seider

Violent protests were not only directed against British officials and soldiers but also against fellow Bostonians who did not adhere to the boycotts. One such protest took place the morning of February 22, 1770, and was directed against the merchant Theophilus Lillie's shop, where English products continued to be sold. A sign that read "IMPORTER" had been placed in front of the shop to shame him. A crowd of young men and boys, including the eleven-year-old Christopher Seider, son of poor German immigrants, marched to Lillie's shop, pulling a cart full of rotten fruit. The purpose of the rotten fruit was obvious to everyone. A custom collector, Ebenezer Richardson, happened to be in the neighborhood. Richardson was despised among the colonists for collecting fees for the British, and for his reputation of low moral standards (this included Richardson violating his sister-in-law and blaming the local minister for the act).

Richardson tried to stop the rioters, but failed. The crowd, which kept growing by the hour, turned their anger towards Richardson, and when rocks and other projectiles started to fly, he and his wife fled to their home to take shelter. This did not stop the protesters. Windows were smashed, and the altercation got worse. After his wife was hit by eggs and stones, Richardson fired shots into the crowd with his musket from a window on the second floor. Two boys were hit. One of the youngsters survived his injuries, but the other boy, Christopher Seider, was hit in the chest and died later that evening.

This event created an outcry in the community and was well covered in the local press. The *Boston Gazette* reported that "a barbarous murder… was committed on the body of a young lad of about eleven years of age." The *Boston Evening Post* described how "the child fell but was taken up and carried into a neighboring house, where all the surgeons within call were assembled, and speedily determined the wounds mortal, as they indeed proved about 9 o'clock that evening." Warren was among the surgeons called to examine the dying boy, and was later asked to perform an autopsy. The autopsy confirmed that the injuries sustained in front of Richardson's house were the cause of death: "his body was opened and in it were found 11…slugs…one which pierced his breast…and passing clear thro' the right lobe of the lungs, lodged in his back."[24]

Richardson was brought to Faneuil Hall, where he had to answer to three magistrates and was charged with murder. Warren testified at the trial and the jury concluded that Seider had been "willfully and feloniously shot by Ebenezer Richardson." Richardson was found guilty and sentenced, but later received a royal pardon on the basis of self-defense. He even got a new job within the customs service. Needless to say, the pardon of Richardson and his continued employment did not improve the feelings between the citizens of Boston and the British.

Christopher Seider's funeral, partly organized by Warren, turned into a big political event masterminded by the Sons of Liberty, and it became a huge manifestation directed against the British. More than two thousand of Boston's approximately fifteen thousand citizens marched in a remarkable procession. John Adams wrote, "My eyes never beheld such a funeral. The procession extended further than can be well imagined." Even Hutchinson was amazed by the size of the funeral, and stated that it was "the largest perhaps ever known in America."[25]

During the immediate aftermath of Christopher Seider's killing and burial, fights between British soldiers and bands of Sons of Liberty became frequent. Insults between the parties often accompanied the skirmishes. Notably, the Sons of Liberty used tarring and feathering to shame British officials. A British officer remarked, "The insolence as well as the utter hatred of the inhabitants to the troops increased daily." The hatred against the soldiers was also fueled by the sentiment that they stole both jobs and women from the Boston men.

On the second day of March, just a week after Seider had been killed, a young, angry man approached an off-duty soldier and asked if he wanted work. When the soldier said he would be interested, the young man answered, "Well, then go and clean my shithouse!" The offended soldier returned to the site with several of his fellow Redcoats, and street fighting erupted, further increasing the agitation in town.

Soldiers spread rumors that many Bostonians "carried weapons concealed under their clothes." Such were the feelings and behavior between the inhabitants of Boston and the British troops. It is not surprising that this atmosphere led to more violence. Only two weeks after Christopher Seider's death, more shots were fired on the streets of Boston, an event that has gone down in history as "the Boston Massacre."

The Boston Massacre

The Boston Massacre on March 5, 1770, resulted in the death of five colonists at the hands of British soldiers, who were under the command of Captain Thomas Preston. [26] Although not at the scene of the event, Warren was part of the subsequent town delegation that went to the State House, requesting that Hutchinson order the removal of the troops from within Boston to Castle William. After initially refusing the request, Hutchinson ultimately ordered the British troops out of the city and had them stationed at Castle William. Although this may have eased the tension somewhat, the Townshend Duties remained in place, and most of the soldiers participating in the Boston Massacre were acquitted at a trial held several months after the event. Consequently, the bad blood between the British authorities and the Bostonians not only remained in place, but kept growing at an even more rapid pace.

When lawyers John Adams and Josiah Quincy Jr., both of whom were involved in the Patriot movement, defended the British soldiers at the trial, the people of Boston were astonished and upset. Adams and Quincy did so, however, because they felt it was important to demonstrate that providing a fair trial was something even enemies deserved. Maybe even more importantly, no other lawyers in Boston wanted to take on the defense of the soldiers and their commander in fear of retribution by the citizens.

Captain Preston and his soldiers were tried separately.[27] Preston was found not guilty by the jury mainly because multiple testimonies provided evidence that he had not given the order to fire and had tried to prevent the soldiers from using their muskets. He was set free, awarded £200 in compensation, and soon left the continent for England, never to return.

Most of the soldiers were also found not guilty on the basis of having acted in self-defense. They had been taunted by the mob with snowballs, stones, and other objects. Only two of the soldiers, who had deliberately fired into the crowd, were found guilty of manslaughter. The English law "plea to clergy" was invoked to save the lives of the two culpable soldiers.

In addition to being part of the delegation pleading with Hutchinson to remove the British soldiers from Boston, Warren would become involved in another aspect of the aftermath to the Boston Massacre. In 1772 and 1775, he was called upon to deliver the annual speech commemorating the massacre. Warren's first annual speech, given at the Old South Meeting House, was his first speech before a large crowd. It gave him prominence among the Bostonians as a great orator, and made people realize that he was evolving into an important figure in the resistance against the British rule.

The annual Boston Massacre speeches were highly anticipated and always drew big crowds. The first Boston Massacre speech was given by Dr. James Lovell on March 5, 1771. Throughout the years, other orators included Joseph Warren, Benjamin Church, and John Hancock.

The Committee of Correspondence

In 1772, a Boston town resolution authorized the formation of a Committee of Correspondence.[28] The early members counted several Patriots, including Samuel Adams, and at least three surgeons: Joseph Warren, Benjamin Church, and Thomas Young. The purpose of the committee was to provide correspondences between the Patriots in Boston and towns elsewhere in Massachusetts, as well as Patriots in other places on the continent, such as New York and Philadelphia. The committee members were busy writing letters and other manifestos that frequently expressed concerns over the relationship between the motherland and the colonies.

One of the initial tasks of the committee was to compose a document comprised of three parts. The first part discussed the rights of the colonists as Englishmen and Christians, and was authored by Samuel Adams. The second part was written by Joseph Warren, and provided a list of twelve injustices and infringements of the rights of the colonists. The third part was written by Benjamin Church, and encouraged other towns in Massachusetts to form their own committees.

During the next couple of years, the Committee of Correspondence would play an important role in laying the groundwork for what would become the American Revolution. The committee was instrumental not only for the opposition against the British in Massachusetts, but also for developing bonds between the different provinces in the political movement.

The Tea Party 1773

Parliament's passing of the 1773 Tea Act caused further outrage among the colonists. To bail out the nearly bankrupt East India Company, the British government removed tariffs paid by the company, and allowed it to sell tea directly to the colonies. People had previously been smuggling cheaper tea into the colonies, but due to the Tea Act, the East India Company's tea became the least expensive. This basically gave the company a monopoly on the American continent. But Parliament also decided that the colonists would have to continue to pay the Townshend tax on the imported tea, something that angered the colonists. Saving the East India Company and collecting money would be a win–win situation for the government.

Tea was a socially important drink and was consumed in large quantities among the colonists. The implementation of the Tea Act became another despised example of the British Parliament's arrogance: introducing new rules and regulations without consulting the people who were affected. The opposition against "taxation without representation" continued to be a pillar in the resistance to British rule.

Boston was the first port of entry, seeing tea arriving from the warehouses in England after the Tea Act had been passed. Because of this, the resistance to the new law became particularly prominent in Boston. Three ships (*Dartmouth, Eleanor,* and *The Beaver*) arrived in Boston in late November and early December, carrying big shipments of tea.[29] The opposition to the Tea Act culminated in the "Destruction of the Tea" (an event that later became known as the "Tea Party") on December 16, 1773. The tea brought to Boston was worth at least one million dollars in today's currency. Therefore, throwing the tea chests into the Boston harbor not only had symbolic meaning, but a great economic impact as well.

The Destruction of the Tea was carried out by Patriots who had first assembled at the Old South Meeting House. A huge crowd of angry Bostonians, including members of the Sons of Liberty, attended the meeting. For days, they had requested that Governor Hutchinson send the ships back to London without unloading the tea, but he had refused. The patience among the colonists was running thin, and the Patriots decided to take things in their own hands. After the meeting at the Old South Meeting House, about 200 Patriots marched down to the harbor, embarked the ships, and threw more than 340 chests of tea into the water. The Patriots participating in the event disguised themselves as Mohawk Indians in order not to be recognized, as they risked severe punishment if caught.

The Patriots were able to carry out their deed without violence. Instead, there seems to have been an almost friendly atmosphere between the perpetrators and the sailors onboard the ships. Several of the Patriots stayed on after the activities and helped clean up the mess they had created.

When the news about the destruction of the tea spread on the continent, many colonists initially condemned it as an act of vandalism. Even

George Washington and Benjamin Franklin expressed their disapproval. Of course, as time went on, the view of the Tea Party changed, and it is now a celebrated event that led up to the American Revolution.

Although Warren's role in the gathering at the Old South Meeting House and the ensuing Destruction of the Tea has not been well documented, he probably played an important role behind the scenes, perhaps orchestrating and organizing the event. He certainly participated in writing letters sent out from the Committee of Correspondence, broadcasting the news about the dumping of the tea to Patriots in other parts of the colonies, including New York and Philadelphia. In the aftermath, the British requested that the East India Company be compensated for its losses. This became a hotly debated issue among the Patriots, who ultimately decided to oppose it. Warren was one the most outspoken rebels against paying for the tea thrown overboard.

Anxiety in Boston after Destruction of the Tea

After fully realizing what had happened at the Destruction of the Tea, people in Boston started to get nervous about what the British's reaction would be. The aftermath to the Tea Party saw increasing tensions between Loyalists and Patriots, and even between different fractions among the Patriots. If there was any hope that the British would try to reduce the antagonism between the freedom-seeking Patriots and the government in London, that hope was quickly crushed during the spring of 1774.

In May of that year, Thomas Gage had arrived in Boston as the newly appointed governor, replacing Thomas Hutchinson. Hutchinson had been recalled to London for "consultations" and never returned to America. Soon after arriving, Governor Gage informed the Bostonians about the Boston Port Act, which would close the harbor on June 1. The British declared that the port would be closed for both imports and exports until the East India Company had been compensated for the destroyed tea and the people in Boston had agreed to adhere to the Townshend duty on tea. The Port Act signified the beginning of a year during which dramatic political and military events would take place, ultimately resulting in the start of the American Revolution. Just about a year remained between the announcement of the Port Act and the Battles of Lexington and Concord and Bunker Hill. Warren was actively involved in most of the events during the twelve months leading up to the Revolutionary War.

The Port Act created strong frictions among the Bostonians. To get the port blockade lifted, most Loyalists and some Patriots wanted to compensate the East India Company for the destructed tea and abide by the Townshend tea taxes. This would help merchants to again conduct their businesses and make a living. In contrast, many colonists wanted to convey a tough stance against the British demands. Along with his mentor Samuel Adams, Warren belonged to the faction among the Patriots that strongly argued for a radical opposition to the British. During the next twelve months, the growing tensions between the British Parliament and the colonists resulted in an escalating radicalization of the Sons of Liberty, and Warren's increased involvement and importance.

Warren's most significant contributions during this time included the writing and distribution, through the Committee of Correspondence, of the Solemn League and Covenant. Until the Port Act was repealed, merchants were asked to swear not to conduct business with the British or anyone who continued to interact with them. The strongly worded document, however, did not achieve what Warren had hoped for. Many merchants, who saw their businesses hurting, did not accept the Solemn League, and the document certainly did not soften the British, who responded by introducing new regulations. In August 1774, the Massachusetts Government Act was announced, and the Administration of Justice Act subsequently followed. These Acts—which, along with the Port Act, were named the Intolerable Acts—took away colonists' remaining influence on the political systems. The introduction of the Intolerable Acts strengthened the resolve of Warren and other Patriots to continue the opposition against the British. During 1774 and 1775, the meetings of the Provincial Congress occupied Warren.[30] Energy also went into preparations for the first Continental Congress, which was scheduled to take place in Philadelphia in September 1774. Along with several other prominent Patriots, including his surgeon colleague Benjamin Church, Warren was elected member of the Massachusetts Committee of Safety and Supplies.[31] Since it was involved in preparing for a possible military conflict, the committee increased the standoff between the colonies and the British.

Warren the Orator

Warren's increasing involvement in the movement against the British made him a prominent person in Boston and strengthened his popularity among the Patriots—as well as the infamy among the British. In addition to his accomplishments as a physician, surgeon, politician, thinker, and proliferative author of polemic newspaper articles and letters, Warren's skills as an orator came to full fruition during his last year. There were at least three public speeches that cemented his fame as a public speaker.

In early September 1774, Warren's oratory skills were an important reason why a bloodbath did not take place in Cambridge. On September 1, Governor Gage ordered British infantry to march to Cambridge, with the mission to seize a cache of gunpowder stored in East Cambridge.[32] After completing the task successfully, the troops returned to Boston. Rumors rapidly spread all over Massachusetts that the military involvement in Cambridge was part of a military strike against the colonists, and an attack on Boston. With amazingly great speed, large numbers of armed militiamen from the inner and western parts of Massachusetts descended on Cambridge. When no British soldiers were found in Cambridge, the mob-like herds of militias instead congregated on "Tory Row" and directed their anger at the luxurious homes on that street, getting ready to ransack and destroy the houses. These were mansions owned by Loyalists, several of whom had been appointed to the Governor's Mandamus Council that replaced the Governor's Council when the Government Act was announced earlier in 1774.

When the situation grew volatile, and the militiamen threatened to plunder and wreck the homes on Tory Row, the governor wanted to send troops back to Cambridge to get the situation under control. The Mandamus counselors, however, declined the assistance from the military, fearing that the arrival of soldiers would escalate the threat of violence.

Warren heard about the standoff in Cambridge and hastily galloped there to try to defuse the situation. In a speech in front of the agitated militia, he succeeded in convincing them to disperse without further unrest. Before leaving, the militia had won a victory by forcing the public resignations of the Mandamus Counselors living on the street. Some of them fled their homes, and hurried to Boston for protection by the British army. They would never return to their estates and comfortable way of living.

The events in Cambridge during the first three days of September 1774 have gone down in history as the "Cambridge Powder Alarm."[33] Warren's successful speech in front of the infuriated militia highlighted his ability to address a big crowd. He understood the importance of the success, both in terms of his evolving role as a Patriot leader, and as somebody who could deliver a public speech in tense situations.

It was only a week after his speech in Cambridge that Warren was again on the stage addressing a big audience. The Suffolk Convention met in Milton, just outside Boston, on September 6. During the next three days, nineteen articles were drafted, all with major input from Warren. The articles ("The Suffolk Resolves") dealt with issues related to the interactions between the British authorities and the Patriots. Although the resolves acknowledged the Colonies' allegiance to the throne of Great Britain, they also listed a number of severe grievances. The language was strong and included statements condemning the "unparalleled usurpation of unconstitutional power, whereby our capital is robbed of the means of life; whereby the streets of Boston are thronged with military executioners." The constitution of Britain was described as "totally wrecked, annulled and vacated." Warren declared that the Suffolk county citizens were free of the numerous British Acts, particularly the authority of the Governor's Mandamus Counselors, the Administration of Justice Act, and the various Tax Acts. Although the articles favored nonviolent opposition to the British government, it was clear that violence could not be avoided if the British did not meet the Patriots' demands.

It was bestowed on Warren to read the resolves aloud to the delegates at the convention. Tradition has it that on September 9, 1774, he read the articles standing in the doorway of Daniel Vose's house in Milton.[34] His oration was met with great enthusiasm and each resolve was unanimously approved by the delegates. The occasion further confirmed Warren's abilities as a great public speaker.

Historians consider the Suffolk Resolves Warren's most important writing. Immediately after the resolves had been approved at Milton, Revere was sent racing down to Philadelphia on horseback to deliver them to the Continental Congress. He arrived in Philadelphia on September

16, and the following day the documents were read to the Congress. The resolves were enthusiastically approved, and the Massachusetts ban of British goods became a unified colonial boycott. The Congress delegates were jubilant. John Adams wrote in his diary, "This was one of the happiest days of my life.... This day convinced me that America will support the Massachusetts or perish with her."[35]

The third event in which Warren's oratory skills were at full display took place on March 6, when he delivered the annual Boston Massacre lecture for a second time (March 5, 1775, fell on a Sunday, which is why the annual oration did not take place on March fifth that year). Warren addressed an Old South Meeting House that was filled to overcapacity with thousands of anticipating Bostonians. He arrived late to the oration after seeing six patients earlier in the day. Like the preceding years, the event was immensely popular, and Warren had to enter through a side window in order to get around the crowds, including forty mean-spirited British officers. Somewhat theatrically, Warren gave his speech robed in a toga.

In his thirty-five minute talk, Warren addressed most of the issues that were on the minds of the citizens, and related to the growing tension between the British and the Patriots. He started by giving a historical review of how and why the Pilgrims had left Europe, and their search for freedom on the American continent. He went on by criticizing Britain for trying to harvest the fruits of the colonists' hard labor without giving them credit or allowing them to fully participate in the governance of the colonies. Warren also provided sharp criticism of the "taxation without representation" imposed on the colonies. He expressed outrage over the presence of armed British forces on the continent, particularly in Boston, and emphasized the importance of individual responsibility in the fight for freedom and opposition to the British authorities.

Despite the fact that Warren's oration took place only about one-and-a-half months before the start of the Revolutionary War, Warren also stated that, "An independence...is not our aim. No, our wish is, that Britain and the colonies may...grow and increase in strength together."[36] It is possible that Warren did not believe this claim himself, because a couple of sentences later he speculated about what would happen "if these pacific measures are ineffectual, and it appears that the only way to safety, is through fields of blood...."

At the time of Warren's oratory, the tensions between the Patriots and the British were at an all-time high. During his speech, Warren painted a picture of the military's abuse of the citizens in strong words, talking about fathers of young children being killed. He did not spare his words when he said, "Take heed, ye orphan babes, lest, whilst your streaming eyes are fixed upon the ghastly corpse, your feet glide on the stones bespattered with your fathers' brains."[37]

During this time, the number of British soldiers patrolling the Boston streets had increased substantially, and altercations between Bostonians and soldiers were common. Rumors suggesting that the British were planning an all-out attack on Boston flourished. The presence of British officers during Warren's speech contributed to the charged atmosphere. It was feared that the speaker would be assassinated, particularly if he was caught saying anything against the king. Allegedly, an officer was prepared to throw an egg in Warren's face, and that would be the signal to massacre Warren, John Hancock, Samuel Adams, and hundreds more. The killings, however, did not happen, and Warren's life was spared—at least for the moment. A freak accident may have prevented the assassination of Warren. It was reported that "he who was deputed to throw the egg fell in going to the church, dislocated his knee, and broke the egg, by which means the scheme failed."[38] Even if the feared killing of Warren was just a rumor, genuine dangers did lurk.

Speeches were not the only time Warren felt threatened. Whenever he walked the streets of Boston, he risked British officers and soldiers insulting and sneering at him. On one occasion, when walking with his apprentice Eustis, he said: "These fellows say we won't fight. Would to heaven I might die knee deep in their blood."

It wouldn't be long before Warren's wish was fulfilled.

The Battles of Lexington and Concord

The political temperature continued rising in Massachusetts and was approaching the boiling point. Governor Gage decided to send troops to Lexington and Concord on April 19, 1775, in order to apprehend John Hancock and Samuel Adams, and lay hands on military supplies that had been stored by the Patriots. This became the match that ignited the Revolutionary War. At the time, John Hancock and Samuel Adams were in Lexington preparing to travel to Philadelphia to attend the second Continental Congress.

Warren had become aware of the British plans, possibly through information provided by Gage's wife Margaret, although he may have had other sources as well.[39] In the evening of April 18, Warren activated the "Alarm," a process by which minutemen and other militia were alerted to the threat and instructed to gather in Lexington to prevent an assault by the British forces. Following the rules set forth by the Provincial Congress, he called the Alarm from the office of his medical practice in Boston. Those rules stipulated that three members of the Committee of Safety needed to be involved in the decision to call the Alarm.[40] Warren also sent Revere and Dawes on their "midnight rides" to reinforce the Alarm along the route Warren suspected the enemy would use to get to Lexington and Concord. Dawes was instructed to leave the city via Boston Neck and then proceed via Roxbury, while Revere was to take a boat across Charles River to Charlestown and then ride on to Lexington and Concord. Warren sent two men in case one of them would be captured by the British. By having rebels signal with lanterns from the steeple of North Church, the freedom fighters stationed in Charlestown would be informed which route the British were coming ("one if by land, two if by sea"). Two lanterns signaled that the British were coming by sea, crossing the Charles in the middle of the night on sloops, and landing in Charlestown. The next morning, when Warren heard that fighting had erupted at Lexington, he left his practice in a hurry and turned the care of his patients over to his apprentice, William Eustis. Then he rode off to the battle scene.

The military expedition became more difficult than the British had anticipated. The soldiers did not find Samuel Adams or John Hancock, both of whom had fled Lexington after Revere and Dawes had warned them about the approaching Redcoats. In Lexington, a band of hastily mobilized colonial militia met the British troops, and during the fight that followed, the "shot heard round the world" left eight militia dead on Lexington Green. It is still uncertain who fired the first shot. The leader of the militia, Captain John Parker, has been quoted as telling his minutemen, "Don't fire unless fired upon, but if they mean to have a war, let it begin here."[41]

From Lexington, the British forces marched on to Concord where initially, they did not meet any significant resistance. They captured or destroyed whatever they could find of cannon, ammunition, flour, and other supplies the rebels had stored in the area. The spoils, however, were much smaller than hoped for, because, after being warned about the approaching Redcoats, the rebels had managed to move much of the supplies to safer places. During the morning hours, thousands of minutemen and militia had been alerted and kept pouring into Concord. Fighting became intense, particularly at the North Bridge. There were losses of lives on both sides, but the largest losses were among the British. After a couple hours of fighting, the Redcoats started to feel threatened and realized they needed to get back to Boston to find protection. The rebels kept harassing the British troops during their retreat, causing additional fatalities. The day ended in a humiliating British defeat, with approximately three hundred dead.

Warren played an important role in the victory over the British troops on that fateful day of April 19, 1775. Not only was he responsible for calling the Alarm, but he was also at the site of the fighting. On the battlefield, he used his surgical skills to attend to wounded rebels, but was also heavily involved in the actual melee. He worked closely with General William Heath, who was a fellow member of the Committee of Safety. Warren was described as "perhaps the most active man in the field" during the day.[42] During the British retreat, Warren participated in the hounding and harassment of the enemy soldiers, and during that effort, he was willing to take great risks. It was said that he "exposed himself recklessly." When a British soldier fired at him, "the bullet came close enough to knock out a pin he wore to keep his hair in place." General Heath was impressed with Warren's courage.

After the Battles of Lexington and Concord, Warren had less than two months to live. These were months filled with hectic activities related to what would become the American Revolution. Warren was engaged in most of the activities in one way or another.

In the immediate aftermath of Lexington and Concord, the anger against the British was palpable, and it became enhanced when people read the description of the events of April 19. A committee was formed on April 23 with the purpose of writing a narrative that would be sent to neighboring colonies and, importantly, to Great Britain. This would hopefully gain support for the Patriots in their fight for freedom, and in what started to look like a war against the English power. Warren was actively involved in crafting the document, and signed the cover letter to the report. The document was a strong contribution to the fight against the British and became an important piece of propaganda supporting the view that the British had initiated the military actions. The letter described how the "Regulars rushed on with great violence, and first began hostilities by firing on said Lexington Company, whereby they killed eight and wounded several others." The British troops' cruelty on the way to Lexington was further emphasized by describing how "a great number of the houses on the road were plundered and rendered unfit for use; several were burnt; women in childbed were driven by the soldiery naked into the streets; old men, peaceably in their houses, were shot dead."

The Siege of Boston

Bolstered by their successes on April 19, many Patriots wanted to immediately attack Boston in order to throw out the British troops and reclaim the city. Understanding the urgency of the situation, the Provincial Congress met early in the morning of Saturday, April 23 with the purpose of mobilizing an army of thirty thousand (!). Warren was the acting president of the proceedings and was instrumental in expanding the rebel army.

John Hancock wrote to Warren: "BOSTON MUST BE ENTERED. The troops must be sent away...."[43] The militia, however, was not yet ready to take on the British, so a more realistic approach was taken. Warren, as Chair of the Committee of Safety and as the de facto president of the Provincial Congress, was responsible for the decision to start a siege of Boston rather than attack the city. The plan was to force the British to give up the occupation of Boston by blockading all exits from and entry into the city, by surrounding it with Patriot militia and Minutemen. The only remaining way for the British to get in and out of Boston was through the harbor.

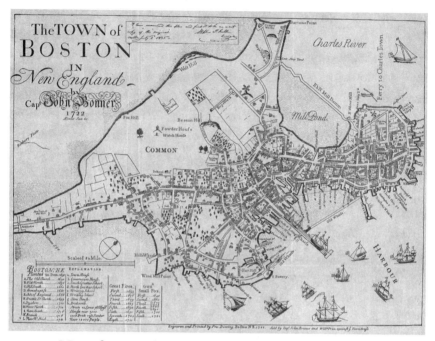

**Map of Boston by Captain John Bonner, 1722. The
population of Boston was about 12,000 when this map
was drawn. It was the largest city of the American colonies
followed by Philadelphia (10,000) and New York (7,000).
At the time of the American Revolution, Boston had grown
to about 15,000. The only land connection of Boston in
the 1700s was the narrow "neck." (Pictures Now)**

The siege resulted in some Patriots getting trapped in the city under
hostile conditions, and some Loyalists being prevented from entering the
city in their search for protection by the British military. To some degree,
a prisoner exchange on June 6, 1775, helped the situation, but the majority
of individuals who wanted to leave or enter Boston remained affected by
the siege. Along with General Putnam, Warren represented the provincials
in the negotiations that resulted in the prisoner exchange.

Warren was involved in many of the events and decisions during the
months that followed the Battles of Lexington and Concord. Some of
those activities reflected his medical and surgical expertise. Together with
Doctors Church, Taylor, Holten, and Dunsmore, he was appointed to a
committee charged with evaluating prospective regimental surgeons. He

supported Dr. Samuel Adams Jr. in obtaining a position as army surgeon. In addition, he was engaged in important political discussions and negotiations about the importance of the military being subordinated a civil government, a principle he considered essential for democracy. Early in May, Warren urged the Continental Congress in Philadelphia to act on this point: "The sword should, in all free States, be subservient to the civil powers; …we tremble at having an Army (although consisting of our own countrymen) established here, without a civil power to provide for and control them."

It is obvious that Warren was a central figure among the Patriots in Massachusetts and that he was destined to play an increasingly important role on the national stage. Then came Bunker Hill.

Bunker Hill

The British had failed their missions at Lexington and Concord and were further humiliated and defeated during their retreat to Boston. In addition, Boston was now under siege. The rebels understood that these circumstances would not go unanswered. The British troops stationed in Boston were being strengthened by the arrival of high-ranking military leaders, including Generals Burgoyne, Howe, and Clinton. At this point, British troops basically occupied Boston, and Royal Naval warships controlled the harbor. To the British, it was frustrating that despite their superiority, they were cut off from access to Boston by land. The only land connection in and out of the city—the Roxbury Neck—was under firm control of the colonial forces, led by General Artemas Ward. By mid-1775, Boston was surrounded by more than fifteen thousand men in what was starting to become a revolutionary army.

Information provided by Boston spies alerted the Patriots that the British planned to try to break the siege by an attack on Charlestown, which would provide an overland opening via the Charlestown Neck. When these plans were discovered, more than one thousand colonists were marched to Charlestown with orders to fortify Bunker Hill and provide a line of defense against the British. The Rebels entered Charlestown on June 16, but instead of gaining control of Bunker Hill (the tallest point on the peninsula), they went up the adjacent Breed's Hill and started construction of fortifications. It remains unclear whether this was a mistake caused by the general confusion and the darkness setting in, or if it was actually a deliberate decision that would put the defense closer to Boston and make it possible to reach the city with the few cannons available.[44] Regardless, a large redoubt was constructed on the crest of Breed's Hill, protected by dirt walls and fence rails.

Warren, whom the Massachusetts Congress had appointed general only four days earlier,[45] was one of the Patriots who went to Charlestown to help with the defense. First, however, he had some medical business to take care of. In the morning of June 17, he visited a woman in labor. After determining that the labor was progressing without problems, he told her that he needed to go to Charlestown "to get a shot at the British" and would return to her in due time—which, of course, he did not. His visit with the pregnant woman may have been one reason why he arrived late to Charlestown. He may have also visited his mother and children before finally getting to the battlefield. When Warren arrived at Bunker Hill, he met with General Israel Putnam and was offered the command of the militia.[46] Warren declined the offer and instead asked to fight side by side with the soldiers. He told General Putnam, "Don't think I came to seek a place of safety, but tell me where the onset will be the most furious."

When informed that the fiercest fighting would occur on Breed's Hill, he decided to go there and be on the front line. When Warren got to Breed's Hill, he was again offered the command of the American forces, this time by William Prescott. Again, he refused and insisted on joining the soldiers.

After the British had bombarded Charlestown with big guns from the warships, setting the town on fire, their onslaught started in the afternoon of June 17. From across the water on rooftops at the shoreline of North End, large numbers of Bostonians watched the battle. Few people believed that the well-trained and well-equipped Redcoats, who came charging up the slopes of Breed's Hill, would meet much resistance. But they did.

The rebels showed a great deal of discipline, and waited till the advancing British soldiers were close before firing their weapons. This created carnage among the British soldiers who, consequently, fell in large numbers. The Americans first took aim at the officers, whom they recognized from their uniforms. Killing the officers created confusion and panic among the soldiers. At the end of the first attack, a colonial officer reported about the British soldiers, "The dead lay as thick as sheep in a fold." The Redcoats were forced to retreat down the hill.

After regrouping, the British launched a second attack, using the same tactics as the first charge. This had the same disastrous outcome. Although the rebels suffered losses as well, it was mainly British soldiers who got slaughtered.

When the Redcoats advanced up Breed's Hill for the third time, Prescott ordered the soldiers, "Don't fire until you see the whites of their eyes," an effort to conserve ammunition.[47] Despite that, the rebels were running out of bullets, and this time the British troops overran the Americans. The Redcoats again came marching up the hill in formation, several lines deep, with infantry soldiers wearing their characteristic tricorne hats and Brown Bess muskets with fixed bayonets, and the feared grenadiers providing support. The grenadiers were large and physically imposing members of the British army. They wore their typical bearskin hats, which made them look even taller and more fearsome. Their main function was to assault the enemy with bayonet charges after the infantry had fired volleys. The grenadiers were ruthless and bloodthirsty, and slaughtered everything in their path. It must have been a horrendous sight for Warren and his rebel soldiers, who were now running out of ammunition, to see the grenadiers emerging from the smoke with their bayonets ready to stab every living enemy in their path.

The Patriots' dire situation was described by a British officer who reported the condition among the Patriots inside the redoubt: "I cannot pretend to describe the Horror of the Scene within the Redoubt when we entered it, 'twas streaming with Blood & strew'd with dead & dying Men the Soldiers stabbing some and dashing out the Brains of others was a sight too dreadful for me to dwell any longer on."[48]

By then, the Rebels had used most of their ammunition and had to fight hand-to-hand, using their bayonets and bare hands, and their muskets as clubs. The British successfully climbed the protective dirt walls and took revenge by slaughtering as many Americans as possible, shooting many and stabbing others with their bayonets. Defenseless Rebels attempted to flee out of the redoubt. A British lieutenant reported, "I was with those two companies, who drove their bayonets into all that opposed them. Nothing could be more shocking than the carnage that followed the storming of this work. We tumbled over the dead to get at the living, who were crowding out of the gorge of the redoubt...the soldiers stabbing some and dashing out the brains of others."

Warren stayed in the redoubt, trying to protect his fellow Americans, who were panicking and trying to flee. The exact circumstances of Warren's death are not known, but tradition has it that Warren, brave in his fighting, was among the last to retreat from the redoubt after covering for as many of the Rebels as possible. Ultimately, trying to flee himself, he was spotted by a British officer and was shot to death at close range by the officer's assistant.

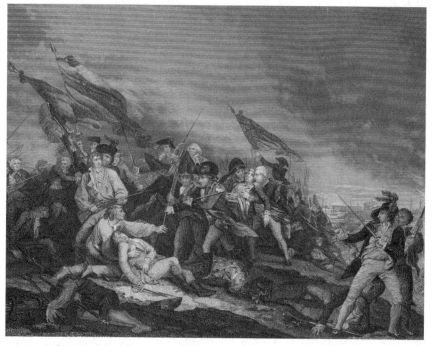

The Death of General Warren at the Battle of Bunker's Hill, 17 June, 1775. Part of this famous painting by John Trumbull ("The Painter of the Revolution") is on the cover of this book. (World History Archive)

Although the battle lasted for only about two hours, the losses were staggering on both sides. A total of 260 British soldiers were killed, and more than 800 were wounded. On the American side, 140 men were killed, and about 300 were wounded. The most severe loss (from the rebels' perspective), or gain (from the British standpoint), was that of Warren. The British general William Howe, who realized the significance of Warren's death, stated that Warren's life was worth the lives of five hundred men.

The agony and suffering at Breed's Hill spilled over to Boston and bloodied its streets. Although the British claimed "the day ended with glory," the evening in Boston turned horrendous when dead and wounded soldiers were brought back to the city. A local man gave the following account: "It was truly a shocking sight and sound, to see the carts loaded with those unfortunate men and to hear the piercing groans of the dying and those whose painful wounds extorted the sigh from the firmest mind."

It is unclear what happened with Warren's body after he was killed. Many stories have been told. Most likely, his body was mutilated and thrown into a grave on the battlefield along with other freedom fighters. A British officer, involved in the burial details later, wrote about Warren that his soldiers "stuffed the scoundrel with another into one hole and there he and his seditious principles may remain."[49]

There were rumors that Warren's body was further abused a couple of days later: "In a day or two after, Drew went upon the Hill again opened the dirt that was thrown over Doct. Warren, spit in his Face jump'd on his Stomach and at last cut off his Head and committed every act of violence upon his Body."

So ended the life of a surgeon, patriot, a potential future signer of the Declaration of Independence, and possibly even commander-in-chief and president of a new country in the process of being born.

Although the Battle of Bunker Hill was a victory for the British, the costs in dead and wounded were high, and these were considered unacceptable by the London powers. The British general William Howe commented, "When I look to the consequences of it, in the loss of so many brave officers, I do it with horror—the success is too dearly bought."[50] The losses cost Gage his position. He was ordered back to England, and General Howe replaced him.

The Postlude

Warren's death created a shock wave among the Patriots. Initially, it was difficult to obtain confirmation about his fate, and many refused to believe that Warren had died. When his brother John realized that a battle was going on at Charlestown, he left his surgical practice in Salem and hurried, together with other militia, to the place of fighting, in the hope of joining the American forces. However, they arrived too late. The battle was over, and the Americans had been defeated. John desperately tried to get information about his brother's fate, but when he attempted to pass the Charlestown neck and enter the town, he was stopped by a British soldier using his bayonet. The confrontation resulted in a scar on John's chest that he showed to his children every now and then during the decades to come.

Many Patriots expressed their deep sorrow and despair when they realized that Warren had died. In a letter to her husband John, who at the time was attending the Second Continental Congress in Philadelphia, Abigail Adams wrote that "our dear Friend Dr. Warren is no more but fell gloriously fighting for his Country."[51] John Adams, in turn, wrote that, "Our dear Warren has fallen with Laurels on his Brows, as fresh and blooming as ever graced and Hero."[52] Elbridge Gerry, one of Warren's fellow members on the Massachusetts Committee of Safety, wrote, "Our good, our beloved Friend Doctor Warren was on Bunker Hill when the Lines were forced and is no more."[53]

News about Warren's death echoed even on the other side of the Atlantic. In a London newspaper article written by a Revolution sympathizer, it was commented that, "he was a man of great courage…learning, and much humanity. It may well be said he is the greatest loss we have sustained."[54] Not surprisingly, the official British view of Warren was different; he was described as a scheming social climber and a reckless rebel against the king's authority. He was also ridiculed as someone who had used his ambition to raise himself from a "bare-legged milk boy" to a major general of an army.

It would take almost a year before Joseph's brothers Ebenezer and John managed to find the grave on Breed's Hill in which Warren's body had been thrown along with other militiamen. Paul Revere accompanied the Warren brothers in the search for Joseph's body. He played an important role in the identification of the body, recognizing a dental prosthesis consisting of two artificial teeth in the left upper jaw that he had made for Warren. This event has been quoted as the first example of forensic medicine being used to identify a body.

Warren's body lay in state at the Massachusetts Provincial State House for several days before being buried at the Old Granary Cemetery. His funeral service took place on April 8, 1776. The eulogy was delivered by Perez Morton, a young lawyer who had been one of Warren's patients. In his speech, Morton described Warren's noble character as a surgeon and physician, and praised him for providing the best care, even to patients who could not afford to pay him: "Whenever he beheld an indigent Object, which claimed his healing Skill, he administered it, without even the Hope of any other Reward than that which resulted from the Reflection of having so far promoted the Happiness of his Fellow-men."

Although other leaders of the revolution, including George Washington, Benjamin Franklin, John Adams, Samuel Adams, and Paul Revere, are now better remembered than Joseph Warren, at the time of the Revolution Warren was regarded as one of the most significant Patriots in the fight for freedom. His fame was widespread not only in Massachusetts, but across the colonies and ocean as well. Several theater plays were produced in Warren's honor, and performed on many stages in the country. In the plays, Warren's role as a general was typically the subject, although his career as a general only lasted four days. John Trumbull's famous painting, *The Death of General Warren at the Battle of Bunker's Hill*, helped preserve Warren's legacy as a soldier and general. This emphasis on Warren's role on the battlefield, and in other sometimes violent acts, made some people concerned that other features of Warren's character had become forgotten. After seeing the play *Bunker Hill: or the Death of General Warren: an Historic Tragedy* in New York City in 1797, John Adams, then the president of the United States, commented: "My Friend, Joseph Warren, was a scholar and a gentleman, but your author has made him a bully and a blackguard."

It is indeed remarkable that a surgeon was able to leave such big footprints in the creation and history of this country, not only as a physician, but also as a writer, politician, Patriot, freedom fighter, and army general.

Had he not died at the Battle of Bunker Hill, it is likely that he would have continued to play a significant role in the American Revolution, and would have become one of the Founding Fathers and leaders of the newborn country.

CHAPTER 2

JOHN WARREN—
Founder of Harvard Medical School

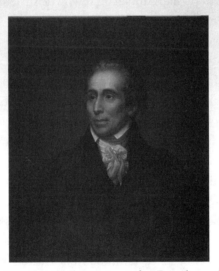

John Warren (1753–1815). Portrait by Rembrandt Peale. John
Warren was with Washington at the Battle of Long Island. Later,
he became a busy surgeon in Boston. He founded Harvard Medical
School in 1782. When John Adams's daughter Nabby underwent
a mastectomy for breast cancer, Warren was the surgeon.

J ohn Warren (1753-1815) was the youngest brother of Joseph Warren,[55] and a Continental Army surgeon during the Revolutionary War. He stands out in the annals of surgery for performing one of the first successful laparotomies in America, and a gruesome mastectomy on then ex-president John Adams's daughter in 1811. He was the founder of Harvard Medical School and was appointed its first Professor of Anatomy and Surgery in 1782.

Childhood

John was only two years old when he witnessed his father fall from an apple tree and carried home to the house dead. Despite his young age, the event was etched into John's memory for the rest of his life.[56] After adding the death of his brother at the Battle of Bunker Hill when John was still a young man, one can perhaps understand why he suffered periodic depressions throughout his life.

John was the youngest of five children. In contrast to his father, John's mother had a long life and died in 1803 at ninety years old. John grew up on the family farm in Roxbury with his brothers Joseph, Samuel, and Ebenezer. His childhood was influenced by strong religious and moral principles, with an emphasis on the importance of justice and family values. Although fatherless from early childhood, John was blessed by a strong and loving mother who provided a family home and traditions. Her children and grandchildren continued to visit when she grew old. She had the entire family for Thanksgiving dinners every year, and, up to the age of eighty, she prepared those dinners herself and always made sure she had cooked enough to allow her guests to take leftovers with them.

Even after her sons reached adulthood, she treated them as children. In a letter dated August 6, 1776, written to John when he was twenty-three and a hospital surgeon in the Continental Army at Cambridge, she started the letter with "Dear Child" and ended it with "Your affectionate mother, Mary Warren."[57]

The Warren brothers became well known in society, as Joseph and John were surgeons and involved in the Revolution, and Ebenezer was a judge in Maine. Samuel was an exception. He was somewhat reclusive and spent most of his time at the family farm, taking care of the orchard and serving as an important support for his mother. He never married, and was described as "shy." Whenever he went into the "big city" to visit with Joseph and his family, he was nervous because he felt that Joseph's wife was more elegant, both in dress and behavior, than he was used to at the farm. Before entering his brother's house, he used to buy gingerbread from vendors in the street and eat the bread before knocking on the door. This helped him to avoid sitting down and eating at the same table as Joseph and his wife.

Education

In the biography written by his son Edward, John Warren was described as a slow starter when it came to learning: "He did not evince any precocious talents for learning."[58] He could not read until he entered Roxbury Latin Grammar School at the age of ten. Once starting school, however, he quickly developed academic proficiency and did well during his school years. After finishing at Roxbury, he followed in the footsteps of Joseph and was admitted to Harvard College at the age of fourteen.

At Harvard, John became a successful scholar and developed a particular interest in the Latin language, something that turned out to be useful later in life when he was communicating with medical colleagues and scholars in Europe. His other passion in college was the study of anatomy. He became a "leading spirit of the Anatomical Club,"[59] the Spunkers, and participated in the illegal, but profitable, retrieval of corpses of executed criminals or newly buried persons, who were snatched from their graves and used for anatomical dissections.

Establishing a Medical Practice in Salem

After graduating from Harvard in 1771, John started studies in medicine as an apprentice with his brother Joseph, who, at that time, was a highly regarded surgeon and one of the most successful physicians in Boston. Following two years' apprenticeship, John established himself as a practitioner in Salem, along with Dr. Edward Holyoke. He chose Salem since

Boston "was well supplied with surgeons,"[60] making the environment quite competitive.

John initially struggled to build a practice in Salem. As a newcomer, he often ended up seeing patients who were less economically fortunate than those seen by the more established Dr. Holyoke. John, therefore, had difficulties generating a substantial income. He was conservative in his economic dealings and was unwilling to take on debts. This was the subject of letters between the Warren brothers.

In January 1775, Joseph wrote a letter to John, asking him for payment of a note most likely issued for medical tuition while John was an apprentice with Joseph. If John was not in an economic position to pay the note, Joseph advised him to give the note to a Dr. Greenleaf for £200, which would be paid in two years. The thought of this, however, scared John, who did not feel that he would be able to pay the sum in so short a time. In a letter to Joseph, John wrote, "It is true I have as good share of business as I could reasonably expect for the time I have been here, but I cannot collect more than money sufficient to defray the charges arising from clothing and other common expenses." He explained that, "I am not able to pay anything towards my board or apothecaries' bill, and am pretty certain that at the expiration of the above mentioned term I shall not be able to satisfy more than these annual demands, not to mention what I shall then be behindhand on these accounts." He understood he would not be able to increase his fees in the foreseeable future. He continued the letter, "A physician who should charge anything nearly sufficient barely to support the dignity of the profession, or should attempt to make any innovations upon the ancient usage of the town, would at once throw himself out of practice. The note has ever laid like the weight upon my mind, but I was always in hopes that you would not have occasion to call upon me to discharge it, till my circumstances should render it easy for me to do it."[61]

John also complained that it would probably take a long time before he would be able to take over the care of patients from his partner: "The principal business is still in the hands of Dr. Holyoke, and will doubtless remain until he is incapable for business, which is not likely to be soon." Little did he know how true this statement would turn out to be. Holyoke did not retire until the age of ninety-nine and lived beyond the age of one hundred! In his biography about his father, Edward wrote, "Dr. Holyoke's place did not soon become vacated. In October, 1828…I had the pleasure of going through the wards and offices of the Massachusetts General Hospital with him, then a hale, active man, in full possession of his faculties of mind and body, one hundred years old the 12ᵗʰ of August preceding. He had retired from business the year before, in 1827."[62]

It is unclear how the issue involving the unpaid note was resolved, but it did not seem to have caused a rift between the brothers. It is likely that the note was never paid. Only five months later, the Battle of Bunker Hill would not only end Joseph's life, but would also change John's career from that of a private surgeon in Salem to a surgeon in the American Continental Army.

While building his practice in Salem, John got involved in the examination of candidate physicians. The experience of one candidate was described as "nerve-wrecking," and during the examination, the aspiring physician was "agitated into a state of perspiration." When at one point, a colleague of John was asked how he would produce a sweat in the treatment of rheumatism, he answered, "I would have him examined before a medical committee."[63]

Drawn into the Military Conflict with England

Only twenty-two years old, John was drawn into the evolving military conflict with England in 1775. Like his older brother Joseph, John longed for the "shackles of British tyranny" to be gone.[64] On April 19, he participated in the Battles of Lexington and Concord together with his brothers Joseph and Samuel. Only two months later, he was at Bunker Hill searching for Joseph, whom he feared dead.

In the afternoon of June 17, while still seeing patients in his Salem practice, John heard the sounds of artillery to the south. When the sun was about to set, smoke from a big fire at Boston (Charlestown was burning!), along with arriving news about a military engagement, made John nervous. He knew that his brother Joseph was likely engaged in the battle, and he felt it was his duty to get involved as well. After a couple of hours' sleep, "in the morning about two o'clock," John "went off on horseback"[65] only to discover that he arrived too late. The battle was over with great losses on both sides, and the British troops ultimately defeating the American freedom fighters. When John realized that Joseph had indeed participated in the battle, he tried to find his brother. He was met with confusing and contradictory information, some of which reported Joseph as dead, some saying he was alive and well. In order to find out himself, John tried to enter Charlestown to look for his brother but was stopped by a British guard and "received a thrust from a bayonet, the scar of which he bore through life."[66] Eventually, John had to come to grips with the thought that Joseph had been killed in the battle.

The Battle of Bunker Hill made the hatred between the British and the Patriots even greater. John used strong words to express his disgust of the English rulers: "Unfeeling wretches!.... ye miscreants! stay your bloody hands...cover your heads with shame, ye guilty wretches."[67] John Warren wanted to give up his surgical career, at least temporarily, and join the Continental Army to fight the enemy on the battlefield. Knowing his medical qualifications, people close to him, however, convinced him to contribute to the freedom fight as a surgeon rather than as a soldier. As a result, Warren was appointed senior surgeon of the army hospital at Cambridge. In the process, he had to give up his growing practice in Salem.

Although Warren was trained as a surgeon, he, like many other surgeons, also had to take care of patients with non-surgical diseases. Fevers and diarrheas, particularly those caused by dysentery, were rampant in the military camps and were often fatal. Warren was concerned about the shortage of willow root that was popular in the treatment of different types of fevers. The shortage of willow root, and its great demand, made it one of the most expensive medicines of the day.

Warren's most important role at the Cambridge Hospital, however, was providing surgical care of wounded soldiers. Wound care and amputations were the most common procedures. The importance of surgeons in the military is exemplified by events taking place on November 22, 1775. On that day, Major General Putnam planned a major attack on British troops stationed at Cobble Hill. Dr. John Morgan (the newly appointed Surgeon-General of the Continental Army) issued the following instructions to "Dr. Warren, or the Orderly Surgeon of the week. As Dr. Foster was Orderly the last week, I take it for granted that Dr. Warren is for the present. The Orderly Surgeon is hereby directed to repair immediately but with all secrecy to Cobble Hill, with five Orderly Mates, a case of amputating instruments to each person, plenty of lint, tow, and bandages, for a brisk action,—at least two or three hundred if in readiness; a case of crooked needles, and a number of compresses. Let a second surgeon and mates be ready to follow if sent for. But at least two surgeons and the remaining mates should stand fast, nor by any means leave the hospital."

It has been speculated that Morgan feared a battle of the same magnitude as Bunker Hill. The Americans were surprised when they found that the British did not make Cobble Hill a battlefield. Washington suspected that the British had something else up their sleeve and were secretly contemplating "some important enterprise."

The Evacuation of Boston

The siege of Boston, initiated after the battles of Lexington and Concord, continued. The British could not get out by land, and the rebels could not get in. Both sides felt something needed to be done.

In early March 1776, Washington outmaneuvered General Howe. With great secrecy, protected by the dark of the night, Washington managed to haul cannons, brought by Henry Knox to Boston from Fort Ticonderoga, up the hills of Dorchester. When Howe woke up one morning, he could see cannons directly overlooking Boston, and threatening the city as well as the ships anchored in the harbor. The city was now at the mercy of Washington. Realizing the gravity of the situation, the British, along with many Loyalists, started to make preparations to abandon the city. On March 17, about 9,000 troops, along with 1,000 of their family members and 1,200 Tories, sailed out of the harbor on more than 120 ships. The day, St. Patrick's Day, is still remembered in Boston as the Evacuation Day.

Many British soldiers were upset they had to leave without time to plunder the city. On March 21, Warren wrote in his journal, "The soldiers, it appears, were much dissatisfied at being obliged to leave the town, without glutting their revengeful tempers with the blood of Yankees."[68]

The Americans were afraid the British would burn the town on their way out, and were surprised it didn't happen. Most likely, the city was spared from destruction as a result of the Americans' restraint from firing at the fleeing ships. Washington suspected that the fleet would sail to New York for continued fight. He was struck by disbelief when he realized the ships had sailed to Halifax in Nova Scotia.[69] By then, he had already ordered American troops to march to New York.

After the British evacuated Boston, the rebels entered the town, fearing massive destruction. They found Boston in better shape than anticipated. Warren wrote in his journal, "The houses I found to be considerably abused inside, where they had been inhabited by the common soldiery; but the external parts of the houses made a tolerable appearance. The streets were clean, and upon the whole, the town looks much better than I expected." Warren gave credit for the reasonable condition of Boston to General Howe, who "had been very careful to prevent his men from committing depredation." Indeed, when Howe understood that looting was going on, he proclaimed that, "The first soldier who is caught plundering will be hanged on the spot."[70]

Everything was not rosy, however, and Warren was outraged to find the medicines "left behind by the British…in great disorder" and poisoned with arsenic, "small amounts of yellow and white arsenic mixed in with them [the medicines]."[71]

After the evacuation of Boston, Warren initially stayed on at the hospital of Cambridge where he, along with other surgeons, tended to large numbers of sick, wounded, and invalids. Then, on May 11, Warren set out on horseback for New York to join Washington and his army.

Warren in the Revolutionary War

It didn't take long before Warren grew busy in New York. Shortly after his arrival, an epidemic of dysentery broke out. Hundreds of soldiers came down with the disease in a short time span. An interesting observation was made—only soldiers lodged in narrow spaces such as garrets or underground rooms contracted the malady—and it was concluded that its cause was the close quarters with the putrid air. One can only imagine the smell and horrible conditions in the narrow rooms filled with men having running diarrhea. Soldiers housed in larger apartments, or outdoors in tents, were not affected by the epidemic to the same degree. Based on these observations, men, both sick and well, were moved to larger and airier habitats. These measures helped stop the epidemic.

Warren also became aware of other events taking place shortly after his arrival in New York, an event that could have resulted in the defeat of the rebels and the end of the Revolution. In the middle of June, a plot engineered by Loyalists was discovered. They were expecting the arrival of British forces in New York, and had planned to work with the British troops on their arrival. The governor of New York, the mayor of New York City, and some of Washington's own bodyguards were involved in a scheme. Washington was the main target and was intended to become the first victim. He received intelligence, however, alerting him to the threats.

Many different stories about how Washington was going to be eliminated and how the revolution would be crushed have circulated through the years. According to one version, Washington was going to be either killed or kidnapped and delivered to General Howe after New York was set on fire. In a different legend, Washington was going to be served green peas poisoned with arsenic. As reported in that story, Washington's housekeeper had learnt that the peas she was about to serve Washington had been poisoned. She grabbed the peas away from the intended victim just before he was about to consume them and threw them out the window. Chickens roaming the street were reported to have died after eating the peas.

The story about Thomas Hickey is more grounded in facts than the story about the green peas. Hickey had deserted from the British army and had become a member of Washington's lifeguard. He started to have second thoughts when he realized that Washington's army could be defeated by the British. He was drawn into the conspiracy to kill Washington, but was discovered. He was court-martialed and found guilty and sentenced to be executed by hanging. Washington wanted to make an example of Hickey and ordered off duty soldiers to watch the execution. At eleven o'clock in the morning of June 28, more than twenty thousand people came to see the hanging of Hickey.

That Warren was aware of these dramatic events is obvious from a letter Ms. Grafton wrote to Warren from Salem on July 6. In the letter, she commented, "The melancholy account you gave me of the late discovery, was very shocking, and had they put their hellish plot into operation, what would have become of us? I sincerely hope that all their wicked desires may be brought to light, and they may receive the punishment due to their great crimes." In the same letter, she expressed her frustration with the conditions on the American continent: "Oh that this unnatural war was at an end, which separates friends and acquaintances."[72]

Warren was put in charge of the General Hospital of New York at Long Island.[73] Patriots anticipated the arrival of British forces and significant military activities, so the hospital was being prepared "for the reception of sick and wounded persons, whose cases may require it; which John Warren, Esq., surgeon in the General Hospital is appointed to superintend and direct." Around the same time, Dr. John Morgan, who had succeeded Dr. Benjamin Church as Surgeon-General of the Continental Army, gave specific instructions to the surgeons about how to treat (and triage) injured soldiers on the battlefield:

> The amputation of a limb, or performance of any capital operation, cannot well take place in the heat of a brisk action. It is seldom possible or requisite, what the surgeon has chiefly to attend to, in cases of persons being much wounded in the field of battle, is to stop any flow of blood, either by tourniquet, ligature, lint and compresses, or a suitable bandage, as the case may require, to remove any extraneous body from the wound; to reduce frac-tured bones; to apply proper dressings to wounds;.... The wounded being thus dressed by the regimental surgeons, are next to be removed to the nearest hospital belonging to the brigade, or to the general hospital, as may be most convenient.... The regimental surgeons ought to call on the officers of the corps to which they belong, to settle with them, what persons are to be employed in carry-ing off the wounded, and for a supply of wheel barrels, or more convenient biers, for conveying them from the field of battle to the place appointed for reception of the wounded, or general hospital.

At this time, the tensions and power struggle between the regimental and hospital surgeons started to frustrate Warren. Although the rank of the regimental surgeons was below that of the hospital surgeons, the regimental surgeons had the right to send patients to the general hospital. The hospital surgeons, therefore, had no control over which patients were admitted to their hospitals. Typically, wounded soldiers were initially admitted to the regimental hospitals, but when they developed fevers, diarrheas (particularly dysentery), or other signs or symptoms of infection, they were sent to the general hospital. Not only were the general hospital surgeons unable to refuse patients sent to them from the regimental hospitals, they could not even admit their own patients without the approval of the regimental surgeons. This created an atmosphere of jealousy and antagonism, where hospital surgeons started to feel useless and unnecessary (even though most of them were better trained and more skillful than the regimental surgeons).

Warren vented his frustration in an August 10, 1776, letter to Morgan. He complained that the situation made him feel "a very useless person" and that his situation was "extremely disagreeable." He even threatened to resign from his position if conditions did not improve. (He was quick to add, however, that he still would remain in the army until he "had served as a volunteer in the apparently decisive battle.")

The Battle of Long Island

Not long after Warren's letter to Morgan, the British showed up at New York—and they showed up in force. They arrived with a huge fleet carrying 30,000–40,000 troops assembled during their stay in Halifax. Because the British were simultaneously involved in conflicts in Europe, there was a shortage of soldiers. To remedy this, the British had hired German mercenaries (the "Hessians") to fill the ranks. The British landed their forces in Long Island in preparation for a major attack on New York City. The activities made Morgan keenly aware of the need for surgeons and surgical equipment. In a letter that history has remembered as the "Razor Letter," Morgan wrote Warren that he had ordered young surgeons to provide assistance, and outlined additional efforts taken to remedy the situation. The young surgeons sent for assistance were to "bring five hundred additional bandages and twelve fracture boxes" containing saws, knives, and other instruments necessary for the treatment of fractures and other injuries— treatments that often consisted of amputations. There was a shortage of scalpels: "I fear they have no scalpels, as whatever I have committed to the hospitals has always been lost. I send you two, in which case, if you want more, use a razor for an incision knife. Let me know, from time to time, at Long Island."[74]

On August 27, the disastrous Battle of Long Island took place. The day before the fighting, Washington emphasized the importance of the upcoming battle and tried to instill courage in his soldiers: "The time is now near at hand, which must...determine whether Americans are to be freemen or slaves." The battle resulted in nearly two thousand Americans killed, wounded, or taken prisoners, and prompted Washington's famous retreat across the East River.

After the Battle of Long Island, Warren followed the army during its retreat. He ended up spending extended time as a hospital surgeon at Hackensack. Another major general hospital was at Newark, headed by Dr. Isaac Foster. At this time, the tensions between the regimental and hospital surgeons seemed to have somewhat eased. According to communications from Morgan, it is clear the regimental surgeons were required to report to Warren or Foster, and to act under them at the hospitals, making them subordinate to the hospital surgeons. The restructuring of the hospitals, and the reinforcement of the rank order between the hospital and regimental surgeons, caused the regimental surgeons' resentment and bitterness towards Morgan, something that did not help him in his power struggle with Shippen.

The surgeons, including Warren, were overworked and exhausted. Warren fell ill and was out of commission for several months. In the biography of his father, Edward Warren wrote that "the fatigue and exposure added to the causes of anxiety and depression, brought on a severe and dangerous illness."[75] Although it is unclear what the nature of Warren's illness was, it created major concerns among his family, friends, and colleagues. His superior, Director-General Morgan, started a letter written on October 4: "Dear Sir,—I have been very anxious about your illness...." Whatever the illness was, Warren improved and, at the end of October, his brother Ebenezer wrote in a letter that "I hope by this time you are perfectly recovered."

At the end of 1776 and during the early months of 1777, when the forces led by Washington continued to retreat, the Rebels' spirit and moral were down. Offered pardon by General Howe, many American soldiers deserted. Overwhelmed by the large number of injured and sick, the surgeons also felt their safety was being ignored. For example, in the evacuation of New York, the medical corps were initially left behind and, as described by Dr. Eustis, "escaped only through the bad firing of the Hessians."

The same type of disregard for the surgeons and other medical personnel was displayed shortly after Washington's famous crossing of the Delaware River, and the capture of Trenton in December 1776. Although the victory at Trenton was a boost for the American morale, the situation for the Rebel army was still critical, and Philadelphia remained threatened by the British. A large contingent of British troops had been left at Princeton under the command of Lord Charles Cornwallis. Washington made secret plans to attack Princeton from Trenton, where American forces were now in control. In order to deceive the British, Washington ordered campfires to be lighted in the evening of January 2, which made the British believe that the American troops were still at Trenton. Only a few men were left behind to manage the campfires while the rest of the American troops, protected by the darkness of the night, sneaked away and marched to Princeton.

Lord Cornwallis probably thought he was in a bad dream when he woke up in the morning and realized that the American campsite at Trenton had been abandoned, and that the Rebels were now threatening Princeton. But equally great was the surprise of Warren and his colleague surgeons, who had not been informed about the plans to attack Princeton and now found themselves alone in Trenton, defenseless against any British troops. They left Trenton in great haste, galloping away on their horses, not knowing which direction to take. After some tense moments, they managed to reach Princeton just in time to start tending to the wounded. Their escape, however, was "a very narrow one."

In early 1777, Congress terminated Morgan from his position as Director-General of the American Hospitals. He was replaced by William Shippen Jr., a personal friend of Washington. The event was followed by a reorganization of the medical administration, and Congress reappointing medical officers. Warren applied for the position of subdirector, and asked to be placed in Rhode Island, close to Boston. Warren was strongly supported by several influential people, including General Greene, who, in a letter directed to John Hancock (then the President of the Continental Congress), wrote that Warren "is a young gentleman of ability, humanity, and great application to business." Despite the support, however, Warren was not successful in his application and did not get the job. This made him anxious and nervous about his future. In a letter directed to Washington, dated February 10, 1777, he wrote, "Sir,—By the suspension of Dr. Morgan from the directorship of the Eastern Department, the commission which I formerly held in the General Hospital is vacated. I am now only employed…by Dr. Shippen, without any positive assurance of an appointment upon the new establishment…. Having served as a senior surgeon in the General Hospital ever since the commencement of the war, I must, consequently, be considered experienced in the business of hospitals, especially as I have, both at Long Island and Hackensack, had the sole direction of the hospitals there established."[76]

In his reply letter, Washington was noncommittal and almost dismissive, basically confirming that Warren was out of luck. One important reason for this development was probably the fact that Warren had been appointed by and worked for Morgan. Any friend of Morgan was now the enemy of Shippen, who may have been actively working against Warren. And, of course, the friendship between Washington and Shippen did not help Warren's situation.

Warren felt he had no other option than to head back to Boston. This probably did not upset him too much. He would now be closer to his family, including his brother's orphaned children. In Boston, Warren was offered the position of superintendent of a military hospital that would be founded by the State of Massachusetts. He was appointed Senior Surgeon of the General Hospital in Boston on July 1, 1777. He had secured a job without the help of Washington and other people in the "establishment," and would play an important role in the advancement of surgery and medicine in Boston and nationwide.

Back in Boston: Love and Marriage

Warren was only twenty-four years old when he returned to Boston. From a professional standpoint, he was busy attending his new job as Senior Surgeon at the General Hospital, and reestablishing a private practice. Both his experiences as a surgeon in the military and his reputation from his time in Salem came in handy and helped him succeed in building a private practice.

Since he was young, good looking, and a successful surgeon, it is not surprising that Warren was interested in and became pursued by attractive women. The woman who excited him the most was only about seventeen when Warren returned to town. Abigail ("Abby") was the daughter of John Collins, the Governor of Rhode Island. When the British took Rhode Island in December 1776, Abigail came to Cambridge to join the family of her cousin, Colonel Thomas Mifflin. During this time, she moved in Washington's inner circles, and her beauty actually caught Washington's eye. She became a protégé of Washington, and lived in the midst of the military and civilian elite. When Mifflin was promoted to general, he moved to Philadelphia, where he and his wife became known for their parties that were attended by many prominent patriots. It is likely that Warren met with Abigail both in Cambridge and Philadelphia at these occasions. It is uncertain whether it was love at first sight, but in love he fell. Abby "excited his interest, and he was fortunate in winning her from the many rivals who surrounded her."

In his biography about John Warren, his son Edward described his mother as possessing "a good deal of beauty; that especially of expression, which is given by strong powers of mind. Her features were fine, her stature rather tall and commanding, and she possessed that delicacy of complexion which the Newport climate was said to promote. In character she formed a remarkable and happy contrast to my father. She was reserved, self-possessed; of acute sensibility indeed, but this sensibility kept under the strictest control. She was one who would bear the sting of a concealed serpent, rather than let the world know she suffered."[77]

John and Abigail were married on November 4, 1777, two years into the Revolutionary War. Edward described his father as someone who held "very old-fashioned notions of marriage. He believed that man and wife actually became one; one in thought, one in feeling, one in interest, one in sympathy, and one in the ownership of property."[78] Warren wanted his wife to share not only his political interests, but also his medical studies and cares. One of the first books she read after her marriage was a treatise on surgery.

As a newlywed couple, John and Abigail had to make do on the young surgeon's limited pay from the General Hospital and his newly built practice. Their love and devotion likely helped them survive any potential financial hardships.

One way by which Warren hoped to generate extra income was to go into business with two colleagues, Doctors Isaac Rand and Lemuel Hayward. In April 1778, they entered a partnership to form a hospital at Sewall's Point in Brookline. They were to inoculate for smallpox, and treat patients with the disease. Reading the contract makes it clear that financial aspects played an important role:

> "Articles of agreement made and concluded this twenty-third of April, 1778, between us…. That we, from this time forward, for the space of fourteen months, do enter in partnership in the business of inoculating for the small-pox at Sewall's Point, in Brookline, and also for patients in the natural small-pox that may be sent to said hospital (except those patients belonging to the army)…. That we will be at equal charges in repairing the barracks, which we shall improve for said inoculation, and all other necessary charges…and that the profits arising therefrom shall be equally divided between us."

As a newlywed with a pregnant wife, Warren was hoping for extra income from the business arrangements with Rand and Hayward.

The couple's firstborn, John Collins, arrived on the first of August, 1778. Warren's continued involvement with the army as senior surgeon at the General Hospital often forced him away from home. He kept in touch with his wife by frequent letters, which he typically started with "My Dear Girl," "My All," or "My Dear Abby." He wrote so many letters that he started numbering them to make it easier for Abby to keep track of them, and to avoid confusion.

Some of the letters were painful, particularly when he realized his beloved wife was not doing well. About three weeks after the birth of John Collins, she seemed to have suffered from mastitis (infection of the breast), commonly caused by breastfeeding. On Saturday evening, August 22, he wrote to Abby that he was concerned about her breast problems, and was also afraid she was concealing some of her symptoms in order not to worry him. He wrote, "If the swelling and hardness of the breast continues, let the enclosed recipe be put up by Dr. Willard, and rub it on three or four times a day. But if anything sudden should take place, immediately procure the best assistance. I feel, if possible, more than you undergo. You call my letters love epistles; I care not what epithet you give them; they speak the sentiments of my heart."

As a consequence of the mastitis, Abby was never able to breastfeed any of her later children.

Financial Crisis at the Hospitals and among the Surgeons

Only a couple of years into the Revolutionary War, hard economic times affected Boston and the colonies in many different ways. Money lost value, especially the paper money. In October 1778, it was reported that "our money is little better than blank paper. It takes forty dollars to purchase a barrel of cider; fifty pounds lawful for a hundred of sugar, and fifty dollars for a hundred of flour; four dollars per day for a laborer and find him, which will amount to four more." So great was the depreciation of the Continental paper money that the nominal value of forty pounds in bills equaled one pound of silver, and even at that rate, paper money was not always accepted.

Injustice and corruption worsened the economic hardship that Warren and other members of the medical profession had to endure. Soldiers and officers started to leave the army because of the deplorable conditions they were asked to put up with, and the decreasing value of their pay. In order to keep the army together, Congress decided that all officers who stayed in service till the end of the war would be paid half their annual salary for the rest of their life (basically providing a pension); they would be compensated for the depreciation of the paper money, and rewarded according to their rank at the close of the war.

To the dismay of Warren and other medical officers, these arrangements and compensations affected only line officers, not the medical officers. This prompted a petition submitted to Congress on October 5, 1779, requesting that members of the Medical Department of the army be treated equally to the line officers. So strong were the feelings about the unfair conditions that medical officers got together and signed a report to Congress, in which they gave an ultimatum and threatened to resign if the injustices were not addressed soon, and by a set deadline:

> "We, the subscribers, officers of the Medical Department in the army of the United States…do hereby mutually and severally engage to one another, that unless the terms of the petition which we have subscribed are complied with by Congress before the first day of January next (1780), we will, on that day, resign our several appointments in said medical department, and will not again serve or do any other part of the duty…until Congress shall have paid a satisfactory attention to said petition…."

Protesting and writing letters and petitions, Warren was on the frontline of the fight for better financial compensation. The corruption he saw in the corridors of power upset him. In a letter to Samuel Adams, Warren wrote, "Gentlemen who are near Congress are extremely artful and assiduous in promoting the interests of themselves and dependents, but surely Congress will not suffer themselves to be so imposed upon by the designing artifices of interested men, as to listen to every proposal of theirs, whilst those who cannot be personally heard are winked out of sight, or forgot."[79]

Warren and his colleagues pointed out that when following the army and providing care for wounded and sick soldiers, they had risked their lives. They certainly subjected themselves to the dangers of death, which was proven by the frequent loss of medical officers. They also ran the risk of being wounded or taken prisoner. Perhaps the greatest risks, however, were those associated with the care of sick and wounded soldiers under relatively primitive conditions: "The daily attendance in a crowded hospital, filled often with putrid and infectious disease, involved equal danger, unaccompanied with the excitement of battle."

Warren felt he was justified to lead the fight for better and more just treatment of the surgeons. As he pointed out in a letter to Timothy Pickering, dated May 8, 1780, "I doubt not you will excuse my informing you that I am the oldest senior surgeon on the continent."[80] At this point, Warren was two months shy of turning twenty-seven.

Although the petition was taken up by Congress, it was not met with success. Several members of Congress suggested that the petition should have instead been submitted to the legislature of Massachusetts.

Not only did the difficult times affect the surgeons' personal financial wellbeing, but they also resulted in severe problems at the hospitals. In a letter addressed to the Governor and the Legislature of Massachusetts, Warren wrote about the difficult conditions:

> Gentlemen,—Though I have frequently represented the distressed conditions of the sick in the Continental Hospital, yet I have never had so ample occasion to deplore their miseries as at present.
>
> For some days, they have not had an ounce of meat; not a stick of wood but what they have taken from the neighboring fences; for near a week not a vegetable; and scarcely any medicine for above a year. In fine, to sum up the whole in a few words, the sick and wounded, many of which are exceedingly dangerous, and some of them in a state which requires immediate amputation, are not furnished by the public with a single article of sustenance except bread alone, and must have perished ere this had not the charitable donations of a few individuals in some measure contributed to their relief.
>
> I have been incessantly making application for these last twelve months to all the departments for supplies, but cannot procure any. During which time the groans of

the sick and wounded, suffering, and perhaps dying, for want of necessities, have been perpetually saluting my ears. I must, therefore, beg your Excellency and Honors' action in this matter, and am with the greatest respect, gentlemen,

Your most obedient servant, J. WARREN.[81]

The troubling state of the American finances created a difficult and interesting dilemma. On one hand, avoiding taxation was one of the main reasons behind the war. On the other hand, more money and soldiers were needed to carry out the war. It was estimated that an advance of £2,000,000 from Massachusetts was needed to cover the cost for recruiting an additional two thousand soldiers and other war-related expenses. And the money was going to be raised by direct taxation! One important difference, of course, was this taxation would be decided by the colonists and not the Parliament.

The Boston and Massachusetts Medical Societies

In 1780, Warren was one of the principal founders of the Boston Medical Society. The founders also included Doctors Samuel Danforth, Isaac Rand, Thomas Kast, and Thomas Bulfinch. Among these individuals, Kast and Bulfinch were particularly well educated. Kast had spent two years in London, attending lectures and training at Guy's Hospital and St. Thomas'. He had established a busy practice in Boston and enjoyed a reputation as a skillful surgeon. Bulfinch had trained under the famous London surgeon William Cheselden, and also established a successful practice after returning to Boston.

The initial aim of the Boston Medical Society was to regulate physicians' fees. This differed from the objective of the Massachusetts Medical Society, founded one year later with Warren's active involvement. The principal charge of the Massachusetts Medical Society was to regulate the licensing of physicians. Members of the society had the authority to "examine all Candidates for the Practice of Physic." Today, the Massachusetts

Medical Society remains the oldest continuously operating medical society in the United States.

In a 1781 written public notice, Warren, who was one of the thirty-one founding members of the Massachusetts Medical Society, described additional important purposes of the society: "The design of the institution is to promote medical and surgical knowledge, inquiries into the animal economy & the promotion & effects of medicine." Dr. Holyoke of Salem was the first president of the Massachusetts Medical Society (1782–1784). Warren had a long tenure as the seventh president (1804–1815).

The Massachusetts Humane Society

The interest in resuscitating dead or dying individuals was not limited to executed criminals. The Massachusetts Humane Society, founded in 1780, had a broader objective: "to promote measures to restore to life persons apparently dead." Warren was one of the founders of this society as well, and, according to Warren's son, the Massachusetts Humane Society "was one of the strongest objects of interest" of his father. The purpose of the society was "for the recovery of all persons who meet with such accidents as to produce in them the appearance of death, and for promoting the cause of humanity by pursuing such means, from time to time, as shall have for their object the preservation of human life, and the alleviation of its miseries." The Humane Society was also a charitable organization, helping poor and unfortunate members of the society.

One of the Humane Society's first actions was awarding twenty-eight shillings to a Mr. Andrew Sloane for saving the life of a boy who had drowned after falling through the ice. Another example was the resuscitation of a child who had fallen into a deep well and seemed to be dead when taken out; however, after "long and continued efforts in the employment of means recommended by the society, animation was restored." This act also resulted in a reward from the Society.

Shipwrecked sailors along the coast of New England were another focus of the Massachusetts Humane Society. In order to help these unfortunate seamen, the Society arranged for the erection of huts along the coast.

Members of the Society inspected the huts on an annual basis. To their dismay, they often found the huts damaged and plundered of their content.

Warren personally participated in the development of lifeboats and life vests. Edward Warren had seen one of the life jackets in his father's house, and described it as "a leather bag made air-tight, to be worn around the body, with shoulder straps and belt, and fitted with a brass cock for filling it with air from the mouth...."[82]

The Society's charitable activities grew as time went on. At a later time point, a committee was formed, coordinating with the medical faculty at the Massachusetts General Hospital, to provide for the sick and poor. Abandoning unwanted infants was a sad reality, reflecting the inability of mothers without means to provide for their babies. Rescuing foundlings, therefore, became an additional important task for the Humane Society.

Another concern attracting the interest of the Society was the many people drowning in Charles River near the colleges. Along with Dr. Dexter, Warren formed a committee that coordinated with the city of Cambridge, and built bathing houses along the river. The Humane Society donated $150 for this purpose.

Warren must have kept quite busy during these years with his time split between his private surgical practice, hospital appointments, surgeries, and the founding of several medical and humane societies. His life, however, would grow even busier.

The American Academy of Arts and Sciences

The American Academy of Arts and Sciences was founded in Boston in 1780. The Academy's members included the most distinguished men in science and literature of the time. Several of the founders were Patriots who were heavily involved in the ongoing Revolution. They included Samuel Adams, John Adams, and John Hancock. Other founders were physicians and surgeons, and Warren was elected a member in August 1781.

The initial priorities of the Academy are quite interesting. Agriculture was number one on the list of purposes because it was well understood that successful farming was essential for the prosperity of the country. Members of the Academy were requested to "examine the various soils and determine what each is best adapted to produce; to ascertain the most suitable manures, and the means of increasing them; to devise methods to secure the fruits of the field and of the trees from the blight, and destructive insects." The second object of the Academy was the study of natural history, followed by the studies of botany, chemistry, astronomy, and mechanical arts and manufactures.

Founding of Harvard Medical School

The first medical schools in America were established in Philadelphia in 1764, and in New York in 1767. About fifteen years later, the Corporation of Harvard College and its president charged Warren to develop plans for a medical school in Boston. The plans were presented to the Harvard Corporation in September 1782, and included the creation of three professorships (similar to the model used in Philadelphia).

Each professorship had specific requirements. The Professor of Anatomy and Surgery should "demonstrate the anatomy of the human body with physiological observations; and explain and perform a complete system of surgical operations."[83] The Professor of Theory and Practice of Physic should "teach their pupils the theory and practice of physic, by… lecturing on the diseases of the human body, and taking with them such as are qualified to visit their patients; making proper observations on the nature of the diseases, the peculiar circumstances attending them, and the method of cure." Finally, the Professor of Chemistry and *Materia Medica* should "explain the theory of Chemistry, and apply its principles in a course of actual experiments." It was stipulated that the professors of the medical school should be equal to the other professors at Harvard. The professors and medical students should also be granted access and use of the library.

After some revisions and amendments, Warren's proposals, constituting twenty-two articles, were approved and confirmed by the Harvard College Corporation and by the Board of Overseers in the fall of 1782. Harvard Medical School had been established!

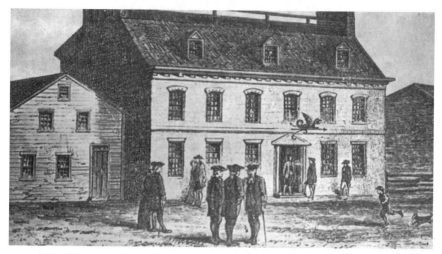

**Building in Cambridge used by Harvard Medical School
in the early years after its founding. (The History of HMS,
https://hms.harvard.edu/about-hms/history-hms)**

Not surprisingly, Warren played an important role at the medical school. He was appointed the first Professor of Anatomy and Surgery on November 22, 1782. In a letter dated December 3, addressed to the Reverend Simon Willard at the Board of Overseers, he expressed his gratitude: "Dear Sir,—The flattering testimony of attention which I yesterday received from the Hon. Board of Overseers of Harvard College in their vote of concurrence with the Corporation in their choice of a Professor of Anatomy and Surgery, demands my warmest return of gratitude...."[84]

Warren worked diligently to make certain the other professorships were filled as soon as possible. On Christmas Eve 1782, Dr. Benjamin Waterhouse was appointed Professor of the Theory and Practice of Physic. Waterhouse was a personal friend of the Warren family. He had received his medical education in England. He was a proliferative author and had penned many medical articles.

In May 1783, Dr. Aaron Dexter, a lifelong friend of Warren, was elected Professor of Chemistry and *Materia Medica*. It was said that Dexter was a better theorist than practical chemist—an important observation since one of his duties as professor was applying the theory of chemistry in a course of actual experiments. He became known for frequently ending his classes with, "Gentlemen, the experiment has failed." However, he told them not to worry since they had been taught the theory, and encouraged them to repeat the experiments in their own rooms "with better probable success."

From his colleagues in Philadelphia, Warren sought advice regarding the organizational aspects of the medical school. One concern was the rank order between the professors, and Warren sought to find out how it was done in Philadelphia: by seniority of age, graduation, or time in medical practice, and whether foreign education would influence the precedence. He was informed that in Philadelphia, the rank order between the professors was determined by the seniority of appointment, and if two professors had been appointed at the same time, they were considered equals. This explanation probably pleased Warren since he was the first professor appointed at Harvard Medical School.

The first several years at Harvard Medical School were primitive and lacking in resources. Lectures were held in apartments and basements rather than lecture halls. Despite the unfavorable conditions, Warren was an enthusiastic lecturer of his subjects, anatomy and surgery. He "interested the students, and held them in fixed attention during lectures of two hours' length; for he did not limit himself to a fixed time." Warren's contemporaries admired his warmth and enthusiasm. His lectures were "not a dry account of bones, muscles, and blood vessels." A student commented "the driest bone of the human body became in his hands...the subject of animated and agreeable description."[85]

In addition to having only relatively small apartments available for lectures, several other problems made the early years of Harvard Medical School challenging. As we have already seen, difficulties finding enough corpses for dissection continued to be of great concern. The lectures were delivered in Cambridge, where the cost of living was higher than in Boston. Consequently, the Professors of Anatomy and Surgery and Chemistry could not afford to reside in Cambridge and had to get to their lectures either by a long travel over land (through Roxbury and Brookline), or by the Charlestown Ferry. Both routes took time and were often slowed by snow and ice. Warren did not only have to endure rough physical conditions; he also had to sacrifice income from his private surgical practice in order to fulfill his duties as Professor of Anatomy and Surgery (unpaid in the era of enlightenment and idealism). Almost three decades after the foundation of Harvard Medical School, a vote was passed by the corporation and overseers that finally allowed the Professors of Anatomy and Surgery and Chemistry to deliver their lectures in Boston. Prior to this, the Professor of Physics lived in Cambridge, and was not interested in moving his lectures to Boston.

During the early years of Harvard Medical School, the historical and religious prejudice against dissections, their associations with unlawful grave robberies, and the lack of corpses continued to be challenges, especially for Warren, the Professor of Anatomy and Surgery. Despite the challenges, the role of dissections in the teaching of anatomy continued to grow. Anatomy kept generating great interest among surgeons and medical students, and the dissections, which were often open for the public, drew big crowds.

During the first several years, only one student graduated from the medical school per year. Remarkably, the first MD degree ever given by Harvard Medical School was awarded in 1783 to Edward A. Holyoke, who, a decade earlier, had been Warren's colleague (and competitor) in Salem.[86] In 1812, the annual number of graduates had risen to three. In comparison, the number of medical students graduating from Harvard was greater than sixteen hundred in 2018.

When Harvard Medical School started to issue the MD degree, there was confusion between the academic degree and the license to practice medicine. This confusion resulted in disputes between Harvard University and the Massachusetts Medical Society. The Society had been charged by the legislature to license candidates for "the practice of physic and surgery," and it was unclear whether an MD degree provided the right to practice medicine. After deliberations between Harvard and the Medical Society, things were clarified, and "the two institutions have henceforth exerted their respective functions in perfect friendship and honor with each other, the one in teaching, and the other in licensing practitioners in medicine."

Another area of tension between Harvard Medical School and the Massachusetts Medical Society was the privileges to admit patients to the almshouse. The professors at Harvard considered care of the patients at the almshouse an important opportunity for the medical students to get bedside experience. The Medical Society opposed the idea of Harvard professors and medical students gaining privileges, because the professors charged high fees for their services. Warren seemed to have been a major offender in this respect, and was described as showing "the worse grace... as his pecuniary demands against the government for his attendance on the State's poor, are more than double any that were ever made in the same period for the same business."[87]

Warren wrote several petitions to the legislature, requesting better pay for his services at the almshouse, but was rejected each time. On one occasion, he called his application, "Another of my useless petitions to obtain my just rights." When negotiations between the medical school and the Board of Overseers of the Poor failed, the opportunity for valuable clinical experience for the medical students was lost.

A Successful Laparotomy for Removal of an Ovarian Tumor in 1785

The agony and suffering of patients undergoing surgical procedures without anesthesia were horrifying. Previously, most of those procedures had consisted of amputations, removal of bladder stones ("stone cutting"), and repair of hernias ("ruptures"). In 1785, Warren reported on a patient who underwent a laparotomy (opening of the abdomen) and survived the procedure.[88] He reported the case to the American Academy of Arts and Sciences as an example of "the perfect safety with which large and free openings may be made under certain circumstances into the abdomen," and entitled his paper "Large tumor in the abdomen containing hair."[89] The procedure was remarkable, not only because it was done without anesthesia, but because of what was found at the surgery.

Warren's patient was a "negro woman" who presented with a large tumor in her abdomen. The tumor had been there for quite some time but had grown in size more recently, and had become fluctuating. Her doctors suspected she had an infected tumor with pus developing. The details of the surgery were described in the biography written by Warren's son:

> An extensive incision was made through the rectus muscle, and about a pint of watery matter immediately issued from it; after which some quantity of pus was discharged.

On introducing two or three fingers into the cavity, a quantity of soft substance was felt within it, much about the consistency of soft soap. This was removed with a table-spoon to the quantity of about a pound, and after three or four successive dressings, about three pounds more were removed.

At each dressing the matter was particularly examined, and found to contain a large quantity of short hair or wool, about three quarters of an inch long, uniformly mixed with it. On careful examination no bone or other foreign substance could be found in the tumor. The matter had evidently been contained in a sac, which firmly adhered to the peritoneum.[90]

The patient was a sensation, and "was visited by many of the practitioners in Boston, and the supposition of an extra-uterine fetus was entertained, but the absence of all the usual signs of pregnancy, and of bone or other foreign matter in the sac, contradicted the supposition. Dr. Warren was inclined to consider it a diseased ovarium adhering to the neighboring part of the uterus as well as to the peritoneum, from the common result of inflammation. The patient recovered perfect health, became moderately corpulent, and had the *catamenia* (menstrual periods) regularly."

Warren's case was only the second documented laparotomy to have been performed in America. The first laparotomy reported in the colonies was performed by Dr. John Bard in 1759, as we will find in a later chapter. It is interesting that historians commonly list Dr. Ephraim McDowell's 1809 laparotomy, which was performed in Danville, Kentucky, as the first. McDowell's patient was also a woman with an abdominal tumor. She underwent a laparotomy on Dr. McDowell's kitchen table, which had been brought into the front room of the surgeon's house. Her tumor was a large ovarian cyst that was successfully removed. She also survived the procedure and lived for several more years. Although McDowell's heroic surgery is typically described as the first laparotomy performed in America, Bard and Warren preceded McDowell by about fifty and twenty-five years, respectively. In addition, two laparotomies for ectopic pregnancies had been performed by the Virginia surgeon, William Baynham, in the 1790s.[91]

Growing Family and Improved Living Quarters

In 1785, Warren had been married for eight years. He and his wife seemed to have a happy marriage and life together. Their family had expanded, and they now had no less than ten children in their household: five of their own and five adopted children, whom Joseph Warren had left behind after his death. By now, Warren was an established and busy surgeon and could afford a bigger home. He bought a house on School Street, with the property facing Washington Street on one side and Tremont Street on the other. Warren's son, Edward, who grew up in the house, described it lovingly in his biography of his father.[92]

The house was a three-story building. The first floor had two parlors, one on each side of the entrance, with one of them used as a dining room. There was also a "medicine room" on the first floor described as an "apothecary's shop in miniature." Warren let his apprentices use the medicine room as a study and reading room, and as a place to prepare medicines and fill prescriptions. Behind the medicine room, Warren had his study where he saw patients and also kept his books and surgical instruments. The first floor was connected to an extension of the house in which the kitchen was located. The hallway between the parlors had doorways into the garden, and also led to a staircase to the second floor. As Warren's financial well-being continued to improve, the hallway was expanded into the garden, with part of it converted into a room for large dinner parties and dancing.

On the second floor, there were four large chambers (bedrooms) furnished with closets, window seats, and fireplaces. One of the chambers on the second floor was called the "nursery"; it could not be used during winter because it was too cold, and was seldom used at other times.

The third floor harbored five chambers. One of these chambers was particularly interesting. It was called the "study" because it was used for that purpose before the medicine room on the first floor had been expanded. During Edward's childhood, the study on the third floor was used as a "fruit and wine room." It had shelves filled with bottles of Madeira on one side, and shelves with the season's fresh fruit on the other. As a minor, Edward was not allowed to enter this room, but was occasionally allowed to peak in. The sight—and probably smell—of Madeira and fresh fruit excited him, and in his mind the room was like heaven.

The house was also equipped with several skylights. Leaking around the skylights was a constant problem, particularly from melting snow during winter and spring, and from heavy rains during other seasons. Warren, however, seemed to take this nuisance with a stride: "…in these days people did not care so much for comfort and luxury, as in later times. The surgeon who had served through all the hardship and privations of the Revolutionary War, thought very little of such minor inconveniences. When in his office, he was too much occupied with keeping his books or preparing his lectures, to find fault with what was, by comparison, real comfort."

Outside, the house was surrounded by gardens. Warren was interested in plants and vegetables, and was often seen wandering around with a pruning knife, caring for his plants. He was a successful gardener and was able to raise "fine peaches, plums, sweet water grapes, abundance of cherries and almonds."[93] During one period a greenhouse was built, which Warren managed to fill with exotic plants, including lemon and orange trees. As Warren's surgical practice grew, and he became increasingly involved in additional activities, gardening had to take a back seat, and part of the garden fell into disrepair. Warren's son described how "the greenhouse was a wreck, the glass gone, and the benches or racks empty."

In addition to Dr. and Mrs. Warren and the ten children, the household had a number of servants, including a cook and a chambermaid. Furthermore, "…a black boy was kept as a footman. Mrs. Mickerson, a black woman, came to assist at the family wash, and black Rose came on Thanksgiving days to make the pies, and preside in the kitchen. Black Abram, also a distinguished character, always came to saw the wood."

There were other occasional staff members adding to the household as well. Although Warren was a surgeon, used to handling sharp instruments, he did not feel comfortable shaving himself. Therefore, in early days, he kept a Black girl who was accustomed to shaving him. Later, a barber came every day for the same purpose and also made Warren's hair.

Although the Warrens were nice to their servants and treated them well, most of the time, they were kept apart from the family. The servants' chambers were disconnected from the rest of the house, and were accessed by a separate staircase from the kitchen.

The country was still almost a hundred years away from the Civil War, but slavery and the slave trade were already a source of consternation for many members of society. Warren had strong sentiments against the enslavement of Black people, and for this reason, he had two engravings proudly displayed in the entrance of one of the parlors. One of the engravings was titled "African Slave Trade" and depicted Africans chained and forced from their families onto slave ships. The other engraving, called "African Hospitality," represented a group of Africans saving white men who had been shipwrecked on the African coast. Warren's wife was opposed to slavery as well, and she called it a "peculiar institution."[94] Still, the family employed several Black servants.

Perkins' Metallic Tractors

Warren was always open to new ideas, although he was sometimes skeptical. The Perkins' metallic tractors were certainly something that made Warren curious. Elisha Perkins was born in Norwich, Connecticut, and was thirty-four years old when the Revolutionary War broke out. He practiced medicine in his hometown, and became successful in the endeavor. What made him famous, however, were his metallic tractors.[95]

The tractors were two three-inch long metal rods, rounded at one end and pointed at the other (the "Point"). By moving these rods over a body part afflicted by pain, Perkins claimed that he could "draw off the noxious fluid that lay at the root of suffering." He reported that the treatment could cure many types of inflammatory conditions, including rheumatism and pain in the head and face. In 1796, he took out a fourteen-year patent for his invention.

Many detractors questioned Perkins integrity and the results he reported. He was consequently expelled from the Connecticut Medical Society, and the tractors were described as a "delusive quackery." Perkins was called a "patentee and user of nostrums." Despite these critical views of Perkins and his tractors, he also had a large number of followers. Perkins reported that his treatment had cured at least five thousand patients, and that this had been certified by professors, physicians, and priests. Several medical institutions took up the use of the tractors as a treatment modality and reported successes. Even abroad, such as in Copenhagen, Denmark, medical faculties embraced Perkins' tractors. In London, the Perkinian Institution was formed.

Warren met with Perkins on several occasions, but did not quite know what to make of him. Although generally considered a warm and passionate person, Warren felt skeptical of Perkins and his tractors. Warren was "too much of a man of practice to enter very warmly into any novelties which did not appeal to reason."

Some prominent individuals were less suspicious than Warren. George Washington himself purchased a set of Perkins' tractors. Perkins' son, Benjamin, wrote that the President of the United States was convinced the tractors were helpful.

Additionally, some of Warren's colleagues seemed to have accepted the healing powers of the tractors. In a certificate found among Warren's papers, a Dr. Abiel Hall wrote:

> I certify that in the course of my practice, I have made frequent experiments with Dr. Perkins' Points, in removing agues, rheumatic pains, headaches, and inflammation of the eyes. One case of rheumatism I will relate.

> Captain J.R., aged forty, was violently seized with rheumatism in his back and knees, which continued forty-eight hours with no remission. I was called in the night, for they were afraid he would not live the night out, his pain was so severe. When I came, I thought best to let blood; but while warming the water to put his feet into, I applied the Points to one of his knees, and so down his leg, which in a few minutes removed the pain, and brought on very free perspiration. I then applied them to the other knee, which had the same effect as on the first; and then applied them to his back with the same success. He then got up

and walked about the room, and the next day went out of doors, and had no more of the complaint.

Hall continued by describing "one case of sore eye." He reported that, "Mr. P.C.'s child, twenty-four hours after birth, was noticed to have an inflammation of one of his eyes. Every method that is prescribed in this complaint was taken with little or no effect, until the child was two years old; then I applied the Points about two minutes, and to my great astonishment, the eye was perfectly well in forty-eight hours."

Although today, it may seem strange that rational and highly educated individuals had embraced the theory behind the metallic tractors, this was not the only questionable "science" that was accepted at the time. Those were the days when Franz Mesmer had just published his ideas about "animal magnetism" and the "Influence of the Planets on the Human Body." During the same era, the Italian scientists Luigi Galvani and Alessandro Volta performed work in the field of galvanism, the influence of electrical currents on bodily functions and health. Put in this context, it is not surprising that the healing power of the metallic tractors was a hot topic for discussions and believed by many to be true.

Impatient and Always in a Hurry

During the years after the Revolutionary War, Warren was involved in both local and national politics. Despite his political engagements, Warren remained first and foremost a physician and surgeon. According to his son Edward, obligations to his patients were his number-one priority, along with keeping abreast of medical knowledge and new developments. He had a warm and generous heart, and constantly felt strongly for society's needy. Edward wrote about his father: "…he never neglected his profession, but continued to labor earnestly for the advance of medical skill and science, and at the same time to lend his aid in the earnest support of every benevolent and charitable purpose."

On the other hand, Warren was a man of fast decisions, and sometimes came across as impatient. "The remarkable rapidity with which he made his visits, the rapidity of his ideas, by which he took in at a glance the whole situation of his patient, enabled him to obtain time for other objects—charitable, scientific, and political."

Not only were the visits with the patients quick, his comings and goings were fast. Warren seemed to be someone who traveled in the fast lane most of the time. Edward wrote: "At this period, my father made most of his visits on horseback; but when he drove in a sulky or chaise, he drove very rapidly; sometimes fearfully so. On one occasion, Dr. Danforth accompanied him to a consultation. He afterwards declared in very strong language that he would never ride with Dr. Warren again. He would sooner ride with the d–l."

Yellow Fever Epidemics

Yellow fever was a feared disease that caused recurring epidemics. Outbreaks afflicted Philadelphia in 1793 and 1798. A yellow fever outbreak hit Boston in 1798. Today, we understand the disease is caused by a virus spread by the *Aedes aegypti* mosquito, but that knowledge was not available in the 1700s. Although it was not known how the disease was spread, it was well known that victims were often clustered in certain areas of the city, making physicians believe it was a contagious disease. An interesting observation was that epidemics typically "subsided on the appearance of the first frosts." Mosquitos, of course, die in subfreezing temperatures, but the connection was still not made.

The disease was feared for good reasons. Individuals who contracted yellow fever went through a painful and devastating period of illness with high fevers. The disease killed people at a high rate. Between three and four thousand deaths were registered in Philadelphia during the 1793 epidemic. People with the means fled yellow fever-afflicted areas and lived in the countryside till the epidemics had subsided. During the epidemic of 1798, Philadelphia was described as "deserted by almost all its inhabitants."

Although the mode of spread was not well understood, the clinical condition of yellow fever patients was well known. In a communication to physicians in Philadelphia, Warren described the 1798 epidemic in Boston[96] and gave a detailed description of patients afflicted by the disease.[97] It is quoted here at some length because it illustrates Warren's clinical observational skills. It also shows that in those days, oftentimes the only thing physicians could do was observe the patient and try to determine in which phase of a condition he was.

Warren reported that:

> The fever was generally ushered in by a chill, but I think by no means equal to that which commonly precedes fevers of the ardent kind, nor in proportion to the violence of its subsequent periods. In a short time, the rigors were succeeded by excessive heat; the pulse, which had been small and contracted, became hard and full; the respiration laborious, from violent oppression at the *scrobiculus cordis;* the tongue assumed a whitish coat, the eyes became highly inflamed, while the pains in the head, back, and legs, became intolerably severe. To these symptoms succeeded nausea and vomiting of a highly bilious matter, seldom attended with diarrhea, but often with a burning at the stomach, tenderness of the abdomen, paucity of urine, and, in one instance, a dysuria, with a great proportion of blood at each evacuation of that fluid.

> These appearances usually continued about forty-eight hours, after which, they suddenly gave place to a very different train of symptoms. The pulse sunk astonishingly and became intermittent, the heat and pains entirely subsided, and the patient supposed himself to be out of danger. From a perfect possession of all his intellectual faculties, with a serenity of mind which, in no other disease, I believe, is so generally observed to accompany its last stages, in about the fifth day from the accession of the fever, he fell into a state of insensibility, and hence sunk gently into the arms of death. In others, this change was less rapid; the pulse became gradually smaller, the distressing symptoms slowly abated, a coolness of the extremities took place, and continued for several days before death, accompanied with clammy sweats, often without

any perceptible pulse in the wrists, for several hours before the fatal termination.

The tongue seldom became much coated, to the last. Delirium was by no means generally attendant, and a yellowness of the skin was far from being universal. Sometimes, however, this appearance was observed within the three first days, often on the fourth and fifth, and I was induced to consider it rather an accident, than a constituent character of the disease.

No effective treatment of yellow fever was available, and physicians often felt helpless before the patients. When treatment was attempted, it typically included bleeding, active purges, and calomel (mercury chloride). Although mercury was part of the armamentarium, it was used with caution because of disturbing side effects including diarrhea, bleedings from the gums and nose, and injuries to the teeth. Warren was well aware of these consequences of mercury and quoted them as "frequently troublesome and at times alarming."[98] As we will see later, Benjamin Rush, another prominent surgeon during the 1700s, also became involved in the yellow fever epidemics in Philadelphia.

The term "yellow fever" reflects the jaundice frequently seen in the patients. As Warren pointed out, however, the "yellowness of the skin was far from being universal." If the patient died and an autopsy was performed, evidence of inflammation, or even necrosis of the liver was frequently observed. Inflammation of the bile ducts was presumed to block the flow of bile from the liver into the bowel. Calomel was used in order to evacuate the intestine but was also believed to increase the flow of bile through the bile duct. The calomel also increased the activity of the salivary glands, and the increased salivation was taken as evidence that the dose of mercury was high enough to treat the yellow fever. In addition to the other side effects, calomel also produced an odor of the patient's breath, and Warren used the smell to gauge the treatment. He did so in a brave and unselfish way: "It is stated that Dr. Warren was in the habit of inhaling the breath of the fever patients, in order to judge the effect of the mercury and its progress towards salivation, it being considered necessary to produce salivation in order to check the disease; and this he did at a time when the disease was considered contagious."

Abigail Adams Smith's Mastectomy in 1811

It would soon be time for Warren to perform yet another heroic surgery. John and Abigail Adams's daughter, Abigail Adams Smith, or "Nabby," had a strained relationship with her mother for many years. One reason was that Mrs. Adams was resentful of Nabby's marriage to William Smith, and never seemed to get over the fact that Nabby had married Smith against her mother's advice.[99] Nabby and William met in London when John Adams was the United States Minister to Great Britain and Smith was serving as Adams's secretary. Smith had participated in the Revolutionary War and seen action in several battles in New York and New Jersey.

Smith was Nabby's senior by ten years. He was a good-looking man-about-town and moved in the higher circles of society. Although Nabby had a fiancé back in America, she fell in love with William shortly after they met, and she subsequently broke up with her betrothed. Nabby and William were married at John and Abigail Adams's London residence on June 12, 1786.

In addition to the age difference, Smith's poor and sometimes disastrous financial decisions, combined with his flamboyant lifestyle, were important reasons why Abigail had a hard time accepting him. His many unwise and speculative decisions finally brought the newlyweds to the brink of poverty. Abigail, therefore, considered her son-in-law "wholly devoid of judgment."

Later in life, Smith also got involved in shady political activities, shipping men and supplies out of New York to support the revolution in Venezuela. Although he claimed to have done this with the knowledge (or even encouragement) of President Thomas Jefferson and Secretary of State James Madison, he was put on trial in New York for violating the Neutrality Act of 1794. He was found not guilty, but as a result of the affair, he was fired from his position as surveyor of the Port of New York and lost the family's steady source of income.

Through all these ordeals, Nabby remained devoted to and supportive of her husband. Impoverished, the Smiths left New York City with their children and moved to a small farm in the central part of the state.

After not hearing from their daughter for some time, John and Abigail received a letter from Nabby in February 1811. She informed her parents that she had been diagnosed with "a cancer in my breast." She was then forty-five years old. She had discovered a lump in her breast almost a year earlier, and despite local doctors' attempts to treat the lump with pills and potions, it had kept growing bigger.

As soon as John and Abigail received the letter, they urged Nabby to come to Boston for medical consultations. By the time she arrived at Braintree with her husband and daughter Caroline, the breast tumor had grown even larger. It was now visible to the naked eye and had distorted the shape of the breast. When Abigail saw it, she found it "alarming."[100]

Her parents took Nabby to several physicians in Boston. The doctors initially tried to reassure her that because the situation and her general health were good, the condition did not "threaten any present danger." They even tried to "poison the disease" with hemlock pills and other drugs. Nabby, however, was not reassured. She had heard about Dr. Benjamin Rush and his experiences treating breast cancer. She also knew Rush was a good friend of her father. She took it upon herself to write a letter to Dr. Rush on September 12, 1811:

"...about May 1810 I first perceived a hardness in my right Breast just above the nipple which occasioned me an uneasy sensation, like a burning sometimes an itching & at time a deep darting pain through the Breast, but without any discolouration at all. It has continued to Contract and the Breast has become much smaller than it was. The tumor appears now about the size of a Cap, and does not appear to adhere but it be loose....

I have consulted several Physicians upon the Subject they have all advised me not to make any outward application to it.... Still I am uneasy upon the Subject—for I think

I observe it becoming harder and a little redness at times on the skin...."

Rush responded to Nabby's letter within a week. In his letter, he addressed her father rather than Nabby (this was probably done not to upset her, as he advised surgery). He wrote:

"I shall begin my letter by replying to your daughter.... After the experience of more than 50 years in cases similar to hers, I must protest against: all local applications, and internal medicines for her relief.... From her account of the moving state of the tumor it is now in a proper situation for the operation. Should she wait 'till it supperates, or even inflames much, it may be too late. The pain of the operation is much less than her fears represent.... I repeat again—let there be no delay in flying to the knife. Her time of life—calls for expedition in this business, for tumors such as hers tend much more rapidly to cancers after 45."[101]

On October 8, 1811, Warren, one of the most renowned surgeons in Boston at the time, and also a friend of the family, was called upon to perform the surgical removal of Nabby's diseased breast. The surgery was performed in one of the upstairs bedrooms of her parents' home.[102] Despite the horrors of undergoing a mastectomy without anesthesia, and fully understanding what was awaiting her, Nabby remained calm and composed during the preparations for the procedure, as well as during the surgery itself. She brought a hymnbook and was singing favorite hymns from it as a distraction. The courage she showed during the affliction astonished her surgeons.

For the procedure, Warren brought a team of assistant surgeons with him. Among the assistants were Doctors Amos Holbrook and Thomas Welsh. Warren's son John Collins Warren, who had returned from training in Edinburgh and joined his father's practice only a couple of years earlier, was also present. The surgical team brought instruments and other equipment to be used during the surgery, including a large wooden-handled knife, a big fork with two six-inch needle-sharp prongs, and a large number of bandages and compresses for dressing the wound. In addition, a thick, heavy iron spatula was heated on burning coals in an oven in a corner of the "operating room." This would be used to cauterize hemorrhaging blood vessels on the chest wall after amputating the breast.

Nabby entered the room dressed in Sunday clothes and was placed in a reclining chair. She was tied down to the chair, preventing any movement of her arms, legs, and body. To further prevent movement, members of the surgical team held up the right arm, pressed her shoulders and neck to the chair, and held her head still in a strong grip.

Although all details of the surgery are not fully known, a historian described the scene in vivid but plausible terms.[103] After Nabby had been belted down to the chair, the writer described how:

> Warren then straddled Nabby's knees, leaned over her semi-reclined body, and went to work. He took the two-pronged fork and thrust it deep into the breast. With his left hand, he held on to the fork and raised up on it, lifting the breast from the chest wall. He reached over for the large razor and started slicing into the base of the breast, moving from the middle of her chest toward her left side. When the breast was completely severed, Warren lifted it away from Nabby's chest with the fork. But the tumor was larger and more widespread than he had anticipated. Hard knots of tumor could be felt in the lymph nodes under her arm. He razored in there as well and pulled out nodes and tumor. Nabby grimaced and groaned, flinching and twisting in the chair, with blood staining her dress and Warren's shirt and pants. Her hair matted in sweat. John, Abigail, William, and Caroline turned away from the gruesome struggle. To stop the bleeding, Warren pulled a red-hot spatula from the oven and applied it several times to the wound, cauterizing the worst bleeding points. With each touch, steamy wisps of smoke hissed into the air and filled the room with the distinct smell of burning flesh. Warren then…bandaged the wound, stepped back from

Nabby, and mercifully told her it was over. The whole procedure had taken less than twenty-five minutes, but it took more than an hour to dress the wounds. Abigail and Caroline then went to the surgical chair and helped Nabby pull her dress back over her…shoulder as modesty demanded. The four surgeons remained astonished that she had endured pains so stoically.

Nabby's recovery was long and painful. The dressing changes caused agony. She remained weak and feeble for several months after her surgery. The movements of her arm and shoulder were impaired, and she had to wear a sling for an extended period of time. Finally, after seven months, she recovered enough to go back to her home in upstate New York, optimistic she had been cured. Dr. Rush even wrote a congratulatory note to John Adams, "…in the happy issue of the operation performed upon Mrs. Smith's breast…her cure will be radical and durable. I consider her as rescued from a premature grave." Unfortunately, it would turn out that Rush was wrong.

Nabby's breast cancer was only one of several trials the Adams family had to endure in 1811. John and Abigail described as "the most afflictive year" of their lives. Other family members suffered from tuberculosis, incurred severe injuries when thrown off a horse, and John Adams himself, now seventy-five, tripped and fell, sustaining a wound to his leg that forced him to be confined to home. The greatest worry, however, was the suffering of Nabby. Her father commented that he felt as if he were living in the Book of Job.

Five days after Nabby's surgery, John Adams made an interesting comment in a letter to Benjamin Rush: "Oh! That a vaccine Inoculation could be discovered for this opprobrium…. The Cancer, This Physical disgrow of Nature!" The concept of a vaccination against cancer was more than two hundred years ahead of its time.

Only a couple of weeks after her return to New York, Nabby started to experience signs and symptoms of recurrent breast cancer. Headaches and pain in her spine and abdomen were initially believed to be "the rheumatism," but when new tumors started to emerge on the chest wall, it became obvious that her cancer was back—with a vengeance. Realizing that she was terminally ill from cancer, Nabby told her husband that she "wanted to die in her father's house."

In July 1813, less than two years after her mastectomy, Nabby undertook the more than three-hundred-mile journey in a carriage. Upon finally reaching Braintree on July 26, Nabby was in terrible shape, gaunt and thin. Nabby's pain was so excruciating and severe that her mother could not bear to watch her suffering. It was John Adams who became the immediate caregiver during Nabby's last days: feeding her, cleaning her, helping her with her natural needs, combing her hair, and holding her hand.

Nabby died on August 9, 1813, two weeks after coming back to her parents' house. She was surrounded by her immediate family when she took her last breath, which John Adams described in a letter to Thomas Jefferson a few days later: "Your Friend, my only Daughter, expired, Yesterday Morning in the Arms of Her Husband, her Son, her Daughter, her Father and Mother, her Husbands two Sisters and two of her Nieces, in the 49th Year of Age, 46 of which She was the healthiest and firmest of Us all: Since which, She has been a monument to Suffering and to Patience."

Family life and Some Anecdotes

Edward Warren's biography of his father gives interesting insights into Warren's character as a person, as well as his family life. Warren and his wife grew a large family. At the turn of the century, sixteen children had been born into the family. Seven of the children died in childhood at between ages sixteen months and nine years. The losses weighed heavily on Warren and his wife.

Warren was a religious man. He and his family attended the Brattle Street Church on a regular basis. Belief in the Trinity, atonement, and other Calvinistic doctrines were important pillars in their lives. The family attended church not only on Sundays, but also on several other days during the week, sometimes even twice per day. On the first Sunday of every month, the family participated in Communion. The Sabbath was strictly observed, and the entire family typically spent Sunday afternoons together, relaxing and reading the Bible. Warren was described as someone who loved the Scriptures and regarded them as the words of God. Every morning, he read family prayers from the Book of Common Prayer.

Although this description of Warren may suggest he was a quiet, peaceful, and maybe even timid person, there were also other sides to his character. Edward described him as "exceedingly impulsive." He was also very principled and was always ready to sacrifice for his country, and for what he believed was a just cause: "like the elder Brutus, he could have sat in judgment upon one of his sons, had the life of the nation depended upon it."

Warren was sensitive to injustices inflicted not only on himself, but also to others. This need for fairness, coupled with his impatience and impulsiveness, got him into trouble on several occasions. Edward told the story about his father and mother riding in a chaise in Roxbury. A truck man was careless and bumped into Warren's vehicle. When Warren protested, the truck man replied in a less than respectful manner. This angered Warren, who lost his temper, jumped down from the chaise, and challenged the truck man without considering that the truck man was bigger and stronger: "It is needless to say that [Warren] had very much the worst of it."

Another incident could have ended much worse. As part of his inheritance, Warren owned a piece of land on Walk Hill. A neighbor, who also happened to be a physician, claimed a portion of the land that Warren believed belonged to him. In addition to this dispute, the two colleagues were opposed to each other in both political and medical affairs. On one occasion, a heated confrontation between Warren and his neighbor ended with his colleague drawing a knife and threatening to stab Warren. A witness to the argument intervened and stopped the fight before the knife came to use.

Warren felt quite disturbed by the altercation. He asked one of his sons to get a set of dueling pistols, and sent a message to his neighbor challenging him to a duel. Warren, when driving to Walk Hill for the duel, drove his sulky so fast that it overturned, and both the pistols and their owner were thrown out onto the road (this was typical of Warren, who often drove too fast). A great crowd gathered to witness the spectacle. The sulky was turned back on its wheels, and Warren rushed on. When he arrived for the duel, Warren found his opponent had refused to accept the challenge. This probably resulted in the loss of Warren's honor, but possibly saved his life.

Warren's personal attributes can be summarized as devoted husband, father, and family man; religious; impatient; quick to lose his temper; always in a hurry; ready to fight for his honor, even risking his life to stop what he perceived as injustices; and, on top of all this, a skillful, brave, and highly regarded surgeon.

The End

After founding Harvard Medical School in 1782, Warren had another thirty-two years to live. Those years saw dramatic events unfold: the Revolutionary War was won; a peace treaty with Britain was signed in Paris; and the American Constitution was written. In addition, a new war with Britain erupted in 1812, and lasted for three years.

Throughout the years, Warren's opinions regarding political events and debates continued to be valued and respected. Most of his time, however, was spent in his busy medical practice and with his family. After seeing several of his children die at a young age, Warren was survived by nine children—five sons and four daughters. One of his sons, John Collins Warren, followed in his father's footsteps and succeeded him as Professor of Anatomy and Surgery at Harvard Medical School. John Collins Warren was instrumental in founding the Massachusetts General Hospital, and became the first surgeon to perform an operation under general anesthesia (induced by ether). He had great respect and admiration for his father, and at one time wrote: "My father, who preceded me, was a much better surgeon than myself."

Although Warren was involved in the American Revolution and the movement around the Patriots, the love for his profession remained his priority. In a way, it even played a role in ending his life.

In addition to performing surgeries, Warren was involved in the caring for patients afflicted with many "nonsurgical" diseases that were common and feared in those days. These included smallpox, yellow fever (as we have seen), dysentery, diphtheria, measles, and consumption (tuberculosis).

For many years, Warren had suffered periodic chest pain—most likely what we would call angina pectoris today.[104] He also had periods of depression. In 1815, he was sixty-two years old and was becoming increasingly feeble and dispirited. This, however, did not stop him from participating in important political events and, more importantly, in the selfless care of his patients.

The winter months of early 1815 were cold and saw significant snow falling on Boston. The 1812–1815 war with England had just ended, and the peace was celebrated with big fireworks in the evening, and the illumination of major buildings. Washington's birthday had been selected for the celebrations. Despite the wintry weather and his deteriorating health, Warren walked the streets and enjoyed the celebrations. When he returned home he said: "Now let me depart in peace, for I have seen the salvation of my country."

It would be another six weeks before Warren departed. During these weeks, he continued to disregard any dangers and inconveniences to himself in order to care for his patients. At about this time, Governor Brooks, who resided in Medford, a short distance outside Boston, fell critically ill. Warren was called upon to care for the governor, and despite "the feebleness of his health," Warren went to see Brooks on a daily basis, sometimes even visiting twice per day. Caring for the governor required traveling in the cold weather by chaise or sleigh. Warren was delighted when he saw Brook's health improve, and the patient recover from his illness.

One evening when Warren returned home, he found a letter from Foxborough, which is approximately twenty-five miles outside of Boston. The letter said that Warren's brother, Ebenezer, had dislocated his shoulder. During the three days since it had happened, local surgeons had been unable to reduce (put in place) the dislocation, and in the letter, Warren was asked to help his brother. He ordered a carriage to take him to Foxborough. His family urged him to at least wait till the morning so he could rest before going there. He brushed that advice aside and immediately set out to see his brother.

When he arrived, he made several attempts to reduce his brother's shoulder dislocation, but finally had to give up further attempts that night. He let his brother rest, but woke him up before morning to make another attempt. Finally, after another couple of hours, he managed to get the shoulder back into its correct position.

He got into his sleigh, and when he returned home, he was exhausted. Despite that, he did not allow himself to rest, but immediately resumed his schedule and went out to visit patients.

After that, Warren's poor health finally caught up with him. He had to stop going out for patient visits, and limited his practice to only seeing patients at his house. One day, when Warren was sick and "laboring under severe illness and confined to the house," Professor Dexter, the friend and colleague at Harvard, took ill and sent for Warren. Against the objections of his wife and family, Warren went to see Dr. Dexter. Warren probably understood that he was risking his life by heeding the request from his colleague.

Warren's health continued to worsen in a rapid and worrisome manner. On March 22, Warren developed fevers and shortness of breath, in addition to his chest pain. In spite of this, he again went out to visit patients, and also received patients in his house on March 23 and 24. These were the last days that he was able to see patients. His fevers continued, and he developed worsening right-sided chest pain, laborious breathing, and occasional coughing. The treatment he received did not help, but probably made the situation worse. He was subjected to a course of calomel and opium and "a copious bleeding," the universal remedy for any type of inflammation. If anything, the bleeding probably hastened his demise. During the next couple of days, "the functions of all the organs appeared to be irrecoverably deranged," his heartbeats became irregular and intermittent, and his breathing continued to be difficult. Early in the morning of April 4, 1815, Warren "expired without any struggle or groan" at the age of sixty-one.

In an autopsy, Warren was found to have chronic and severe disease of his coronary arteries, explaining his long-standing symptoms of chest pain. In addition, the lungs were affected by acute inflammation, and pneumonia was considered the immediate cause of death.

CHAPTER 3

BENJAMIN CHURCH—
Patriot Turned British Spy

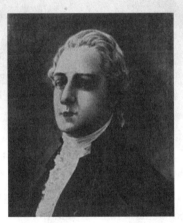

Benjamin Church (1734–1778). Initially one of the leading Revolutionary Surgeons. Was found guilty of treason only three months after his appointment as the first Surgeon-General of the Continental Army. Only a very few images of Church have been saved for history. (Wikipedia, Benjamin Church, physician)

Although most remember Benjamin Church for being a British spy and traitor, he was initially regarded as one of the leaders of the American Revolution. He was a surgeon by training but also a writer and politician. He was part of the inner circle of the Patriots,[105] and a good friend to most of them, belonging to the same clubs and organizations and serving with them on numerous committees, including the Committee of Safety and Supply and the Committee of Correspondence. He was a member of the Sons of Liberty. Ultimately, he was accused of being a spy for the British. Church's motives for providing secret information to the British have never been conclusively settled. He never admitted to being a spy or committing any other crime, and continued to claim that he had provided information to the British to save the colonies from a bloody war. Nevertheless, he was found guilty in the eyes of the public and, importantly, by George Washington. His role as an informant therefore became his legacy.

The Early Years

Benjamin Church Jr. (1734–1778?) was born in Newport, Rhode Island. When Benjamin was six years old, his family moved to Boston. At that time, his father was thirty-six and his mother twenty-five years of age. After moving to Boston, Benjamin's father became a prominent figure in town and filled many different positions during the years, including those of constable, assessor, and deacon in his church. His other positions included those of town warden, and one of four auctioneers in Boston. He was a member of a committee charged with locating and registering Boston's streetlights. (Streetlamps, lighted by oil and available by subscription, were not introduced in Boston until 1773.)

Growing up, Benjamin accompanied his father on many occasions to auctions and other events related to Church Sr.'s positions. Furniture, household goods, clothes, books, chocolate, real estate, and many other items were sold. His father also auctioned slaves at least twice in 1751.

Benjamin entered Boston Latin School in 1745. Boston Latin, the oldest public school in the United States still in use, was founded in 1635, one year before the establishment of Harvard College. Interestingly, five of the fifty-six signers of the Declaration of Independence attended Boston Latin School: Samuel Adams, John Hancock, Robert Treat Paine, William Hooper, and Benjamin Franklin.[106]

In July 1750, Church, about to turn sixteen, was admitted to Harvard College. In those days, admission to Harvard College was based on an entrance examination requiring a solid knowledge of Greek and Latin, as well as good moral standing. When he graduated from Harvard in 1754, Church decided to pursue a career in medicine. He apprenticed for a couple of years in the medical profession in Boston, and then served for a short time as a surgeon onboard the war ship *Prince of Wales*.

At the time, no formal system existed for physicians to be licensed. Few physicians practiced exclusively as surgeons, and most doctors primarily interested in surgery also provided services as obstetricians, internists, and general practitioners. Upon graduating from college, students who wanted to pursue careers in surgery had two options. They could undergo an apprenticeship with an established surgeon in the colonies, or travel abroad for more formal training under a famous surgeon. This was most commonly done in London or Edinburgh.

Church's Voyage to London

Church traveled to London in 1757. In those days, London was considered one of the most important cities in the world for medical and surgical training, rivaled only by Edinburgh and Paris. Seeking surgical training in London not only allowed Church to become a highly regarded and famous physician upon his 1759 return to Boston (he would soon become known as the best-trained Boston surgeon at that time); it also allowed him to come home with an English wife.

It must have been exciting, and probably overwhelming, for Church to arrive in London at the young age of twenty-three. He had left Boston, a small town of approximately fifteen thousand inhabitants, and arrived in a metropolis with a population of more than seven hundred thousand. London was growing rapidly, and was buzzing and hectic. Large numbers of people were moving from the countryside to the city for work and other opportunities, and people and businesses were migrating to London from other countries as well.

The purpose of Church's stay in London, of course, was to improve his medical and surgical training, and for this he enrolled as a medical student at the London Hospital to train under the renowned Dr. Charles Pynchon. Along with five other hospitals, the London Hospital, initially called the London Infirmary, was founded in 1740 to provide care for indigent patients. The name was changed to the London Hospital around 1748. Because the hospital became rundown and unfit, funds were raised to build a new place for the sick, and in September 1757, the year Church arrived, patients and staff moved into a new hospital located at Whitechapel Mount. Church and other medical students, therefore, received their training in facilities that would have been modern for the time.

Medical students who trained under the staff of the London Hospital were registered as private students. It was not until 1785 that The London Hospital Medical College was founded. Private medical schools had already existed, but the London Hospital Medical College was the first private school directly affiliated with a hospital.

Although Church worked and studied hard during his time in London, he had time for some romance as well. Soon after arriving in London, he fell in love with Sarah Hill of Ross-on-Wye, Herefordshire. Sarah was a sister of one of his fellow medical students. Church and Sarah were married in 1758, only a year after Church's arrival in London.[107] After Church finished his training, Sarah Hill accompanied her husband back to Boston where they built a family and had three children. When Sarah left England with Church in 1759, she could not have imagined that she would one day return to her home country with her husband in jail for treason, begging the British government for financial support.

It is not known exactly how the training of surgeons occurred at the London Hospital when Church was there, but based on information from other medical students who were studying in London at the same time, Church probably had long days divided between lectures; work on the floor taking care of sick patients; assisting senior surgeons performing operations; and anatomic dissections. The time and money spent in London were well invested, because when Church returned home he could claim that he was better educated and trained than most practicing Boston surgeons at the time.

Surgical Practice in Boston

When Church reentered the Boston scene in 1759, he brought drugs and medicine with him, as well as books in surgery and midwifery. He advertised in the local press about the sale of these items.[108] Church's reputation as a skilled and well-educated surgeon was enhanced by his public lectures on anatomy. Obstetrics and eye surgery (mainly surgery for cataract) were among the services Dr. Church provided in his practice.

On June 10, 1773, the journal *Massachusetts Spy* reported on a successful operation that Church performed on a fifty-six-year-old woman. Mrs. Hodges had been blind for several years from cataracts. After Church performed "couching upon the eyes," she immediately distinguished color, and every day her sight continued to improve.[109]

On one occasion, while in Philadelphia delivering a message to Congress in July 1775, Church met with John Adams and interacted with him not only as a representative of the Massachusetts Provincial Congress, but also as a private physician. John Adams at the time was suffering from problems with his eyes. Church treated him with an eye lotion that, according to a letter John wrote to his wife, Abigail, was quite helpful.

During the smallpox epidemic of 1764, Church, along with Joseph Warren and several other doctors in Boston, was one of the physicians Governor Bernard commissioned to provide inoculations at Castle William to the general population. Announced in an ad published in *Boston Gazette* on March 5, 1764,[110] inoculations were available from that day to the middle of May. John Adams was one of the individuals inoculated at Castle William in April 1764.

Treating diarrhea is another example of a nonsurgical skill that Church needed to perform. In a prescription sent to Elbridge Gerry (then a merchant in Marblehead, Massachusetts) on September 8, 1775, Church gave the following dietary advice to treat Gerry's diarrhea: "Light mutton or chicken broth or gruel or ale must be your diet to-morrow, in general weak chocolate with a proper proportion of milk will serve you; milk and water boiled together is a good draught for you, the Hartshorn Decoction is good with brown biskett after the operation of the physic, rice in every form suitable, wine and water, ripe fruits, chamomile tea may be used with discretion—proceed in this way my dear sir, make haste to recover."[111]

The patient suffering from the diarrhea survived his illness and went on to become Governor of Massachusetts (1810–1811) and Vice President of the United States (1813–1814). Thus, if Church's recommendations helped Gerry recover, it can be argued that diarrhea and its treatment can have interesting political ramifications. Interestingly, the term "gerrymander" is derived from Gerry's name and the word "salamander." At the time Gerry was governor of Massachusetts, one of the election districts had the shape of a salamander.

Church the Writer

In addition to his medical career, Church was a proliferative writer, and quite acclaimed at the time. He started writing poems when he was a student at Harvard. Church and his fellow Harvard students wrote satiric poems, mocking Harvard personalities and events. Church was known for being particularly vicious in these writings.

One of Church's best-known literary works is the poem "The Choice." It was penned before Church left Harvard, but was not published until 1757, three years after his graduation. In it, he described how he envisioned his future and his hopes for a peaceful and virtuous life: "Whatever station be for me designed / May virtue be the mistress of my mind." These lines are ironic (and tragic), considering the types of activities Church would participate in later in life.

Church had a reputation for being a womanizer, and he probably had several paramours on the side of his marriage. Around the start of the Revolutionary War, he actually lived with his pregnant mistress in Cambridge while his wife and children were living in Boston. His lover would ultimately play a role in the events that led to Church's arrest and conviction.

It is clear Church was recognized as a writer in his earlier years, as he was invited to contribute to a volume of poems commemorating King George II after his death in 1760. The volume, *Pietas et Gratulatio Collegii Cantabrigiensis Apud Novanglus,* contained thirty-two poems, two of which were written by Church. Church also wrote about the new king, George III, in the poem, "To the King":

Long live the great George our King, in peace and harmony,
Of his fame we will sing, if we have liberty;
But if cut short of that, we cannot raise our voice,
For hearts full of regret sure never can rejoice.

In the poem, one can sense the conflicting feelings that Church had: on one hand, admiring Britain and her king, and on the other hand, desiring more freedom and independence from England. It seems obvious that Church felt that the continued support for the king was dependent on the king's willingness to allow liberty for the colonies.

In some of his poems, there were hints regarding at least one of the reasons why Church became a spy later in life, namely his ambition and desire to achieve great reputation and recognition. In a poem "Fame," Church described fame as something that may be "but an inconstant Good" and that "we soonest lose," but still he wrote that "This urges me to fight and fires my Mind / To leave a memorable Name behind."

Church's successful career as a physician and surgeon supports the view that he was indeed an ambitious man and also enjoyed fame. He crossed the Atlantic and spent two years in London to improve his surgical skills and become more competitive. He was at the forefront of medicine, daring to challenge the medical establishment with regards to inoculating against smallpox. He adopted a new method to treat cataract disease, and advertised in the press that he was able to perform cataract surgery by removing the opaque lens rather than couching the lens to the bottom of the eye. Church performed this surgery about a decade after Jacques Daviel, a French surgeon, successfully performed the first removal of the lens from a cataract patient.

One of Church's best pieces of political propaganda was a poem published in 1765. The poem, "Liberty and Property Vindicated and the St-pm-n Burnt" is commonly considered a masterpiece of irony and satire. However, because the irony in the poem was not understood by all readers, it was not as successful as some of his later political poems in which the irony and satire were more obvious and easier to understand. In a number of poems written through the early 1770s, Church particularly satirized and criticized Governor Bernard and various Loyalists. His attacks on

Governor Bernard were particularly vicious, something that made Church immensely popular among Whigs, and hated and cursed among Tories.

Some of Church's writing was in the form of articles published in Whig newspapers. Interestingly, some of the articles published in the Tory press "responding" to Church's articles may have also been authored by Church himself. As Church's brother-in-law, John Fleming (married to Church's sister, Alice), was a printer and publisher of the Tory newspaper *Boston Chronicle,* this made it easier for Church to play double, and publish pro-British articles in the *Chronicle.*

Church and the Boston Massacre

The years leading up to the Boston Massacre on March 5, 1770, saw increasing tensions between the patrolling British soldiers and the citizens of Boston. Many policies and regulations imposed on the colonies by Parliament, including the Sugar Act of 1764 and, importantly, the Stamp Act of 1765, were immensely unpopular among the colonists and contributed to the rising tensions. In the year of the Boston Massacre, the city was occupied by about four thousand British soldiers who had been deployed in 1768 to keep the rebellious Bostonians in check.

The hostile feelings culminated on March 5, 1770, when British soldiers under the command of Captain Preston were attacked by a mob throwing stones, chunks of ice, and other objects. When the soldiers were struck, they responded by firing their muskets into the crowd, killing five civilians and wounding several others, an event that has gone down in history as the "Boston Massacre." It remains unclear whether the first shots were fired on Preston's command before his soldiers had been harassed, or whether his soldiers fired after being pelted by objects from the mob in an act of self-defense.

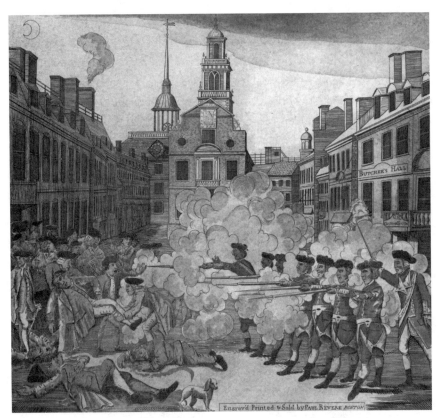

**Boston Massacre, also known as the Incident on King
Street, March 5, 1770. Paul Revere's historic engraving
"The Bloody Massacre in King-Street" was used as
propaganda against the British. (GL Archive)**

Church became involved in the Boston Massacre and its aftermath
in several ways. He arrived early and attended to the wounded. After
the Massacre, he was appointed to a committee that met with Governor
Hutchinson, asking him to remove the troops from Boston to prevent
further violence. The governor's initial response was no. Troops could be
withdrawn if there was a military reason, but not merely to appease the
people. Ultimately, however, the soldiers were removed from the city and
stationed at William Castle in order to defuse the situation.

In addition, Church was requested to perform an autopsy of Crispus
Attucks, the first casualty of the Massacre.[112] Crispus Attucks was a colored man who called himself "Michael Johnson." He is often referred to as

the first martyr of the American Revolution. More details about Crispus Attucks, including who he was and where he came from, are not completely known. He was born around 1723 in Framingham, Massachusetts, and may have been a runaway slave or a freedman. He worked on the docks of Boston, and may have been a sailor as well. His father allegedly was an African-born slave and his mother a Native American.

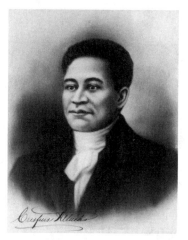

Crispus Attucks, the first victim at the Boston Massacre. Benjamin Church performed an autopsy after Attucks's death at King Street. (The History Collection)

After the autopsy, Church issued the following report (quoted by John Nagy in his excellent book *Dr. Benjamin Church, Spy*):[113]

> I Benjamin Church, jun[ior] of lawful age; testify and say, that being requested by Mr. Robert Pierpont the Coroner, to assist in examining the body of Crispus Attucks, who was supposed to be murdered by the soldiers on Monday evening the 5th instant, I found two wounds in the region of the thorax, the one on the right side, which entered through the second true rib within an inch and an half of the sternum, dividing the rib, and separating the cartilaginous extremity from the sternum, the ball pasted [passed] obliquely downward through the diaphragm, and entering through the large lobe of the liver and the

gallbladder, still keeping its oblique direction, divides the aorta descendens just above its division into the iliac, from thence it made its exit on the left side of the spine. This wound, I apprehended was the immediate cause of his death. The other ball entered the fourth of the false ribs, about five inches from the linea alba; and descending obliquely passed through the second false rib, at the distance of about eight inches from the linea alba, from the oblique direction of the wounds, I apprehend the gun must have been discharged from some elevation, and further the deponent saith not.

Benj[amin] Church, Jun[ior]

Suffolk, ss. Boston, March 22, 1770, Benjamin Church, jun[ior], above mentioned, after due examination made oath to the truth of the aforesaid affidavit taken to perpetuate the remembrance of the thing. Before John Ruddock, Just[ice of the] Peace and of Quorum. John Hill, Just[ice of the] Peace.

From Church's autopsy report, it appears that Attucks was shot at least twice at close range. The injuries described would probably not have been survivable even with modern care of trauma victims. In particular, the transection of the aorta, caused by the bullet that had first traveled through the chest, diaphragm, liver, and gallbladder, must have resulted in rapid exsanguination, killing Attucks within minutes. The trajectories of the bullets suggest that they entered Attucks's body from above, either because Attucks had been knocked to the ground at the moment of impact, or because they were shot from a higher elevation. After the event, a young boy hiding on the second floor of a nearby building attested that he had been forced by a British soldier to use the soldier's musket and shoot into the rebellious crowd through a window.

Of note, Church was not the only patriot who became involved with the Boston Massacre and its aftermath. The actions of Joseph Warren have already been described. John Adams, who, along with Josiah Quincy, defended Captain Preston and the eight soldiers participating in the Massacre at trials held in late 1770,[114] had a radically different view of the situation that he would voice only a few years later. In 1770, when defending Preston and his soldiers, Adams referred to Attucks as a member of "a motley rabble of saucy boys, negroes and mulattoes, Irish teagues and outlandish jack tars."

The Annual Orations

Church was given the honor of giving the third annual oration commemorating the Boston Massacre on March 5, 1773. At the time, Church was quite popular among the Bostonians and was well known as a captivating speaker. It was not surprising, therefore, that the event drew a big crowd. The oration was given at the Old South Meeting House, which was filled over capacity with more than five thousand men, women, and children. The Meeting House was so full that John Hancock, who introduced Church and served as the moderator (and would be selected to give the annual oration lecture in 1774), had to climb through a side window in order to get in and make it to the platform.[115]

That Church was chosen to give the third annual oration confirms the standing he had among the colonists at this time. His identity as a true Patriot was reinforced when at the end of the speech, he appealed to resist the British: "to rouse the luke-warm into noble zeal, to fire the zealous into manly rage; against the foul oppression, of quartering troops, in populous cities, in times of peace."[116] Even though he was a highly esteemed Patriot in the eyes of the people, it is likely that Church had already begun his activities as an informant for the British, providing them with secret information about the Patriots and their plans.

Church the Patriot

Church was involved in most of the events leading up to the Revolution. He was a close friend with most of the prominent Patriots, and was considered a hero and freedom fighter. Church was an active participant in the First and Second Massachusetts Provincial Congresses held on October

12, 1774, and February 1, 1775, respectively. He participated actively at the congresses and was appointed to several important committees, giving him insight and knowledge that would be important for the British.

In the fall of 1774, a secret committee, the Massachusetts Committee of Safety and Supplies, was formed to monitor the movements of British soldiers and to gather information about the activities of the Tories, many of whom were Loyalists. Thus, the committee promoted spying against the British. The committee consisted of about thirty members, including Church, who was one of the most prominent participants. It held its meetings at the Green Dragon Tavern, located in the North End of Boston. It soon became evident that information from the meetings was being leaked to General Gage. Initially, it was suspected that Green Dragon's staff overheard the discussions, but when the leaks continued even after the meetings were moved to another location, the committee members started to suspect each other. Many historians believe that Church was the culprit.

Most of the committees to which Church was appointed included other prominent Patriots, including Samuel Adams, John Hancock, and Joseph Warren. In addition to information about Tories and British soldiers and their activities, details about the growing number of rebels, and their equipment and supplies, were also discussed at the committee meetings. This made it possible for Church to gather information about the size of the Massachusetts militia, and how prepared they were to potentially face the British in combat – which, of course, they would.

Among the Patriots, Church expressed opposition to many of the Acts and taxes that the British Parliament imposed on the colonies. Given what would happen to Church later in his life, it is remarkable that, during the years prior to the Revolution, he worked closely with many of the leading Patriots. These associations and friendships make it hard to believe he was later accused of being a traitor. At the same time, his involvement in meetings and decision-making gave him insight into deliberations and plans—knowledge that is valuable to anybody interested in selling secrets.

In early 1775, Church allegedly provided General Gage with information about the buildup of the rebel militia, and the locations of their stored weapons and ammunition. It was based on this information that Gage sent a British military force to Lexington and Concord to "seize and destroy all artillery and ammunition provisions…and other military stores."[117] The military was also charged with finding and arresting Samuel Adams and John Hancock, who were currently in Lexington, preparing to journey to Philadelphia for the second Continental Congress scheduled to convene in May. The troops were instructed that "if any body of men dares to oppose you with arms you will warn them to disperse or attack them."[118] As we previously saw in the chapter on Joseph Warren, this resulted in the Battles of Lexington and Concord on April 19, 1775, which would signify the start of the American Revolutionary War. The day resulted in an embarrassing defeat for the British, who had to rush back to Boston to avoid a complete disaster. Joseph Warren's activation of the Alarm and the midnight rides of Revere and Dawes resulted in a rapid response by thousands of militia and minutemen.[119]

After Church was accused as a traitor, Paul Revere recalled that he had seen Church the day after Lexington and Concord. Church's stockings were stained with blood, and when questioned, he told Revere that he had participated in the battles the day before and had been splattered with blood from a man next to him, who was killed by the British. Remembering this encounter, Revere commented that "if a man will risk his life to a cause, he must be a friend to that cause; and I never suspected him after 'till he was charged with being a traitor."[120]

That Church was not yet suspected was further illustrated by his assignment at the Massachusetts Provincial Congress on May 16, 1775. Church would go to Philadelphia and deliver a request to the Continental Congress to take control of, and pay the bills for, the troops that were laying siege to Boston. On May 24, one day before he set out on his trip to Philadelphia, Church wrote a secret letter to General Gage, informing him about his travels and the purpose of the trip. He also informed Gage that the trip to Philadelphia would "prevent my writing for some time." He ended the letter by proclaiming his loyalty to England and stated, "May I never see the day when I shall not dare call myself a British American."[121] The statement suggests that money was not the only reason why Church became an informant for the British. In his heart, he was probably a Loyalist, not a Patriot. When history was written, the number of colonists who were opposed to a separation from England may have been understated.

Governing seems to have been done through committees, and Church was on many of them. One interesting committee was formed on July 5, 1775, and consisted of three members, including Church. The purpose of the committee was to meet with Washington and find out what kind of food he desired for his table. Newly appointed Commander-in-Chief of the Continental Army, Washington had arrived at Cambridge on July 2 to establish his headquarter and was met with great respect. He was granted many privileges, including spacious and comfortable living quarters and the option to decide the menus for his meals.

A Medical and Surgical Expert during the Early American Revolution

During the early days of the Revolution, Church was involved in organizing hospitals and other aspects of health care delivery that would be needed during the anticipated war. On February 21, 1775, the Committee of Safety and Supplies instructed Church and his surgeon colleague Joseph Warren "to bring in an inventory of what is necessary in the way of their profession for the...army to take the field."[122] Church was also appointed to a committee that was tracking down fifteen doctors' chests for the newly formed army. Along with Warren, Church was given £500 to purchase medical supplies for the provincial medical chests.

Another of Church's committees was assigned to take all the Massachusetts militia's medicines, medical stores, and instruments into custody. The committee also requested that chests with medicines that had been dispensed to the military be returned. The purpose was to make certain that medicine and supplies were not wasted, but were instead allocated for appropriate use.

In July 1775, about three months after the start of the Revolutionary War, the Continental Congress discussed the question of establishing a hospital system (Medical Department) for the Continental Army. There hadn't been much progress in the planning of the hospital, in part because of infighting between surgeons. Washington was frustrated and wrote to Congress on July 20 on this matter: "I have made inquiry with respect to the establishment of the hospital and find it in a very unsettled condition.

There is no principal director, or any subordination among the surgeons; of consequence disputes and contentions have arisen and must continue until it is reduced to some system. I could wish that it was immediately taken into consideration as the lives and health of both officers and soldiers so much depend upon a due regulation of this department."[123]

On July 27, the Continental Congress appointed Church as Surgeon-General of the Continental Army and Director and Chief Physician of the first American army hospital, which was established in Cambridge. For this position, Church was paid four dollars a day and was also given the authority to hire four surgeons and numerous other medical personnel. The four surgeons recruited by Church to Cambridge Hospital were Doctors Isaac Foster Jr., John Warren, Samuel Adams Jr. (Samuel Adams's son), and Charles McKnight. Dr. Benjamin Allen was appointed as apothecary. Little did people know how short Church's tenure would be.

At the time the Cambridge Hospital was established, St. Thomas Hospital in Roxbury was also being used for the care of officers and soldiers. The surgeons in charge of the hospital in Roxbury were Doctors William Aginwall, Lemuel Hayward, and Elisha Perkins. Although there was some confusion with regards to the formal appointments of the surgeons at the Roxbury hospital (Church had not yet been given authority to appoint physicians at that hospital, but his charge was limited to the hospital in Cambridge), the Roxbury surgeons were working hard and were quite successful in their efforts. Dr. Hayward reported that at least six hundred patients had been cared for at the Roxbury hospital from June 10 to the middle of October 1775, with all but forty patients surviving.

During this time, the most common causes for hospital admissions were fevers, dysentery, and, of course, wounds and other injuries sustained by soldiers during fighting around Boston. This included the battles of Lexington and Concord on April 19, 1775, and the Battle of Bunker Hill on June 17.

Church's Accusation

There is evidence that Church provided the British with secret information both before (maybe even from 1772) and during the early months of the

Revolutionary War. Indeed, Church never denied that he had informed the British about the build-up of the rebel army, but what is not clear is his motives. Because Church received payments for his services and the information given to the British was considered damaging, Church was ultimately found guilty of criminal activities during his trials. Church himself, however, continued to profess his innocence to the end. By providing the British with secrets, he claimed that he was preventing a bloody war on the American continent, and impressing on the British that a military attack on the colonies would not succeed and would ultimately result in the loss of the American colonies. Historians have suggested that Church viewed himself as an arbitrator who could help restore friendly relations between the colonies and the motherland. Church's arguments, however, were rejected, and Church was convicted of "communicating with the enemy."

Although the exact point when Church started his activities as an informant is not known, it is clear that he began providing the British with sensitive information several years before the start of the Revolution. Interestingly, at the time, Americans were split with regards to their opinion about England and the continued British rule of the American colonies. The Loyalists, who wanted to keep ties with England, constituted a relatively large segment of the society. Only a few seemed to believe that the British would actually use military force to quell the opposition.

Church was not alone in his attempts to prevent an outright war. Other prominent revolutionaries also initially expressed desires to try to avoid hostilities, and were surprised by the way things evolved. John Adams has been quoted as saying, "There was not a moment during the revolution when I would not have given everything I possessed for a restoration to the state of things before the contest began, provided we could have had a sufficient security for its continuance." Along the same lines, Jefferson commented, "Before the commencement of hostilities, I never heard a whisper of a disposition to separate from Great Britain, and after that, its possibility was contemplated with affliction by all." Reflecting the same sentiment, Benjamin Franklin stated "that he never had heard in any conversation from any person, drunk or sober, the least expression of a wish for a separation, or a hint that such a thing would be advantageous to America."[124]

Important exceptions to these more peaceful opinions were ideas strongly favored by John Hancock and, in particular, John Adams's cousin Samuel Adams. Prompted by the strong opposition to the Stamp Act in 1765, Adams and Hancock founded the Sons of Liberty, a secret organization that rapidly spread to all thirteen colonies. The Sons of Liberty became increasingly vocal and active in the opposition to the British, and were responsible for several acts of violence against both people and private property. When the revolutionary sentiment on the continent became more widespread and a fight for independence seemed inevitable, the Sons of Liberty were joined by increasing numbers of Patriots, including James Otis, Paul Revere, and Patrick Henry (who was best known for the quotation "Give me liberty, or give me death"). As we have already seen, several prominent surgeons were also among the members, including Joseph Warren, Benjamin Rush, and Thomas Young.

In addition to Church's claim that he was trying to prevent a war between England and the American colonies, another reason why Church "communicated with the enemy" was money—or rather lack thereof. In 1768, Church had built an expensive summerhouse on Nippahonsit Pond in Raynham, located about thirty miles south of Boston. At that time, Church was known to be short of cash, and this may have been an important reason why Church started his activities as an informant. Three years after building his summerhouse, Church bought a home in an expensive part of Boston, located on the north side of Marlborough Street with elegant homes owned by wealthy people—an additional reason why Church needed money to support his lifestyle.

Church's plans to establish a royal maritime hospital in Boston with himself as director may have also motivated him to provide the British with secret information. It has been speculated that Church was hoping to get approval and financial support for a hospital from then Governor Hutchinson by supplying anonymous papers to the government.

A further reason for Church becoming an informant may be that in the early 1770s, it was considered highly unlikely that the colonies would be able to form a union and fight the British in unity. The colonies at that time had become quite hostile towards each other, with ugly name-calling occurring frequently. For example, in New York, Boston was called "the Common Sewer of America," and in Boston, the neighboring colony to the south was referred to as "the filthy, nasty, dirty colony of Rhode Island."[125] By collaborating with the British, Church was hedging the bets, hoping to be on the winning side (which appeared to be England at the time).

Having an English wife and a Tory brother-in-law have been suggested as additional reasons why Church began communicating with the British. Thus, multiple factors probably pushed Church to become a spy.

Church seems to have been particularly active in providing the British with secrets during the months preceding the Battles of Lexington and Concord. On several occasions during March and early April 1775, the British took depositions from somebody who clearly had insight into the inner workings of the Patriots. Researchers generally agree that the person providing the British with the information during these sessions was Benjamin Church. There is evidence that General Gage was personally involved in the meetings with Church.

The information handed over to the British was indeed damaging to the American side. It included details about the size of the of militia in Massachusetts; locations where weapons and ammunition were stored; deliberations at meetings of the Committee of Safety and Supplies and the Massachusetts Provincial Congresses; plans to engage additional colonies in New England in the fight against the British so that the revolt spread to New Hampshire and Rhode Island; and plans to put more soldiers under arms.

A couple of episodes illustrate Church's need for money at the time. After the British were defeated at Concord, Church expressed the concern that Gage would think that he had led him into a trap, and stop the stream of money. Another telling episode related to Church's need for money is that of Church possibly stealing £125 from Rachel Revere. Three days after the Battle at Lexington and Concord, on Saturday morning, April 22, Church went into Boston, which was then a city under siege and blocked off by the rebels. In order to enter the city, Church had requested a letter from his surgeon colleague, Joseph Warren, to General Gage. Carrying this letter opened doors and allowed Church into Boston. In the letter, Warren informed Gage that wounded British officers and soldiers being held in Cambridge had requested being treated by British rather than American surgeons, and Warren promised the safety of British surgeons who left Boston to treat the wounds of the British soldiers. The letter from Warren to Gage gave Church an opportunity to again meet with the British General, and this was probably Church's motive for going into Boston to begin with.

In Boston, Revere's wife, Rachel, gave Church a letter to her husband (who was then in Cambridge), along with £125. In the letter, Rachel wrote:

> My Dear by Doctor Church I send a hundred and twenty five pounds and beg you will take the best care of yourself and not attempt coming in to this town again and if I have an opportunity of coming or sending out anything or any of the children I shall do it pray keep up your spirits and trust your self and us in the hands of a good God who will take care of us tis all my dependence for vain is the help of man adieu my Love from your affectionate R. Revere.[126]

Neither the letter nor money was delivered to Revere. Church turned the letter over to the British authorities, and probably kept the money for himself.

It is remarkable to see two surgeons, Joseph Warren and Benjamin Church, so involved in the events surrounding the start of the Revolutionary War. One surgeon unknowingly provided cover for the other, a traitor who continued his collaboration with the British, seemingly to a great extent because of greed.

The Ciphered Letter

Although Church was highly regarded as both a Patriot and surgeon during the time preceding the Revolutionary War and the first couple of months after its start, his standing in the Revolution would soon change. Central to Church's fall was the infamous ciphered letter written by Church to a "Major Cane."[127]

Descriptions of the events taking place around the time of Church's conviction read like a spy novel, and include many of the components commonly associated with spy activities: suspense, greed, money, search for power and influence, risks, adultery, and sex. After Church wrote the letter on July 25, 1775, things happened at an escalating pace and resulted in Church's conviction in less than four months.

The letter to Major Cane contained secrets about the American army, including its strength, positions, and places where weapons and ammunition were stored—information that was of extreme value for the British. At the end of July 1775, Church asked his pregnant mistress, Mary Wenwood (with whom he was living in Cambridge at the time), to carry the letter to Newport, Rhode Island, and deliver it to Captain James Wallace. On the way to Newport, Church had instructed Mary to keep the letter hidden inside her stockings between her legs. She must have been aware of the fact that the letter contained secret information and could not fall in wrong hands. Probably because she did not know how to find Captain Wallace, she instead delivered the letter to Godfrey Wenwood, her ex-husband. Mary and Godfrey had divorced in September of 1774, after an almost ten-year marriage. She had left him in August, and, in a note published in *Newport Mercury,* Godfrey announced that his wife "(for reasons to me unknown) has eloped from my bed and board." According to surviving reports, Mary seemed to have been a woman of questionable character and reputation, described by several contemporaries as "an infamous hussy" and a "Girl of Pleasure."[128] Godfrey called her "a very lusty Woman." When Mary left Godfrey, she moved to the Boston area, where she met Church. In a letter to John Adams, John Warren wrote, "The Doctor (Church) having formed an infamous connection with an infamous hussy to the disgrace of his own reputation, and probably ruin of his family, wrote this letter (the ciphered letter) last July, and sent it by her to Newport."[129]

Mary asked Godfrey to secretly deliver the letter to Captain Wallace, who was on the British warship *HMS Rose,* stationed at Newport. The plan was to have the letter taken to Boston on the ship, the only way to get things into the city. Godfrey, who was not happy to see Mary back in Newport, felt uncomfortable about the letter, which he suspected contained illicit information. He and a friend of his, Adam Maxwell, opened the letter and found it to be ciphered, which increased their suspicions. They decided not to deliver the letter, and instead tried to find a decipherer to determine the content of the letter. This turned out to be difficult, and the letter remained in Godfrey Wenwood's possession for almost two months.

Meanwhile, Church started to get anxious about whether the letter had indeed reached Boston, and was concerned the letter may have fallen in wrong hands. On September 20, he wrote to Washington, asking to be allowed to resign from the Continental Army. He claimed that he needed to spend more time with his family. Washington denied the request, but allowed Church to extend his furlough and spend a few more days at home with his family. It is suspected that Church used that time to destroy any damaging evidence against himself.

Suspecting they might have an illicit letter in their possession, Wenwood and Maxwell started to get nervous. They decided to take the letter to Henry Ward, Secretary of State of the Whig government of Rhode Island. Ward advised Wenwood and Maxwell to bring the letter to General Nathanael Greene, commander of the Rhode Island contingent of the Continental Army surrounding Boston. On September 26, they left Rhode Island, carrying the ciphered letter, along with a letter of introduction from Ward to Greene suggesting that "the strictest inquiry ought to be made".

Suspecting the letter contained military intelligence, Greene passed it on to General Washington at his headquarter in Cambridge. At this point, it was understood that Mary Wenwood had brought the letter to Newport. Washington sent Godfrey Wenwood to Mary, trying to get information about who had written the letter. She initially refused to give up that information, but after she was brought to Washington and interrogated and threatened, she named Church as the author of the letter.

Washington acted quickly. On September 28, he had Church arrested and placed under house arrest. After an intensive search for decipherers, Washington obtained a translated version of the letter on October 3. The letter read:

> To Major Cane in Boston
>
> On His Magisty's Sarvice—
>
> I hope this will reach you. Three attempts have been made without success. In effecting the last, the man was discovered in attempting his escape; but fortunately my letter was sewed in the waistband of his breeches. He was

confined a few days, during which time you may guess my feelings; but a little art and a little cash settled the matter.

Tis a month since my return from Philadelphia; I went by the way of Providence, to visit mother. The Committee for warlike stores made me a formal tender of twelve pieces of cannon, eighteen and twenty-four pounders; they having taken a previous resolution to make the offer to Gen[eral] Ward. To make a merit of my services, I sent them down; and when they received them, they sent them to Stoughton, to be out of danger, even though they had formed the resolution, as I before hinted, of fortifying Bunker's Hill, which together with the cowardice of the clumsy Colonel [Samuel] Gerrish and Colonel [James] Scammons, was the lucky occasion for their defeat. This affair happened before my return from Philapelphia. We lost one hundred and sixty-five killed then, and since dead of their wounds; one hundred and twenty now lie wounded; the chief will recover. They boast you have fourteen hundred killed and wounded in that action. You say the Rebels lost fifteen hundred, I suppose with equal truth.

The people of Connecticut are raving in the cause of liberty. A number from this Colony, from the Town of Stamford, robbed the King's stores at New-York, with some small assistance the New-Yorkers lent them; these were growing turbulent. I counted two hundred and eight pieces of cannon, from twenty-four to three-pounders, at Kingsbridge, which the Committee had secured for the use of the Colonies. The Jerseys are not a whit behind Connecticut in zeal. The Philadelphians exceed them both. I saw twenty-two hundred men in review by General [Charles] Lee, consisting of Quakers and other inhabitants, in uniform, with one thousand Riflemen and forty Horse, who, together, made a most warlike appearance.

I mingled freely and frequently with the members of the Continental Congress; they were united, determined in opposition, and appeared assured of success. Now, to come home. The opposition is become formidable.

Eighteen thousand men, brave and determined, with Washington and Lee at their head, are no contemptible enemy. Adjutant Gen[eral Horatio] Gates is indefatigable in arranging the Army. Provisions are very plenty; clothes are manufacturing in almost every Town for the soldiers. Twenty tons of powder lately arrived at Philadelphia, Connecticut, and Providence; upwards of twenty tons are now in camp. Saltpetre is made in every Colony. Powder Mills are erected, and constantly employed, in Philadelphia and New-York. Volunteers, of the first fortunes, are daily flocking to the camp; one thousand Riflemen in two or three days. Recruits are now levying, to augment the Army to twenty-two thousand men. Ten thousand Militia are appointed in this Government, to appear on the first summons.

The bills of all the Colonies circulate freely, and are readily exchanged for cash; add to this, that unless some plan of accommodation takes place immediately, these harbours will swarm with privateers; an army will be raised in the Middle Provinces, to take possession of Canada. For the sake of the miserable convulsed Empire, solicit peace, repeal the acts, or Britain is undone. This advice is the result of warm affection to my King [George III] and the Realm. Remember I never deceived you; every article here sent you is sacredly true.

The papers will announce to you that I am again a Member for Boston; you will there see our Motley Council. A general arrangement of officers will take place, except the chief, which will be suspended but for a little while, to see what part Britain takes in consequence of the late Continental petition.

A view to independence gr[ows] more and more general. Should Britain declare war against the Colonies, they are lost forever. Should Spain declare against England, the Colonies will declare a neutrality, which will doubtless produce an offensive and defensive league between them. For God' sake, prevent it by speedy accommodation. Writing this has employed a day. I have been to Salem to reconnoitre, but could not escape the geese of the capitol; to-morrow I set out for Newport, on purpose to send you this. I write you fully, it being scarcely possible to escape discovery. I am out of place here, by choice, and therefore out of pay, and determined to be so unless something is offered in my way. I wish you could contrive to write me largely in cipher, by the way of Newport, addressed to Thomas Richards, merchant. Enclose it in a cover to me, intimating that I am a perfect stranger to you; but being recommended to you as a gentleman of honour, you took the liberty to enclose that letter, entreating me to deliver it as directed; the person, as you are informed, being at Cambridge. Sign some fictitious name. This you may send to some confidential friend at Newport, to be delivered to me at Watertown. Make use of every precaution, or I perish.[130]

The Trials

After receiving the deciphered letter, Washington again acted quickly. On the same day, October 3, 1775, he called a Council of War at the headquarters in Cambridge. The following day, Church was summoned to appear before the Council.[131]

When questioned, Church acknowledged that he was indeed the author of the letter, but declared his innocence of wrongful activities. His line of defense was that he had written the letter to impress the British enemy of the size of the American army in order to convince them not to attack, thereby avoiding unnecessary bloodshed. This argument, however, did not impress the members of the war council, and Church was swiftly found guilty of "criminal correspondence with the enemy." He was returned to confinement and remained under house arrest, awaiting the decision about his punishment.

On October 5, Washington sent a letter to the Continental Congress asking for advice.[132] He also requested that changes be made in the Code of Laws to introduce clearer and more appropriate guidance when it came to dealing with similar situations.

Washington's letter was read in Congress on October 13. Interestingly, John Adams's initial reaction to the letter to a certain extent mirrored what Church was using in his defense. Adams wrote, "There are so many lies in it [Church's ciphered letter], calculated to give the enemy an high idea of our power and importance, as well as so many truths tending to do us good that one knows not how to think him treacherous: yet, there are several strokes which cannot be accounted for at least by me without the supposition of iniquity."[133] At this point, Adams was withholding his judgment.

Congress, however, was convinced that Church's behavior was at least suspicious and, on October 14, dismissed him from his positions as Surgeon-General of the Continental Army and Chief Physician of the Hospital in Massachusetts. A couple of days later, Dr. John Morgan of Philadelphia replaced Church as the new Surgeon-General of the Army.

The news about Church's betrayal was met with disbelief, disappointment, and outrage. John Adams, in particular, seems to have had a hard time to cope with the news and, as mentioned, initially did not seem to know what to believe. He had known Church for many years in Boston, and spent much time with him. Church had participated in John Adams's inoculation against smallpox in 1764. They had spent time together on various committees and shared other activities as Patriots. They were both members of the Sons of Liberty. Church had also recently treated an eye condition that Adams was suffering from.

As a result of Church's fall, John Adams understood that one had to be on guard when dealing with other people. In letters to his wife, Adams encouraged her to be watchful in her correspondence, and explained that from now on he would not share secret information in correspondence, because he felt he could not trust the post or private travelers, who he feared would either lose the letters or turn out to be British spies.[134]

When Church was discussed at the Continental Congress in Philadelphia, the Massachusetts House of Representatives was meeting at the First Parish Church Meeting House in Watertown. Watertown, a suburb of today's Boston, had just become the de facto capital of Massachusetts. The House requested that Washington explain why Church, who was a member of the House, had been arrested and placed under house arrest. A response to this request was delivered in the form of a letter from Washington. The letter also included a copy of the deciphered letter and a report of the proceedings of the War Council held on October 3–5, where Church had been found guilty of conducting criminal correspondence with the enemy.

The House of Representatives requested that Church be brought from his place of confinement to the House for trial, and if found guilty, be expelled from the House. On October 22, Washington agreed to let Church be released to the House for trial and punishment, but also determined that no actions should be taken until the Continental Congress had sent its recommendations.

The following day, Church sent a letter of resignation to the House of Representatives, hoping that if his resignation were approved, he would not have to appear before the House. His request was declined, and instead it was decided to find "a proper method for bringing Dr. Church before the House."[135] That method turned out to be a spectacle.

At 10 o'clock in the morning of October 27, High Sheriff William Howe and Adjutant General Horatio Gates of the Continental Army, accompanied by a group of soldiers, arrived at Church's place of confinement. Church was summoned to immediately appear before the House. After changing clothes, Church was brought the four miles from Cambridge to Watertown under conditions that probably looked like a parade. Church was riding in a chaise with the sheriff in the middle of a guard of twenty soldiers, and with drums and fifes playing.

After waiting at the door until called, Church was brought into the building. The meeting was open to the public, and the galleries were packed with curious spectators. Church was informed that a hearing was going to be conducted about whether to accept his resignation, or expel him.

During the initial part of the hearings, Church complained bitterly that he had been placed under house arrest for unjustified and unproven reasons, poorly and disrespectfully treated, and isolated from his family and friends. He also complained about the method used to bring him to the House, and that he had been summoned totally unexpectedly. He expressed concern about his poor health that he claimed was the result of being "harassed and sickening with painful suspense, aggravated vexations, rigorous imprisonment, and a load of sorrows no longer supportable."[136] Church also declared that he had not been given any explanations about his arrest until shortly before, when he was informed that he had been convicted by the General Court Martial on October 4 of criminal correspondence with the enemy.

After again admitting that the deciphered letter was basically an accurate translation of his letter to Major Cane, Church continued to profess his innocence, and he denied being a spy. He continued to argue that the letter was written to avoid bloodshed and a disastrous war that the English were sure to lose. In the letter, he was therefore pleading to the British to offer "a speedy accommodation" or the colonies "will be lost forever."[137] He was also stating that in the letter he had exaggerated the strength of the American army "to effect a union, to disarm a parricide, to restore peace to my distracted country." He also said that he wanted to put an "end to the work of death" so "where…is the crime?… I had no suspicion of evil, because I meant none."[138] Church ended his response by pleading to the House members: "To your wisdom, gentlemen, to your justice, to your tenderness, I cheerfully submit my fate."[139] When the hearing was over, Sheriff Howe returned Church under guard to his confinement, where he was to stay until a verdict had been reached.

A committee was formed to review Church's actions and provide recommendations to the House about the next steps. The committee reported to the House on November 2. It concluded that the secret correspondence by Church in July, communicating intelligence to the enemy, was "most injurious and destructive to this and all the United American Colonies," representing "wicked and detestable practices" and "deceitful conduct, horrible ingratitude, and breach of trust." It was therefore resolved that

Church would be expelled from the House, and that the House would not provide the protection that House members were otherwise entitled to.[140]

On November 7, Church was again brought to the House; this time to be notified about the verdict. Also at this time, the transport of Church to the House involved a military escort, fifes, and drums. Once he arrived at the House, Church was informed that he had been expelled from his seat as the elected representative from Boston in the Massachusetts Provincial Congress. The House also decided that the selection of punishment would be deferred to the Continental Congress. While waiting for that decision, Church was to be held in close confinement, with no person allowed to visit him except by special permission.

It should be noted that if Church actually wrote the ciphered letter to prevent an attack by the British, a bloody war, and the separation of the American colonies from England, he was not unique in his opinions. This may also explain why even John Adams initially felt ambivalent when the news about the ciphered letter first reached the Continental Congress.

It is interesting that "secret correspondence with the enemy"[141] is what Church was officially convicted of. Other suspicious activities taking place before the start of the Revolutionary War were not discussed during George Washington's October 3 and 4 council, or during the trial before the Massachusetts House of Representatives, from October 27 to November 2. They were also not part of the deliberations at the Continental Congress.

The different institutions trying Church were not the only ones who found him guilty of treacherous behavior; he was also found guilty in the eyes of the general population. So strong were the people of Massachusetts's feelings against Church that on one occasion he had to flee the mob by jumping out the window of a bedroom he was occupying.

On further consideration of facts that emerged about Church and his activities, even John Adams became convinced that Church indeed was a traitor, and expressed that in very strong words in the fall 1775:

> A Man of Genius, of Learning, of Family, of Character:
> A Writer of Liberty Songs, and good ones too:
> A Speaker of Liberty Orations:
> A Member of the Boston Committee of Correspondence:

A Member of the Massachusetts Congress:
An Agent from that Congress to the Continental Congress:
A Member of the House:
A Director-General of the Hospital and Surgeon General:
Surgeon General! Good God! What shall we say of
Human Nature?
What shall we say of American Patriots?

It is worth noting that although Church was found guilty of treason in the eyes of Washington, the Continental Congress, the Massachusetts House of Representatives, and, ultimately, in the eyes of John Adams, his guilt has remained questioned by some historians throughout the centuries. In one of the most extensive works on surgeons and health care during the American Revolution, published about 150 years after the war,[142] the author concluded that "at this day it is difficult to say what, if any, was his degree of guilt."

The End

Washington, who probably would have recommended Church's execution by hanging, did not feel he could do so in the absence of rules guiding the handling of a spy and traitor. Although Washington requested instructions, the Continental Congress also found it difficult to decide what to do. Instead of determining a punishment, Congress postponed the subject, and decided to put Church in jail under strict confinement. In order to prevent Church getting in contact with people he knew in Massachusetts, he was brought to Connecticut and put in jail in Norwich on November 21. Because of declining health, Church was ultimately allowed to be returned to Boston on May 27, 1776. When Church passed through Watertown and Waltham on the way to his new prison in Boston, the local population expressed outrage against Church and almost lynched him.

To put a closure to the affair, a plan was developed to allow Church to be set free on the issuance of bond. Church, however, did not have money for the bond, so he remained in jail. Another plan was to exchange Church for the prisoner Dr. James McHenry, who had been captured by the British during fighting at Fort Washington on York (present day Manhattan).

That deal fell through when, on October 2, 1777, General Heath, who was leading the defense of Boston, refused to approve the prisoner exchange. Heath feared that Church would bring secrets with him and share them with the British.

As time went on, it became obvious that the continued incarceration of Church under strict conditions was becoming an expensive affair, and the authorities started to make plans to get rid of him. On January 9, 1778, the Massachusetts House of Representatives decided to allow—or more likely force—Church to leave America on the sloop *Welcome,* bound for the Island of Martinico (presently known as Martinique) in the Caribbean.[143] In mid-February 1778, two years and four months after his arrest, Church boarded *Welcome* and set sail for Martinico. Somehow, Church disappeared and never surfaced on the pages of history again. The exact circumstances surrounding Church's disappearance remain unknown and are somewhat mysterious. Although a shipwreck caused by a storm seems to be the most common theory, it has also been speculated that Church was thrown overboard by the sailors shortly after leaving Boston.[144]

Church's imprisonment gravely affected his family. His father, Benjamin Church Sr., made several attempts to have his son freed, or at least treated more humanely. He paid a high price for the support of his son, and saw his home ransacked and robbed of everything of value by rebels.

In July 1777, with Church still in prison, his wife, Sarah, boarded a ship along with their three children in order to sail to England. Only a couple of days after sailing out of Boston, the ship was captured by an American warship and brought to Rhode Island. After two weeks delay, the ship was finally allowed to continue its voyage. Upon arriving in England, Sarah filed a request for a pension, claiming her husband had provided service to the British government. Officials supported her claims. The fact that the British government provided Mrs. Church with a pension because of her husband's efforts on its behalf provides further support that Church had indeed been a spy and worked for the British—no matter what Church had claimed.

CHAPTER 4

JOHN MORGAN—
Founder of the First Medical
School in the Colonies

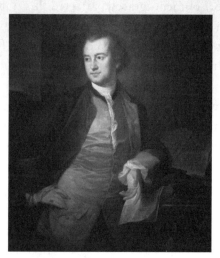

John Morgan (1735–1789). Depicted here at the time of his return from England following five years of medical and surgical training. By many, he was considered haughty and arrogant. He soon became entangled in a bitter fight with his previous friend, William Shippen, Jr., because of rivalry around the founding of the Medical School in Philadelphia. (Niday Picture Library)

J ohn Morgan (1735–1789) was born into a prosperous Philadelphia Quaker family. His father, Evan, had emigrated from Wales and made his wealth on real estate and iron. Benjamin Franklin was a neighbor and good friend of the family.

The Early Years

Morgan graduated from the College of Philadelphia in 1757. During the last couple of years in college, he also served an apprenticeship with Dr. John Redman, an influential practitioner in Philadelphia. After graduating from college, Morgan joined the British Army in the French and Indian War, giving him firsthand insight into military medicine and surgery. This was an experience that would influence his future career as Surgeon-General of the Continental Army during the Revolutionary War.

Training in London and Edinburgh

After two years in the French and Indian War army, Morgan resigned and traveled to Europe for additional medical and surgical training. He arrived in London in 1760, and "walked" the hospitals of London for a year. During his time in the capital, Morgan had the opportunity to meet with many prominent individuals, both in and outside the medical profession. Being a good friend of Benjamin Franklin helped open doors and gave him access to influential members of the society. Attending the Hunter brothers' renowned anatomical school, and lectures with public dissections, gave Morgan a solid insight into the human anatomy and its importance in successful surgeries.

In order to improve his academic standing and gain a medical degree, Morgan left for Edinburgh after a year in London. He received his MD from the University of Edinburgh in 1763 after presenting his thesis in Latin on the formation of pus, "*De Puopoiesi*." The thesis put forward the hypothesis that purulence begins in the blood vessels.

Morgan was successful in Edinburgh and became a shining star among his contemporary trainees.[145] He achieved both clinical and academic acclaims, and became somewhat of a celebrity. His standing in society was also helped by support from influential individuals, including William Cullen, one of the leading physicians and medical teachers in Edinburgh at the time.

After graduating from Edinburgh, Morgan left for the continent. He first spent time in Paris, observing French medical practices and studying anatomy under the famous anatomist Jean-Joseph Sue. Morgan also gave lectures, mainly about suppuration and the methods employed by the Hunter brothers to inject and preserve human anatomic specimens. The time in Paris was followed by Morgan's "Grand Tour" of Europe, an approximately ten-month journey through southern France, northern Italy, and parts of Switzerland.

Morgan's Grand Tour of Europe

In early 1764, Morgan and his close friend and fellow Philadelphian, Samuel Powel, set out from Paris on what would become the travel of their lifetime. Morgan wrote a detailed journal during his travel (*The Journal of Dr. John Morgan of Philadelphia: From the City of Rome to the City of London, 1764*), but like most of his other private papers, only a fragment of the writing has survived. The existing part of the journal covers the period from the 6th of July to the 31st of October 1764.[146] It is full of details that give wonderful insight into not only into the people Morgan met, but also the European living conditions during the 1700s. Morgan provided a rich picture of how people traveled at the time, including road conditions, inns and other places to sleep, taverns, weather, and places worth seeing.

Morgan and Powel planned to travel all the way to Venice before turning around, returning to London, and ultimately sailing back to Philadelphia. The journey took the travelers to many of the European metropolises, including Rome, Bologna, Padua, Venice, Milan, and Geneva. Most of the time, the means of transportation was a chaise, typically pulled by one, but sometimes several, horses. The travel offered exciting experiences, both pleasant and not so pleasant, and was often tiring. The roads were not very comfortable, which was particularly noticeable when bumping around in a chaise. Flooded roads, and roads not passable for other reasons, resulted in detours and long delays. On several occasions, chaise wheels broke down. On one such instance, the accident happened after dark, stranding Morgan and his company roadside, with the travelers waiting for sunrise when help finally arrived. To avoid the sun and heat during summertime, travel in southern Europe was often not commenced until the evening.

Although inns were readily available along the roads, the quality varied. Four days after leaving Rome, Morgan and Powel arrived at nine o'clock in the evening at Macerata, "a pretty little town situated 153 miles from Rome on a pleasant rising ground or hill with a pretty Country about it. Here, for the first time since we left Rome, we met with a tolerable Inn and accommodations, & no bad attendance—a thing not very Common in the Inns of Italy."[147]

Morgan was twenty-nine at the time of his European tour. He was a good-looking bachelor who kept his eyes open for pretty women. On a couple of occasions, he made interesting observations and comments in his travel journal about the women in Italy. About a week after leaving Rome, he arrived at the town of Fanno, which was said "to be remarkable for some of the beautifullest women in Italy."[148] In a somewhat disappointed tone, he added, "What I saw of them were generally handsome, but I did not see many of them who might be supposed to surpass the Italian ladies in other places." Later, when in Milan, he commented that many women were sitting "at the Doors & Windows without veils, have more liberty than common in Italy w'ch to deprive them of is only to make them more licentious, & to seek hidden opportunities, w'ch they are seldom at a loss for. The Ladies here appear tolerably handsome."[149]

Later in the journey, Morgan and Powel spent two weeks at Turin. This gave them the opportunity to gain insights into the higher society's habits. On the 31st of August, they were introduced to "Mad'm la Comtesse de St.Gill," who lived in a palace, appeared to be about forty years of age, and was "handsome eno'." The room where she received Morgan and Powel was darkened "for Coolness & she was in a very light loose dress, thro' which we could see her limbs very easily, & the more so as she spoke much & accompany'd it with a great deal of Action." It is unclear what her relationship with her husband was. Morgan reported that he seemed several years older than his wife, and was not first present when she met with Morgan, but came in and was introduced to the visitors a while later. At the time of Morgan's visit, a number of "English Gentlemen" were living in Turin, and much of the conversation between the *Comtesse* and Morgan related to the "intriguing" by the English gentlemen, in particular with married women. The *Comtesse* did not seem to be upset with their intriguing, but condemned the fact that it was not always carried on with "sufficient prudence and spirit." Morgan commented on the frequent extramarital affairs: "This is not strange in Italy where it is a much greater Wonder to hear of a marry'd Woman, especially amongst those of fashion, that does not intrigue than it is in some other places to hear of marry'd Women who do."

Although Morgan had the privilege of being introduced to a number of exceedingly influential people during his travel, including Pope Clemente, the King of Sardinia, the Duke of York, and the French philosopher Voltaire, the most lasting impressions from a professional standpoint were those from his meetings with Morgagni in Padua, and his visit to the hospitals in Milan.

On the 24th of July, the travelers reached Padua, which was described by Morgan as "a very large, fortified & ancient City; seems very populous; but the Buildings in general old & ruinous. The Streets very unevenly pav'd with stone, w'h makes riding in a Carriage very disagreeable."[150] The travelers' main purpose of visiting Padua was getting the opportunity to meet with the celebrated Professor of Anatomy, Giovanni Battista Morgagni.

After arriving at Padua, Morgan spared no time in seeing Morgagni. Following three hours travel from the town of Ferrara, Morgan and Powel reached Padua at ten o'clock in the morning. In the afternoon of the same day, Morgan went to pay his respects to Morgagni. In his chronicle, Morgan provided a detailed description of the encounter. He brought a letter of introduction from Dr. Serrati, Professor of Medicine at the University of Bologna, with whom Morgan had met a couple of days earlier. Support from Benjamin Franklin and Dr. Cullen at Edinburgh also helped Morgan get the audience.

Morgan was well received by Morgagni, who was vital and energetic, and looked and behaved younger than his age: "He received me with the greatest Politeness imaginable, & shew'd me abundant Civilities with a very good grace. He is now 82 y'rs of age, yet reads without spectacles & is as alert as a Man of 50."[151]

As a gift, Morgan brought Morgagni a piece of a human kidney that he had subjected to corrosion for display of the blood vessels. With this technique, which Morgan had learned in London from the Hunter brothers, all the kidney tissue except the blood vessels were corroded. Morgagni was impressed by the technique that was unfamiliar to him and "acknowledg'd he had never seen any preparation before in w'h the Vessels were so minutely filled."

Morgagni countered with a gift of his own, a new edition of *de Sede et Causis Morborum*, in two volumes. This was the third edition published in three years of his immensely popular and successful textbook about diseases and their causes, sold all over Europe and with "all ye Copies of the last Edition already bought up."

Morgan spent several interesting hours with Morgagni that afternoon. Among other things, Morgagni showed his collection of bones, and how they developed in fetuses from a few weeks up to nine months, and then from birth to adulthood. Morgagni seemed to be particularly proud of a skeleton from a six-to-seven-months-old fetus with spina bifida (a congenital malformation with incomplete development and closure of the posterior aspect of the vertebrae), and who lacked a brain and spinal cord.

Morgagni also had a couple of examples in his collection of stones formed in the urinary bladder around a foreign body. In both cases, the foreign body seemed somewhat strange. One of the specimens was the bladder of a man who had inserted a needle up into his bladder through the urethra, and "a Calculus had form'd on the needle." The other case was a calculus formed on the tip of a corking pin that a woman had inserted into her bladder through the urethra "so as to lay ye foundation of a Calculus of w'h she dy'd." Morgan did not explain or comment on why the objects had been "slipped up the urethra" in any of these cases, but it is tempting to speculate that the purpose was to dislodge an obstructing bladder stone that was stuck at the internal orifice of the urethra, making it impossible to urinate. It is possible that the person lost control of the needle or pin and that it slipped up into the bladder where it was retained and became the nidus for the formation of additional bladder stones.

Morgagni also proudly exhibited several anatomical preparations of the ear, showing the detailed bony structures of the inner ear with the three semicircular canals accounting for hearing and balance. In addition, he had detailed preparations of the bones in the middle ear (malleus, incus, and stapes of the hammer, anvil, and stirrup), with details that "his Master in Anatomy, Valsalva, could never find until he show'd it to him."[152]

In addition to anatomical artifacts, Morgagni had a collection of portraits. Some of the portraits were of old anatomists and famous professors at Bologna. Two of the portraits were of a more personal character—and somewhat tragic.

Morgagni had fifteen children, five of who had died at young age. Among the ten surviving children, eight were daughters. All the daughters became nuns when they grew up. By pairs, they entered four different convents. After their periods of probation, they had to decide whether they wanted to live in the world or take the veil. All eight daughters decided to lead the rest of their lives as nuns. The two youngest joined the strict Franciscan Order, in which they had to go barefooted and always be veiled. They were locked up in the convent, without outside contacts for the remainder of their lives—including contact with their parents. A good friend of the Morgagni family, the famous paintress, Rosalba Carriera, drew portraits of the two youngest daughters and gifted them to Morgagni, so he would remember what they had once looked like. Showing these portraits to Morgan must have been an emotional moment for Morgagni.

Later, when Morgan returned from Venice, he again traveled through Padua and met with Morgagni for a second time. At this time, he was also well received and "entertained very politely & agreeably."

On the way back to London, Morgan and Powel traveled through Milan, where they arrived on the August 15th and stayed for four days. In his diary, Morgan gave a detailed account of what was probably the most memorable experience in the city: the visit to the General Hospital of Milan. Although it was still under construction, Morgan was enormously impressed and wrote, "Tis even now beyond comparison, the finest & largest Hospital I have ever seen in any Country."[153] At the time of Morgan's visit, the hospital was occupied by more than one thousand patients. In addition, thousands of patients were cared for in an outpatient clinic in the countryside.

The General Hospital was well known and attracted people from many different nations; relatively few patients were local. Similar to other countries, babies that could not be taken care of by their mothers were often abandoned and left at the doorstep of the hospital: "They have received about 120 foundlings this last year, whom they send into the country immediately to proper Nurses to take Care of."

With the large number of patients being treated at the hospital, the need for medication and other supplies must have been enormous. Morgan wrote that the "Apothecharys Shop & Quantity of Medic'nes large." The number of physicians taking care of the more than one thousand patients was surprisingly small: "The Number of Physic'ns in daily attend'ce 15, 10 in the Morning & all 15 in the afternoon, of Surgeons in daily attendance 10 besides 70 young Surgeons or Dressers, who all eat at one Table & sleep at one Room. Some of the Surgeons, the extraordinary ones, live at home; some of the others have Rooms in the House."

The hospital also served as a teaching institution with lectures "in Anatomy-Surg'ry-Med'ne & care given to the Pupils in the Hospital but to no others." The hospital's obligations to the patients extended even beyond death. Morgan described how the hospital had a "large & curious place of Burial given by a Benefactor of ye Hospital." What Morgan saw in Milan gave him additional ideas for the medical school he planned to establish after returning to the colonies.

Morgan and Powel reached the final destination of their European tour, London, a couple of months after their stay in Milan. During those months, they again visited Turin, Geneva, and Paris. In Geneva, they met with Voltaire and spent an evening of learned discussions at a reception in Voltaire's residence, the Chateau de Fernay. They were well received: "Mons'r Voltaire himself received us on the steps." During the evening, several interesting topics were discussed, including Benjamin Franklin's thoughts on electricity and Voltaire's opinion of religion. Voltaire explained that "I hate Churches & Priests & Masses."

When Morgan and Powel were about to leave the reception, Voltaire addressed the rest of the company and said, "Behold two Amiable Young Men Lovers of Truth & Inquirers into Nature. They are not satisfy'd with mear Appearances, they love Investigation & Truth, & despize Superstition—I commend You Gentlemen—go on, love Truth & search diligently after it."

On the 29th of October, in the afternoon after finishing dinner, Morgan and Powel left Calais to cross the English Chanel in a packet boat. Thirteen hours later, after "a stormy rough rainey & disagreeable Passage," they finally set foot on English soil again. In the evening of the 31st of October, they reached London. By then, Morgan had been away from London more than three years, and they were "thankfull to Heaven once more to get into the Circle of Friends and acquaintances."

They had planned to leave for America shortly after their return to London, but weather became a factor. Fall and winter storms would have made the voyage across the Atlantic both unpleasant and risky. Morgan was not able to return to the colonies until the following spring.

Morgan Returns to Philadelphia and Establishes the first American Medical School

When Morgan returned to Philadelphia in 1765, he could look back at five successful and exciting years in Europe, including his Grand Tour. He had become well known in Europe and was starting to be treated like a celebrity. His return to Philadelphia was described in a letter from George Roberts to Samuel Powel (who had remained in London) in the following way: "Morgan comes home flushed with honors and is treated by his friends with all due respect to his merit."[154] Dr. Benjamin Rush, a renowned physician at the time, wrote about Morgan: "He returned to Philadelphia loaded with literary honors, and was received with open arms by his fellow citizens. They felt an interest in him for having advanced in every part of Europe the honor of the American name." He was not necessarily easy to get along with, and although he was "informed, able," he was also "strong willed;...unable to get along with people, and too inclined to overvalue his rank and name."[155]

During his time in Europe, Morgan had often pondered the need for a medical school in the colonies. Some of those thoughts and ideas had been shared with William Shippen.[156] He and Morgan had both been in England for training, and had become friends and gotten to know each other. Together, they had discussed plans for a medical school in Philadelphia. Shippen had returned to the colonies ahead of Morgan, and was eagerly awaiting Morgan's arrival to resume their friendship and put their plan for the medical school into action. Soon after returning home, however, Morgan took things in his own hands and alone approached the Board of Trustees of the College of Philadelphia with plans for the establishment of a medical school. His proposal was supported by recommendations from several prominent British medical educators, and was approved without much deliberation. The foundation of the first medical school in the colonies had been laid. As we will see, Shippen considered Morgan's single-handed actions a betrayal, creating long-lasting resentment between the two surgeons.

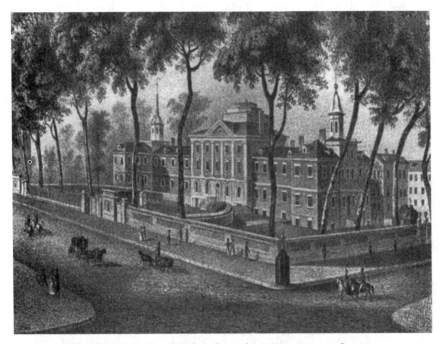

The first Medical School in the American colonies, established at Philadelphia in 1765. Morgan was the founder of the Medical School and was appointed its first Professor of the Theory and Practice of Physic.

On May 3, 1765, Morgan was appointed Professor of the Theory and Practice of Physic. This made him the first medical professor on the American continent. A couple of weeks later, at the Commencement of the College of Philadelphia, Morgan delivered an important speech on medical education, "A Discourse upon the institution of medical schools in America." The system he had been exposed to in Edinburgh heavily influenced the medical school he envisioned.

It was only when Morgan's plans for the medical school had been approved, but not until then, did he recommend Shippen as Professor of Anatomy and Surgery. Although he accepted the position, Shippen was resentful that Morgan had taken charge of the plans for America's first medical school without allowing him to play a significant role. Moreover, Morgan never acknowledged the fact that he and Shippen had jointly developed the scheme for the medical school while in England. These events were never forgotten, nor forgiven, by Shippen, and so started a decade of bitter rivalry, anger, and intrigues. This not only affected Shippen's and Morgan's lives, but also weakened the medical school in Philadelphia and the Medical Department of the Continental Army. The hard feelings between the two men would continue to grow over the coming years, resulting in suspicion and hatred and ultimately paving the way to tragic events that affected both rivals.

There were probably several reasons why Morgan was successful in establishing a medical school by himself. Morgan was somewhat of an academic superstar when he returned to Philadelphia in 1765. He was an early graduate of the College of Philadelphia, the institution he approached to create a medical school. He had the support of many influential individuals in town, several of who were members of the Board of Trustees at the College of Philadelphia. Among them was John Redman, a "commanding figure in the medical world of that day" and with whom Morgan had spent a six-year apprenticeship before his training in Europe. William Smithy, who was the first provost of the College of Philadelphia, and who had been Morgan's mentor, was also supportive.

The Medical School officially opened on November 14, 1765, with Shippen starting a course on anatomy. Morgan's lectures began the following week and were later published as *Materia Medica with Some Useful Observations on Medicine and the Proper Manner of Conducting the Study of Physic*.

The years 1764 and 1765 were banner years for Morgan. After traveling to parts of the European continent during 1764 as a rising star in surgery, he had returned to Philadelphia in 1765 as a hero, managed to establish the first medical school on the American continent, and become the first professor in medicine. On top of all this, he found out that his love, Mary, had been waiting for him. They had been engaged shortly before Morgan sailed for Europe five years earlier, and were subsequently married in September 1765. Mary was described as "possessing extraordinary charms of character, disposition, and manner. She was witty, unaffected, musically gifted far beyond the average, extremely vivacious, graceful, and fascinating."

Although some felt that the successes went to Morgan's head, others described him as "charming and polished in manner, of distinguished bearing, always well dressed, extremely good looking...." He made an elegant appearance on the streets of Philadelphia. Tradition has it that Morgan carried the first umbrella ever seen in Philadelphia and "that until the townsfolk grew accustomed to the sight, crowds of curious and amazed people followed him through the streets."[157]

Morgan's good fortunes continued after founding the medical school. The next ten years were the best of his life. He spent a considerable amount of time and effort on the medical school and its mission. He contributed significantly to the teaching of Physic and was an early proponent of specialization of medicine. From Europe, he also brought back the importance of separating pharmacy and surgery from the practice of physicians (internal medicine). Despite his surgical training in Europe, he decided not to pursue surgery, but to strictly and only be a physician. Ironically, not too long after this he became known as the most elevated surgeon on the continent.

Morgan continued to build a busy and lucrative practice. During this time, both Morgan and Shippen were heavily involved in the Medical School, and both wanted it to be successful. Although Shippen remained resentful towards Morgan, the animosity between the two men did not seem to prevent the successes of either. The bad blood between Shippen and Morgan would explode into open daylight at a later time point.

Morgan Appointed Surgeon-General of the Continental Army

Morgan was appointed Surgeon-General of the Continental Army and Physician-in-Chief of the Army Hospital in October 1775. He replaced Benjamin Church, who had been dismissed in disgrace after less than three months in the position. Morgan considered the appointment yet another honorable recognition in his successful life. He accepted the appointment despite having to give up his large and profitable practice in Philadelphia. His advancement was looked upon with favor by many influential colleagues and politicians of the time. For example, in the book *Medical Men of the Revolution,* Dr. J.M. Toner wrote: "The success which had attended the medical department of the College of Philadelphia under his guidance was of itself a first-class endorsement. His ability as a surgeon, his character as a man, his patriotism, and his influence as a citizen were well known to the public."

In a letter from John Adams to his wife on October 20, 1775, Adams wrote:

> Congress has appointed instead of Church, Dr. Morgan of this city, whose character I will pourtray to your satisfaction. The gentleman appointed Director and Superintendent of the Hospitals is John Morgan, M.D. Fellow of the Royal Society of London, Correspondent of the Royal Academy of Surgery in Paris; Member of the Arcadian Belle Lettres Society at Rome; Licentiate of the Royal Colleges of Physicians in London and in Edinburg, and Professor of the Theory and Practice of Medicine in the College in this City and served an apprenticeship of six years with Dr. John Redman...Dr. Morgan's moral character is very good and his manner is civil, decent, and agreeable.[158]

Adams also wrote a supportive letter to James Warren.[159]

Shortly after his appointment, Morgan and his wife triumphantly traveled to Cambridge, outside of Boston, to report to Washington. In those days, journeying from Philadelphia to Boston meant several days on horseback and in carriages, but Dr. and Mrs. Morgan were in good spirits during the travel, enjoying the moment and the honor bestowed upon him. As Morgan's wife reported in a letter written to her mother, they were well received when they arrived in Cambridge: "There came six or eight of the gentlemen of the faculty to wait upon Dr. Morgan and escort us to the Camp, some of them on horseback and some of them in carriages. I do assure you we had no small cavalcade... Since I have begun this letter I have had the honour of a visit from four Generals—Genl. Washington, Genl. Putnam, Gen. Gates & Gen. Lee." Happy days were spent in the spotlight and in the presence of important people. "There were tea-drinkings, visitings to and fro, and military reviews...." At the time, Morgan and his wife did not understand that these could actually have been the last truly happy days in their lives. Clouds soon started to appear at the horizon. They assembled rapidly and never lifted.

As a new Surgeon-General of the Army, Morgan had to invest time and energy in reinforcing rules for interactions between the surgeons at the regimental and the surgeons at general hospitals. Despite his efforts, the regimental surgeons continued to display insubordination and kept bullying the surgeons at the general hospitals. The situation gave Morgan enemies among the regimental surgeons, something that would haunt him when he was challenged in the not-too-distant future.

Morgan soon realized that the Medical Department of the Revolutionary Army was terribly disorganized and lacked resources. He found wretched sanitary conditions in the hospitals under his care. Despite the obstacles, Morgan tried to reform the system immediately after his appointment. Initially, he seemed to be successful, but he soon understood that he had strong forces against him that not even Washington's support could overcome. He was not given the resources he requested, in great part because of the indecision of the Continental Congress—which, of course, had many other pressing issues at hand during this early phase of what would become the Revolutionary War. More sadly, infighting and jealousy between surgeons in the army also hampered Morgan. When conditions in the medical system continued to be poor despite Morgan's hard work and tireless efforts to improve the situation, he became a scapegoat, and accusations against his leadership started to grow. Morgan also became increasingly convinced that he had many envious detractors actively campaigning against him. High on the list of suspects were Shippen and his supporters. Shippen still bore a grudge against Morgan for the events surrounding the founding of the medical school in Philadelphia—and his feelings were not helped by the fact that it was Morgan, not Shippen, who was selected to become Surgeon-General.

Complaints against Morgan started to be filed with Congress. To clear his name and bring some justice to the situation, Morgan requested an investigation of the affairs of the Medical Department, but members of the Congress, including John Adams, refused to start an inquiry, in part because the threatening collapse of the Revolution did not leave time for such an endeavor. Instead, Morgan's enemies managed to further discredit him, and on January 9, 1777, less than fifteen months after his appointment as Surgeon-General of the Army, he was dismissed from the position by Congress. Three months later, Shippen was appointed to replace Morgan, a turn of events that strengthened Morgan's suspicions that Shippen was behind the calumny against him, and his ultimate dismissal from the army.

Morgan was now a broken man. Although he went back to Philadelphia and took up his medical practice and hospital appointments, his life was never the same. He continued to ask Congress to investigate the circumstances surrounding his dismissal from the military. He prepared a widely circulated paper, "Vindication of his Public Character in the Station of Director-General of the Military Hospital and Physician in Chief to the American Army," rebutting the charges against him. In the opening sections, he wrote, "That a mean and insidious set of men have looked upon my elevation…with an evil eye, and long been concerting my removal, is a matter of which I have too substantial proof to doubt."

It took Congress two full years to finally appoint a committee charged to examine Morgan's conduct and the complaints made against him before he was dismissed. In the report issued by the committee on June 12, 1779, Morgan was honorably acquitted from all charges against him.[160] Although this provided some comfort to Morgan, his spirit remained broken. He continued to hope for revenge against his detractors, particularly Shippen, and his efforts towards that goal ultimately resulted in the court martial of Shippen.

The Court Martial of Shippen

Several factors played important roles in the events leading up to the court martial of Shippen in 1780. Morgan, together with Benjamin Rush, was the accuser and also functioned as the formal prosecutor during the trial.

Not long after Shippen replaced Morgan as Surgeon-General, he started to be subjected to the same criticism that Morgan had received. He was accused of being incompetent and, more importantly, he was also accused of fraud and neglect of his hospital duties, and lack of compassion in the treatment of the wounded soldiers. Dr. Benjamin Rush of Philadelphia initially brought the accusations forward.

Rush expressed his concerns in a letter to John Adams in October 1777, writing that Shippen was "both ignorant and negligent of his duty."[161] In a letter to another member of Congress he complained that the medical system under Shippen's directorship "is a mass of corruption and tyranny."[162] Rush even turned to General Washington, describing the poor hospital conditions and the high death rates among the soldiers in the Revolutionary Army. Washington turned to Congress for advice, but Congress did not seem willing to take actions. Rush gave up and did not make any further moves. Instead, Morgan took over as the principal accuser of Shippen. In June 1779, Morgan started his campaign to force Shippen from office by formally addressing Congress: "I do hereby charge Dr. William Shippen junr. in the service of the United States with Malpractices and Misconduct in Office."[163] Morgan also requested that Shippen be tried by a court martial, and declared his readiness "to give before the proper Court having Jurisdiction the necessary Evidence in the premises against the said Dr. Wm. Shippen." By then, Morgan and Rush had become allies in the attacks on Shippen.

Increasingly understanding that things were not right, Washington ordered Shippen to be brought to trial. In anticipation of a court martial, Morgan crisscrossed Pennsylvania during the winter months of 1779–1780, taking testimonies from individuals who had served in the army and experienced the dreadful conditions in the military hospitals. The court martial started on March 14, 1780, and would last four months. The trial was based on five charges that Morgan brought forward.

The first charge claimed that Shippen had sold hospital stores as his own. He had put himself in a dangerous position by stocking his personal wines in the same cellars that were used for storage of the public's wine and other supplies. Mixing his personal goods with the public's created a situation that could easily lead to temptation and abuse.

The second charge accused Shippen of speculating in goods required by the hospitals. It also included the accusation that Shippen had used public funds to purchase wines and other goods for private use. Shippen was also suspected of being involved in adulterating wine with water, and providing surgeons with less than the amounts they had requested for their patients.

The third charge accused the Director-General of sloppy—or nonexistent—bookkeeping. It is unclear whether his enemies were implying that Shippen had calculatingly neglected bookkeeping to prevent detection of illegal activities, or whether they implied that Shippen was lazy and tried to avoid the hard work needed to keep accurate records. Strangely enough, the court never requested Shippen to produce his records, something historians have interpreted as evidence that the court was biased in favor of Shippen.

The fourth charge against Shippen was that his neglect of duty had caused severe pain and distress and, ultimately, death among wounded soldiers. To support the charges, many individuals were called as witnesses. The testimonies described how "the sick and wounded bounced and jolted in farm wagons over rutted frozen roads in midwinter, lying in unheated buildings without shirts, shoes, or blankets, covered with vermin, their wounds undressed, without medicines, without water, sometimes with nothing to gnaw but the straw they lay on." The impact of these reports was magnified by the description of how hospital surgeons at the same time were kept warm, dry, and safe, and were housed in private homes, "gulping liquor brought 'in buckets-ful' from the hospital stores, dancing and frolicking together till midnight and sometimes till one or two o'clock in the morning." The fourth charge also included accusations that Shippen filed falsified reports to Congress regarding the conditions in the hospitals.

Some of the first four charges were the same that Rush had already made against Shippen in 1778. Rush repeated the accusations during the court martial, including the overcrowded hospitals where soldiers died because of lack of food, clothing, and medicine. Rush also accused Shippen of using wine and sugar from the public stores for his personal trading. He described how wounded soldiers suffered from the "dreaded putrid fever of the hospitals" which made the hospitals look "like slaughter houses."[164]

Astonishingly, the court acquitted Shippen on all initial four charges except the second. The second charge, that Shippen had bought and sold sugar and wine on his own account using government money, resulted in a statement by the court that this behavior was "highly improper and justly reprehensible." One reason why Shippen was not acquitted on the second charge may have been that he was found to have done some of the business under a pseudonym, proving that Shippen was well aware what he was doing was wrong.

The fifth charge was Morgan's personal accusation that Shippen had been intriguing and used "scandalous and infamous practices" to get Morgan ousted as Director-General. Because Morgan, as the prosecutor, could not have presented this charge without strong personal bias, the court considered this charge groundless and refused to hear it. Instead, they turned against Morgan and deemed the charge malicious.

The outcome of the court martial was considered a scandal by many. Some of the events surrounding the trial were also scandalous. The most aggravating occurrence was when Shippen tried to influence the court proceedings by inviting members of the court to a party at which "wines, fruits, and other delicacies brought from Philadelphia" were served and during which he entertained his guests with an evil-spirited imitation of Morgan.

As a result of the acquittal, Shippen was reinstituted as Surgeon-General. At this time, however, he was tired and sick of the acrimony surrounding the position, and retired from it on January 3, 1781. Congress nominated Morgan to succeed Shippen, but Morgan was equally tired of the mudslinging and did not want the post. Dr. John Cochran's appointment to succeed Shippen finally brought some harmony to the position of Surgeon-General.

Morgan's Final Years

Although Congress officially cleared Morgan in 1779, he remained stricken by grief and disappointment during the rest of his life. His bitterness, of course, was not helped by Shippen's acquittal from all except one of the charges brought against him at the court martial. Morgan continued his medical practice in Philadelphia and maintained teaching obligations but withdrew from most social interactions and spent many days in quiet study and reflection. Adding to his tragedy, most of his personal papers had been destroyed during the war when British troops burned down his home in Philadelphia. His wife of twenty years, Mary Hopkinson Morgan, died in 1785, leaving no children. Morgan followed her five years later. So ended a life that had started so brilliantly, filled with both national and international successes, and that was ruined at the end "by the envious jealousy of contemporaries and the dilatory justice of a distracted government."

CHAPTER 5

WILLIAM SHIPPEN, JR.—
Jealousy, Rivalry, Court Martial

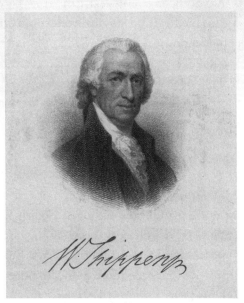

**William Shippen, Jr. (1736–1808). Court-martialed
during his tenure as Surgeon-General, accused of
"Malpractices and Misconduct in Office." He was
acquitted and returned to Philadelphia to rebuild both his
reputation and medical practice. (Historic Images)**

Although William Shippen, Jr. (1736–1808) experienced many successes in his life, and is remembered as a pioneer in American medical education and an early advocate of male midwifery (obstetrics), he certainly also had his share of disappointments and failures. His inability to generate support for the first medical school in America, and become its founder, weighed heavily on him during most of his professional life. His feuds with John Morgan and Benjamin Rush, which ultimately resulted in court martial and resignation from his position as Surgeon-General of the Continental Army, embittered him for years.

Shippen was not a proliferative writer and left only few documents behind, mostly letters. He did not leave any scientific publications (other than his doctoral thesis) for the afterworld. Because of the paucity of writings, his life has not been abundantly described, and no comprehensive biography has been published. An important source of information about Shippen, however, was published in 1951 by Betsy Copping Corner.[165] It contains insights into Shippen's early years; the time he spent in London and Edinburgh for his medical and surgical education; him learning from the famous surgeon–anatomists John and William Hunter; his experiences at St. Thomas Hospital in London; his academic endeavors, resulting in an MD degree from the University of Edinburgh; and his prominent career as anatomist, obstetrician, surgeon, and medical educator.

The Early Years

Shippen's great-grandfather, Edward Shippen, had arrived in America in 1669 from Yorkshire, England. He initially settled in Boston. When he married a Quaker woman, he was persecuted by the puritan Bostonians, and decided to abandon Massachusetts for the City of Brotherly Love. The Philadelphians appreciated Edward more than the citizens of Boston and made him Philadelphia's first mayor in 1701.

Shippen's father was a successful physician with a large and lucrative practice in Philadelphia. He was an admired member of society, with a reputation for being generous to the poor with both his time and money. He was actively involved in the American Revolution, and was elected to the Continental Congress in 1778 and reelected in 1779. Benjamin

Franklin was one of his close friends. Shippen Sr. was the first physician to the Pennsylvania Hospital and was one of the founders of the University of Pennsylvania. He was also a founder of the College of New Jersey (the future Princeton), something that would influence the choice of college for his son. When he entered the world, it is obvious that William Shippen Jr. had big shoes to fill.

When it was time for school, Shippen Jr. was sent to a boarding school in West Nottingham under the direction of Dr. Samuel Finley, a Presbyterian clergyman. The years living in Dr. Finley's country house were formative, and instilled in young William not only knowledge, but discipline as well. The headmaster was strict, and known for being "as punctilious about table manners as Latin grammar."[166] However, he also had a softer side and included various outdoor activities in the curriculum, such as fishing, hunting, and riding.

After boarding school, William went on to the College of New Jersey, at the time located in Newark. When he graduated from college in 1754, some considerations were entertained for Shippen to go into ministry. His father, however, made sure Shippen chose medicine, and took on his son as an apprentice. The four years in training under his father's tutelage went fast, and were followed by four years of continued medical and surgical training abroad. In 1758, at the age of twenty-two, Shippen set sail for England and did not return to Philadelphia until 1762.

Going to London

Knowing foreign training would be costly, Shippen's father started raising funds, and explained in a letter to his older brother, Edward (a successful and wealthy merchant in Lancaster outside Philadelphia), that he was "casting around to raise a sum of money for Billey's improvement abroad."[167] It is possible that Edward helped out with financial support, because, in a subsequent letter to his brother, Shippen Sr. wrote that his son would exercise "Genteel frugality in his Expenses and Living." In the same letter, he outlined the plans for William's journey: "Billey goes on board Capt Dingo's fine ship bound to Liverpool, from hence to London" where he will be met by people "of great reputation" who will help him to behave "as friendly & as sincerely as well as judiciously as any man in London." Shippen Sr. continued by describing his son's awaiting curriculum: "He is to spend this winter in London with the finest Anatomist for Dissections, Injections, &c in England, at the same time visit the Hospitals daily, to attend Lectures of Midwifery with a Gentleman who will make that branch as familiar to him as he can want or wish to have it."

After arriving in London, William wrote a letter to his uncle, reassuring him that he would be careful with his finances, study hard, avoid all sinful temptations in the big city, and be sure to follow his uncle's wise advice. In the letter, dated March 10, 1759, Shippen wrote: "Dear and hon'd Uncle, After an unpleasant and dangerous voyage of 7½ weeks I arrived at Belfast in the North of Ireland. The last week I was put to an allowance of a Quart of Water per diem and Salt Meat, which much enhanced the pleasure of the Irish Shore."[168] Following his dreadful experience at sea, he was tired of that means of transportation, and explained that "to avoid the pleasure of sailing more I took horse to Dublin about 120 miles from Belfast" and then continued on to London.

Shippen continued his letter by declaring that "I find the ways of Vice and Wickedness as many and as various as I expected, but can with pleasure and without boasting say, I find very little Difficulty shunning them" because he would just work and study hard and have no time for follies, and that would only require "a little Resolution and a constant call to more necessary Business." He also expressed that he would be helped by the fact that "Dr Hunter's anatomical lectures begin at the same time, and I hope I shall always have the good sense to make Pleasure give way to Business." In order to further reassure his uncle, Shippen added, "I do not spend [time] trifling about Play Houses, Operas, reading idle romantic Tales or trifling Newspapers at Coffee Houses, &c, &c, as I find many have done before me." Instead, he would use the time to learn "Surgery and Anatomy." As we will see, Shippen did not always live up to his promises.

Finally, in his letter, Shippen addressed the issue of frugality: "Your instructing lessons upon the frugal use of Time and Money are always in my mind and influence my conduct much.... My Money I think I spend very cautiously, yet as you observed, it melts faster than I imagined."

Before departing for London, William had met with his uncle, and received warnings about scoundrels that he might encounter in the big city. In a Nota Bene, added after he had signed the March 1759, letter, Shippen commented: "I find as many fools in England as America, and your remarks are all just."

The Diary

During a six-month period, starting on July 19, 1759, Shippen kept a diary with almost daily entries. Although the notes were short and to the point, "stripped down to the bare bone of fact, as if, unconsciously, he had transferred the techniques acquired in the anatomy laboratory to his task of writing, and had made his record a clean-cut dissection of events," they tell the story of a disciplined medical student with good work ethic. They also give examples of an interesting and expanding social life, and reveal pleasures and interactions with a growing circle of friends. The diary had been buried under layers of dust in an attic for almost two hundred years before relatives working on Shippen's medical library found it by chance.

When the diary starts, Shippen had already been in London for more than half a year. He remained awestruck by the size of the city, at the time having a population of almost seven hundred thousand (compared with less than forty thousand in his hometown), and commented that he had been in the big city for several months but still had "not seen the half of it."[169]

The first three months covered by the diary were spent at St. Thomas' Hospital, although Shippen also interacted with physicians and surgeons and fellow trainees at Guy's Hospital across the street from St. Thomas'. During this period, Shippen lived in a boardinghouse close to the hospital, together with other students.

Shippen was an early riser. Many of the daily entries in the diary start with "rose at 7 breakfasted at 8 and went to Hospital at 91/2." If he overslept, he felt guilty: "Rose at 8 being lazy."[170]

The weeks at St. Thomas' were structured around Tuesdays and Thursdays. Tuesday was "Physician's Day" and Thursday was "Taking in Day" (when new patients were admitted to the hospital). St. Thomas' was a busy place, and a robust number of patients were admitted each Taking in Day. For example, on Thursday, July 26, "Dr. Milner took in the

Patients being 49," and on Thursday, August 9, "57 were taken in by Dr. Reeve, and Mr Baker." On Saturdays, the physicians and surgeons made what would be called teaching rounds today. Seeing patients on the floors and discussing their diagnoses and treatments provided valuable learning opportunities for Shippen and his fellow students.

The time at St. Thomas' offered Shippen a vast clinical experience. Like today's surgical residents, Shippen initially learned from observing and assisting surgeons, and was then given increasing responsibilities and independence. He took notes of all "remarkable cases and prescriptions." On Tuesdays, Physician's Days, the trainees attended the physicians and surgeons in their outpatient clinics. On one Tuesday in July, Shippen "attended Drs. Reeves and Akenside in their Examinations and Prescriptions of all the Patients in St. Thomas, which lasted till 1." Other days, he observed surgical procedures, frequently amputations, for example, when "Mr. Paul took off a mans [*sic*] leg very elegantly," or when the same surgeon on another occasion took "off a man's leg that was mashed to pieces between 2 carts."[171] On August 4, Shippen observed "Mr. Way surgeon to Guy's Hospital amputate a leg above knee very dexterously 3 ligatures...."

In those days, surgeons were true general surgeons, mastering a wide variety of procedures. In addition to "taking off" legs, they also performed eye procedures. Shippen described how he "saw Mr Way and Paul couch 2 men in old way by depression," the old-fashioned way of treating cataract, by pushing the opaque lens to the bottom of the eyeball and out of the line of vision. More up-to-date surgeons had abandoned couching for the extraction operation, where the lens was instead removed through a small incision made in the cornea, a method described by the French surgeon Jacques Daviel in 1745 (and discussed earlier in the book). Other experiences that must have been exciting were when Shippen "saw Mr. Baker perform 3 operations, a leg, Breast & Tumor from Girl's lower Jaw inside, very well operated," and on the same day, "Mr. Warner extracted a large Stone from Urethra of a man and pinn'd the incision up as a Harelip." Cutting for the stone (removal of bladder stones) was a common operation in the 1700s, which Shippen had opportunities to observe and assist in.

Considering Shippen's future interest in obstetrics, his experiences in London were particularly useful. "Male midwifery" was controversial. Untrained midwives handled most deliveries, and it seems Shippen was given more independence in this field than in other aspects of medical and surgical care. He was, however, supervised by Dr. Colin Mackenzie in these endeavors. Along with Doctors William Smellie and William Hunter, Mackenzie was a well-known pioneer in the field of male midwifery. It is possible that the "real surgeons" at St. Thomas' Hospital considered deliveries below their dignity, and therefore let trainees handle many of these cases more or less on their own.

On several occasions, Shippen was called to attend women in labor. On Monday, August 13, he was awakened at seven and asked to attend his barber's maid who was in labor, "continued with her till 2oClock, when I delivered her of a Daughter."[172] A couple of weeks later, Shippen "rose at 6 to a Labour which lasted till night." After resting a couple of hours in his own living quarter, he returned to the woman and "spent afternoon and Evening till 5 in morning at Labour."

In the 1700s, London was a city with high crime rates and violence. People were injured or killed during fights and robberies in the streets. This resulted in traumatized and dead patients arriving at the doorsteps of the hospitals. On Saturday, July 28, Shippen saw a patient with a "fractured skull." Only two days later, Shippen spent two hours performing an autopsy of a man who had "died suddenly, his os humeri [upper arm bone] was broke...."

Smallpox was also a constant threat in London, as it was in the colonies. In 1759, the number of deaths from smallpox in London was about 2,600.[173] The high mortality rate from the disease is illustrated by the diary entry on September 5: "Examined particulars in Hospital several small pox 3 out of 4 die...."[174]

Attending Hunter's Anatomical School

On October 1st, Shippen packed his belongings and moved to John Hunter's house at the Great Piazza, Covent Garden. This was the place where Hunter gave his famous lectures in anatomy, performed dissections of human cadavers, and was creating a huge collection of anatomical and pathological specimens that served as teaching objects.

Covent Garden had been an area of the rich and famous during the 1600s. Early in the 1700s, however, the character of Covent Garden changed, as the nobility and gentry started to move to the west side of London with its new glitzy districts. This led to a Covent Garden mainly inhabited by vendors and bohemians. The area had started to be occupied by businesses of less reputable character, such as taverns, ale houses, supper clubs, gaming houses, and "bathing houses," a common cover name for brothels.[175]

As a result of these changes, property prices started to decline around Covent Garden. This was a reason why the Hunter brothers could afford to buy a house at the Great Piazza in 1749. It was a big house, reminiscent of the golden age of the past, and fitting for an anatomical school; the rooms were large enough for laboratories and spaces for dissections, and the upstairs was used to board the medical students.

Even though Shippen and his fellow students lived in the second floor, they were treated as members of the anatomist's household. During the "autumn course," beginning in early October, Shippen had to get used to a strict schedule with days starting at six or seven, long hours of lectures and dissections, and the days often not ending until nine or ten.

The schedule at the Hunter's Anatomical School was intensive, with daily (and day long) dissections and injections, followed by Hunter's lectures between five and seven-thirty. In the evening, there was time for dinner, reading of medical texts, and, sometimes, continued discussions of anatomical issues with the Master.

John Hunter was energetic and enthusiastic, and had a seemingly unquenchable thirst for new knowledge. He differed from his elder brother William, who was more cautious and less expressive. John set a good example for the students with his tireless activities, and was always generous with his time. On October 16, Shippen wrote, "Dissected till 5 Lecture till 7 ½. Chatted till 10 with Mr Hunter upon anatomical points bedded at 10 ½."[176]

Most of the bodies used for dissection were those of criminals and poor people, who had either died from natural causes or had been executed. Among the general population, there was always the suspicion that bodies dissected at the anatomical schools had been illegally obtained by grave robbery. The cadavers were used to learn gross anatomy, such as the anatomy of muscles, bones, brain, and abdominal organs. The corpses were also used to practice surgical operations, and to perform "anatomical injections" (injection of blood vessels with colored substances to visualize the vasculature of different organs).

Leisure Time and Pleasures

Although Shippen was a devoted and disciplined student during his time in London, his life was not only lectures, studies, operations, and dissections; there was also room for a social life. Even if Shippen had reassured his uncle in Lancaster that he would "always have the good sense to make Pleasure give way to Business" and be able to "shun the ways of Vice and Wickedness,"[177] Shippen did allow himself to participate in a robust social life and some escapades, as well.

He had frequent dinners with friends, and sometimes described elaborate and delicate menus. For example, on July 30, he had "Lobsters for supper" (although lobster may still have been considered a poor man's food in the 1700s). On August 14, he enjoyed "roasted Lamb and french [*sic*] Beans," and four days later, he was "dining with Mr. Mrs. & Miss Huthwaite upon Veal and Ham, Ducks etc very elegant."

Dancing parties were also popular. Some of Shippen's diary entries suggest that the parties sometimes lasted into the wee hours. During these occasions, Shippen kept his eyes open for beautiful women, and often offered his assessments of them. For example, on August 6, Shippen spent "the Evening at the Assembly, where we had 30 brilliant Ladies...."[178] A couple of weeks later, Shippen attended "the Fair [regularly held late in August]...in Company 15, amongst the rest was Miss Watson a very pretty young Lady mere Beauty, Miss Sweet, Still Huthwaite, Matt. etc etc; Mr. L played upon Flute Miss Jeffreys and I sung [*sic*]. We danced all minutes and in short spent the afternoon as merrily as you please." On Monday, September 10, Shippen "went to a dance in the Borrough and danced with Miss S. Church a very pretty soft agreable [*sic*] Girl. We were very merry till 3 next morning. Went to bed at 5 slept till 1 oClock Tuesday afternoon." Three days later, it was time to party again: "Danced in the Evening with Miss Huthwaite and Miss Spencer, till 12, then retired home much pleased; and slept till 8 oClock." He ended the note with a laconic statement, "40 Ladies."

On September 5, Shippen "Dressed in the afternoon for Camberwell Assembly where were 40 young Ladies most of them pretty and genteel...I danced with Miss Jeffery of Peckham, went to bed...about 4 slep't till 9." On December 18, after dissecting human cadavers the whole day and attending a lecture that started at four, Shippen "went to a Ball in City... danced with Miss Knox an agreable [*sic*] Lady and good Dancer. 35 Ladies genteely dress'd etc. Bed at 2."

Coffeehouses had been around since the mid-1600s, and were still popular a century later.[179] They were places where people could not only enjoy a good cup of coffee, but could also read newspapers, meet with friends, and gossip. Unlike alehouses, no alcohol was served at the coffee houses (although there were exceptions). The coffeehouses also functioned as post offices, where letters and packets were received or dispatched. Letters between London and Philadelphia took seven to eight weeks. A couple of diary entries reflect Shippen's use of coffee houses as a post office. On Friday, August 10, he wrote: "Spent the Forenoon and afternoon at my own appartment [*sic*] writing Letters Home and examining my Hospital Book. In the evening carried my Letters to the coffee house." It was always exciting to receive something from back home. On October 13, he "Went to coffee H. where to my great Joy, I found a Pacquet [*sic*] from Philadelphia." Unfortunately, he did not let us know what was in the packet.

Attending Church

To balance the life of studies, lectures, surgeries, and dissections—and parties—Shippen spent Sundays more peacefully. He attended church, sometimes both in the morning and evening. The Tabernacle, where dissenting preachers taught the doctrine of Calvinism, was Shippen's spiritual home. Reverend George Whitefield headed the Tabernacle. Whitefield was no stranger to Shippen. The preacher had visited the colonies on several occasions to conduct preaching tours along the East Coast, and to help raise funds for various charities, including an orphanage in Georgia.[180] His preaching tours resulted in an awakening that swept the colonies (and also generated many controversies). When Whitefield visited Philadelphia in 1740 (Shippen was only four at the time), he drew such large crowds to his sermons that a special building, "one hundred feet long and seventy feet broad, about the size of Westminster Hall," had to be constructed at Fourth Street. Benjamin Franklin's financial support was needed for the building. Franklin was a great admirer of Whitefield, not only for his "integrity, disinterestedness and indefatigable zeal in prosecuting every good work," but also for his imposing presence and strong voice: "This preacher with his outdoor sermons could reach without vocal strain the ears of 30,000 listeners."[181]

During his travels to America, Whitefield had become a close friend to the Shippen family, which gave him the opportunity to observe William grow up and mature into a good-looking, academically successful young man. Curiously, their paths crossed again in 1754 at the commencement exercises of the College of New Jersey. On that occasion, Whitefield was a distinguished guest, and received an honorary MA degree. Shippen graduated at the same time, and was the class valedictorian. He delivered his valedictory in Latin in a way that prompted Whitefield to publicly declare that "he had never heard better speaking," and he compared Shippen to the Roman orators.[182]

In London, it was natural for Shippen to continue his family's custom of attending church on Sundays, and it was a given that he would do so at Whitefield's Tabernacle. Unfortunately, during most of the summer of 1759, Whitefield was away from London, preaching in Scotland. Shippen, therefore, had to make do with substitutes, some of whom he felt less favorable about. For example, on one Sunday evening, when summarizing the events of the day, he complained about the morning service at which he had "heard Mr Stevens preach or rather Grunt. Miserable!" A couple of weeks later, Shippen again had critical comments about a preacher: "Afternoon Mr. Condor a scholar and bad preacher." Nevertheless, Shippen continued to attend services at the Tabernacle, and was able to have dinner with Reverend Whitefield on a couple of occasions after the preacher's return from Scotland.

Frequent Theater Visits

On October 2, Shippen's first day at Hunters Anatomical School, he wrote in his diary that after "Dr. Hunter's Lecture at 5 till 7½ went to the Play to see Tom [the Irish actor Thomas King] in Conscious Lovers…."[183] This was the first in a string of sixteen performances Shippen attended during the four-month period from October to January. He averaged at least one performance per week, and attended two performances some weeks.

Shippen's diary leaves no doubt that he enjoyed the distractions at the playhouse greatly. Because Hunter delivered his lectures between five and seven-thirty p.m., Shippen sometimes missed the first of the evening's two plays (which also meant he was able to get a cheaper ticket). Other days, Shippen skipped the lecture and saw the entire show.

Shippen was not the only student who enjoyed the theater. Because increasing numbers of theater-hungry students played truant from Hunter's lectures, empty seats in the lecture room became a source of concern (and irritation) for Hunter, who was ultimately forced to change his lectures from five to two o'clock.

Theater was an entertainment that was growing in popularity, although only a small minority of Londoners could afford to see plays and had the cultural inclination to attend. That several theaters were located close to Covent Garden, of course, increased the lure for Shippen and his fellow students to skip lectures and go see plays. At the time Shippen attended the anatomical school, the greatest star on the theater scene was the actor David Garrick (who was also Shippen's favorite). The theaters put on both comedies and tragedies, but Londoners were particularly fond of comedies. Garrick was good at both, and one critic gave the following assessment: "A master of both comedy and tragedy, though I liked him most in comedy."

The popularity of the theaters (and other "sinful" activities in the area around Covent Garden) concerned the clergy. Late in 1759, Reverend Whitefield spoke out against theater-going, which he felt "stirred a nest of hornets." Whitefield's preaching created controversy, and was ridiculed in a play entitled *The Minor*. In the play, Whitefield was caricatured as "Dr. Squintum," and other preachers were mocked with names like Shift and Smirk.

Interestingly, Whitefield's view of the theater did not decrease Shippen's interest in the plays, and he continued to see performances almost every week. Whitefield's role as a moral guide in Shippen's life seemed to diminish with Shippen's growing interest in theater and other Covent Garden activities.

Americans visiting the motherland always seemed to attract special interest, and individuals from the colonies were popular. Shippen probably enjoyed the attention. Corner commented in her book, "As a young man Shippen evidently attracted attention in England with his handsome chiseled feature…. Even the gruff Mark Akenside, disliked and caricatured for bearish ways with patients and colleagues, became 'kind and judicious' on rounds with William Shippen at St Thomas's. In compliment to the young man's easy social grace his company was much sought."

The attention that Shippen probably enjoyed the most was that of Benjamin Franklin, the best-known American in Europe at the time. On two occasions, Shippen got to experience something that only the most privileged had a chance to do. On January 3, Franklin invited Shippen to accompany him to the Royal Society, and although "no papers of special interest" were given that evening, Shippen must have realized how lucky he was to be able to attend such an illustrious organization, already a century old when Shippen visited.

Even more remarkable was Franklin's invitation to join him for a visit to the court so he could see the Royal family. After the amazing experience, Franklin took young Shippen out on the town. Shippen noted in his dairy that the partying "lasted till 2," and although he did not give any other details, he finished the entry in the diary by adding "lost my Hat and…."

1759: An "Annus Mirabilis" in England

Shippen had picked a good year for his stay in London. 1759 was a time of victories and celebrations. After years of setbacks in the Seven Years' War (the French and Indian War on the American continent), England finally enjoyed several important victories (although the war would continue for another four years). The British were hungry for some uplifting celebrations and, indeed, "London church bells were ringing almost constantly that summer of 1759 to celebrate English victories." Cities and towns were illuminated, and even though Shippen thought the illuminations he saw in London were "paltry" compared with what he had seen in Philadelphia, others were quite impressed: "Every house is illuminated, every street has two bonfires, every bonfire has two hundred squibs, and the poor charming moon yonder that never looked so well in her life is not at all minded, but seems only staring out of a great window at the frantic doings all over town."[184]

A particularly important victory was the British capture of Quebec. The Capital of the French empire in North America fell to the English on September 13, 1759. The news reached London on October 16, and was made public the following day in the *London Gazette*.[185] On that day, Shippen had probably not yet heard about the news. He reported in his diary on Wednesday, October 17, "Rose at 7 dissected till 5...." On the next day, however, he commented, "Pleased with the news of taking Quebec Illuminations etc." Then, of course, back to business as usual, and he continued the day's entry in his diary, "Dissected till 9. Went to the Hospital at 10 till 1 to College of Physicians at 2 to hear Dr. Akenside's Oration on the immortal Harvey, very entertaining. Lecture at 5 till 7½. Bed at 10."

The year of 1759 was referred to as "the glorious and ever-memorable year" in the press. Others called it the "ever-warm and victorious year" because even the weather seemed to be celebrating: "One would think we had plundered East and West Indies of sunshine. Our bells are worn threadbare with ringing for victories."

Going to Edinburgh

Having finished both the autumn and spring courses at the Hunter's Anatomical School, it was time for Shippen to move on to Edinburgh. Although established only thirty-four years earlier, the Medical School at Edinburgh had already gained a reputation of being a center of the highest academic quality for medical education. The combined experience in London and Edinburgh was a common model used by young American physicians and surgeons. Whereas the time in London provided "hands on" training, which included taking care of patients at St. Thomas' and other hospitals, and dissecting human cadavers with the Hunter brothers, the education at Edinburgh was more academic and theoretical, and provided an MD degree for successful students. London physician John Fothergill recommended splitting the time between London and Edinburgh, and this was adhered to by many surgeons who later became involved in the American Revolution, including John Morgan and Benjamin Rush. Shippen arrived in Edinburgh in the early summer of 1760.

He was eagerly looking forward to lectures given by such prominent teachers as William Cullen and the Monros. William Cullen (1710–1790) was one of the most revered lecturers at the medical school. He was a proliferative author, and had published several authoritative textbooks. He became an influential character in the lives of Shippen, Morgan, Rush, and many other surgeons in training. Cullen was also a standard-bearer of the Scottish Enlightenment.

Alexander Monro primus (1697–1767) and his son, Alexander secundus (1733–1817), were members of a remarkable lineage of physicians and surgeon–anatomists. Secundus may have been an even more outstanding anatomist than his father, and has several anatomical structures named after him, such as the "foramen Monro" (a connection between the third and lateral ventricles in the brain).

With famous people like these teaching at the medical school, it is not surprising that Shippen was excited upon his Edinburgh arrival. He would spend fifteen months there, immersed in academia and working diligently on his doctoral thesis. The hard work paid off with an MD degree in September 1761. Although most of Shippen's time in Edinburgh was devoted to theoretical learning, he also participated in some animal experiments and human dissections. After all, he had just spent one-and-a-half years with the Hunter brothers at their Anatomical School in London and could, based on that, easily claim a spot at the dissection table.

At the time, dissections of cadavers were quite controversial in Scotland. Since the early 1700s, rumors flourished among people and in the press about illegal activities surrounding the procurement of bodies to be "anatomized." Grave robberies, and even murders, for the purpose of making money on corpses, made for good, scary stories.

Executed criminals were an important source of cadavers in Edinburgh, as in London. A couple of decades before Shippen arrived at Edinburgh, a gruesome story circulated in the local press. "The body dissected was that of David Myles, who had been convicted of incest with his sister; she was also hanged for killing the infant subsequently produced."[186] The costs associated with the procurement of the body were also documented in the report: "Incidental expenses incurred by the Incorporation [of Surgeons and Barbers of Edinburgh] includes £18s 6d 'to ye officers & trone men for carrying David Mylle's corps', and 9s 6d for weights for weighting the body."

Shippen must have been keenly aware of the shady business surrounding the human dissections. The rumors swirling around the activities made the profession concerned about its reputation, and in 1725, a disclaimer was published in one of Edinburgh's newspapers: "The Incorporation of Surgeons considering, that several malicious and evil-disposed persons, have industriously raised and spread calumnious Reports, importing, That the Bodies of the Dead have been by them or their apprentices, raised from their graves, to be dissected…. Which reports have met with such great credit among credulous and unthinking people; in so much that they created uneasiness in their minds; and of late have been artfully improven by factious designing men, into Tumults and disturbances in the City. Therefore the Incorporation…Enact, that each apprentice who should be convicted of raising or attempting to raise the Dead from their Graves, should forfeit their freedom and all Privilege competent to them by their indentures, and be extruded their master's service."[187]

An even more-publicized scandal related to illegal procurement of cadavers was still about seventy years in the future. In 1828, sixteen people were murdered in Edinburgh by two accomplices, William Burke and William Hare, who sold the bodies to the famous Scottish anatomist and physician Robert Knox for dissections at his anatomy lectures.[188] Although Knox claimed he did not know how the corpses had been obtained, few believed in his innocence.

Shippen's Doctoral Thesis

Shippen's doctoral thesis[189] was, to a large extent, based on experiments and dissections accomplished in London by the Hunter brothers and

Colin Mackenzie. The writing of the thesis was supervised by the Monros. The thesis, *"De Placentae cum utero nexus"* ("On the connection of the placenta with the uterus") was a twenty-seven page document written in "flowing Latin." It was dedicated to a group of "Skillful physicians of the Pennsylvania Hospital...and to the best of fathers, WILLIAM SHIPPEN, a most expert physician of the same Hospital."[190] Shippen also dedicated a copy to Benjamin Franklin, a copy that ultimately ended up in the Library of the American Philosophical Society.

The doctoral thesis reflected Shippen's interest in obstetrics. It addressed two specific questions:

1) What is the relationship between the blood circulation of the fetus and that of the mother?
2) How does the fetus receive its nourishment from the mother?

At the time, there was disagreement among anatomists about the relationship between the blood circulation of the fetus and that of the mother. One school of observers believed that the circulation of the fetus and mother were directly connected by "anastomoses" in the placenta, providing a "continuous passage between mother and fetus" with "the blood propelled by the vital power of the mother into placental veins." In contrast, others held the opinion that the blood circulation of the fetus and mother represented two systems separated by a membrane that "infolds itself between the lobules of the placenta just as the pia mater enwraps the lobes of the brain."

In his thesis, Shippen described a number of observations and experiments that he argued "have finally shown beyond doubt that the uterine and placental vessels are not continuous with one another." One of the observations supporting his view was that, when the umbilical cord was cut, there was no continuous flow of blood "from the cut end of the umbilical cord as long as the placenta remained attached to the uterus. On the contrary...we never observe the loss of more blood than is contained in the cord."

Another observation Shippen claimed supported his thesis was the discrepancy in size between the blood vessels of the uterus, "so widely patent during pregnancy that a goose quill can be inserted into them,"[191] and the size of the blood vessels in the placenta being "one-twelfth of an inch—in fact the difference between them is even greater—by what mathematical rule, I ask can the tube...¼ inch in diameter, be continuous with the tube being so much smaller?" He went on to ask, "Who will say this can be done?" At this point, Shippen felt convinced he had "refuted...all the arguments used to support the hypothesis that the arteries of the uterus are continuous with the veins of the placenta."

Shippen then went on to describe what seemed to have been the only experiment he performed himself during his thesis work. He "bled a pregnant bitch to death" and found that the vessels of the pups remained "full of blood" even after the death of their mother. He and Monro secundus, who was present during the experiment, concluded that "not a drop of blood passed [from the pups] to the mother," proving that the blood vessels of the placenta were not directly connected with those of the mother.

Less than a fifth of the thesis was devoted to the second aim of the writing, "to consider how the fetus is nourished after the placenta becomes attached to the uterus." Without understanding the mechanism and or being able to perform experiments to prove his theory, he concluded "in all likelihood the vessels which enter the placental lobes function as absorbents and receive the part of the blood which is suitable for nourishing the fetus." It is remarkable how similar Shippen's theory was to today's understanding of the nourishment of the fetus. Although there were many facts he was not aware of, such as the diffusion of oxygen across the placenta, the transfer of certain waste products from the fetus to the mother, and hormonal and immunological functions of the placenta, it is fair to say that more than 250 years ago, Shippen's theories of the nourishment of the fetus pointed us in the right direction.

In the last paragraph of the thesis, Shippen expressed his gratitude "to the very learned professors of this most flourishing institution for their great generosity and benevolence to me." He ended by promising "as far as I am able the greatest diligence and labor in the healing art, that I may not be unworthy of them nor do harm to the sick. Finis."

What a noble ending of his treatise!

Back in London

Shippen's doctoral thesis earned him the MD degree on September 16, 1761. Perhaps tired of all the theoretical studies and his thesis writing, Shippen hurried back to London after the academic honor had been bestowed upon him. He arrived in the big city just in time to get a chance to join the crowds celebrating the coronation of England's new king, George III. Interestingly, John Morgan was also in London, and joined Shippen in the festivities. Morgan wrote in a letter to Shippen's cousin, Joseph, "Dr Shippen (who arrived from Scotland but the day before) and myself with a couple of Ladies were happy to have a good sight of the Procession...."[192]

Shippen and Morgan knew each other well. They had been schoolmates at Dr. Finley's boarding school in West Nottingham, and now they were having a good time in London. Together, they were discussing the future of medicine and surgery in the colonies, and were dreaming about establishing the first medical school on the continent. Little did they know that awaiting was a future of jealousy, bitterness, and ruined friendship.

After returning from Edinburgh, it would be another year before Shippen sailed back to the colonies. During that year, he continued to study medical practices and surgical procedures at the London hospitals. He also continued to interact with John Morgan and had time for a short visit to France in early 1762.

The most important event of the year for Shippen, however, was getting married. His bride, Alice Lee, was from Virginia but was living with cousins in London. The young couple tied the knot in April 1762. Curiously, Alice's name was not mentioned in Shippen's diary, but it is, of course, still possible that she had caught his eye at some time during the period covered by the daybook. She may have been at one of the many dancing parties as one of the "ladies genteely dress'd." On Wednesday, November 21, 1759, Shippen mentioned a lady who seemed to be special to him: "Dissected till Lecture at 5 till 7½. Spent the Evening with a young Lady."

So when Shippen returned to Philadelphia after four years of absence, he had both an MD degree and a wife.

Return to Philadelphia

Shippen's arrival in Philadelphia in May 1762 was presaged by a letter from John Fothergill, written in April of the same year to James Pemberton, the famous Philadelphian Quaker and pacifist. In the letter, Fothergill gave Pemberton heads-up about a gift to Pennsylvania Hospital that Shippen was going to bring when returning from London. The gift consisted of seven cases, containing a skeleton, a fetus, casts, and most impressively, a number of "pretty accurate Anatomical Drawings" by the Dutch artist Jan van Rymsdyk (who at the time was working with William Hunter on *The Anatomy of the Gravid Uterus*). Fothergill thought that the donation would be "a present of some intrinsick [*sic*] value" because "the knowledge of Anatomy is of exceeding great use to Practitioners in Physick and Surgery and…means of procuring Subjects [cadavers] with you are not easy."[193] Fothergill stipulated that the anatomical drawings were to be kept at the Pennsylvania Hospital, to be viewed by students of anatomy or during lecturers of the subject.

To make arrangements for the delivery of Fothergill's gift, Shippen met with the managers and treasurer of the Pennsylvania Hospital on November 8, 1762. Shippen also took the opportunity to remind the hospital executives about additional issues that Fothergill had mentioned in his letter to Pemberton. First, Fothergill had written that he "recommended it to Dr Shippen to give a Course of Anatomical Lectures…he is very well qualified for the subject & will soon be followed by an able Assistant Dr Morgan." Even more importantly, Fothergill had suggested that the two returning young surgeons, "if suitably countenanced by the Legislature will be able to erect a School of Physick." Fothergill argued that the establishment of a medical school in Philadelphia would "furnish…a better Idea of the Rudiments of…[the] Profession than they have at present on your Side of the Water."[194]

No actions were taken at this point by the managers at Pennsylvania Hospital, with regard to Fothergill's idea of creating a medical school. The managers instead got busy unpacking the seven cases gifted by Fothergill, and deposited their contents "in the North Room on Second Floor." They understood the value of the gifts, and decided to have the room locked.

When students or professors wanted to view the collection, they had to sign out the key for a fee.

Anatomical School

Meanwhile, Shippen was busy making plans for an anatomical school, similar to what he had seen in London. Three days after his initial meeting with the hospital managers, Shippen advertised in the *Pennsylvania Gazette* about the school, and explained that the lectures would be "for the advantage of young gentlemen now engaged in the study of physick [*sic*] in this and the neighboring provinces whose circumstances and connections will not admit of their going abroad for improvement to the anatomical schools in Europe."[195] Shippen explained the curriculum as being designed to "demonstrate the situation, figure and structure of all parts of the Human body...their respective uses and as far as a course of anatomy will permit their diseases with the indications and methods of cure." For surgery, Shippen promised that there would be ample opportunities to practice "all the necessary operations...performed on cadavers." Finally, the anatomical school would also provide "directions in the study and practice of midwifery," and teach about the "examination of the gravid uterus."

Tickets for the course would be sold for "five pistoles each." Pistoles were used in the colonies, where they were sometimes referred to as the "French gold louis d'or" or "French guinea." Because the colonists were not allowed to mint their own money, they had to use foreign coins. The anatomical courses were to be held in a building at the Shippen family home. Shippen's father was supportive of the endeavor, and provided both financial and practical encouragement.

The course became a success and was well attended. Curiously, one of the early students was Benjamin Rush, who, at the time, was an apprentice with Dr. Redman in Philadelphia. So, at this time, Shippen had met two colleagues, John Morgan and Benjamin Rush, who would become his worst enemies in the not-too-distant future.

Like in England and Scotland, the teaching of human anatomy, in particular when including dissections of cadavers, was quite controversial. Angry mobs stormed the building where Shippen was performing dissections; they threw stones and smashed windows. On one occasion, Shippen had to flee for his life while being bombarded with rocks and "a shower of other missiles a musket ball through the center of it."[196]

In order to quiet things down, Shippen published letters in newspapers explaining to the public what was going on at the anatomical school. He wanted to reassure the readers that "the reports of his raids on cemeteries were absolutely false and that the subjects he dissected were either suicides or criminals."

School of Midwifery

After a couple of years, the controversies surrounding the human dissections had subsided, and Shippen was now ready to move on to another project close to his heart. His interactions in London with Colin Mackenzie and William Hunter had convinced him about the need for male midwives. On January 31, 1765, Shippen announced in the *Pennsylvania Gazette,* "Doctor Shippen, Junior, Proposes to begin his first course on Midwifery as soon as a number of pupils sufficient to defray the necessary expense shall apply."[197] The course was going to be open for both sexes. He gave a description of the course that would "consist of about twenty lectures" concerning the anatomy of the female pelvis, the uterus, placenta, and the circulation and nutrition of the fetus (subjects for which he could certainly claim expertise based on his doctoral thesis in Edinburgh). To increase the appeal of the course and the hands-on experience for the students, Shippen would arrange for "a convenient lodging...of a few poor women who otherwise might suffer for want of the common necessities on those occasions." In addition to paying for the lodging, Shippen would pay the cost for making sure the women were "to be under the care of a sober, honest matron, well acquainted with lying-in women." With these arrangements, he hoped that "each of his students might handle at least one natural labour."

In his first lecture at the midwifery school, Shippen emphasized some ethical aspects for the future midwives. He wanted to improve society's view on male midwifery. He warned against being greedy and said "charge no one extravagantly, and every one in proportion to their abilities," and he also warned against "the danger of acquiring the habit of alcoholism."[198]

Shippen was now a busy man, dividing his time between the anatomical school, the school of midwifery, and a growing surgical practice. Consequently, his reputation in Philadelphia was on the rise. He was also looking forward to his friend John Morgan's return from London, and was realizing his dreams of establishing a Philadelphia medical school.

The First Medical School in America—Disappointments and Jealousy

John Morgan returned to Philadelphia in the spring of 1765. He was eagerly awaited by Shippen, who was hoping to reconnect with his old comrade, and to revisit their plans to establish a medical school in Philadelphia. Although, at the initial meetings with the board of the Pennsylvania Hospital in 1762, Shippen had mentioned the plans for a medical school as proposed by John Fothergill, the idea at that time had fallen on deaf ears.[199] Shippen seemed to accept that the plans for the first medical school in the colonies would have to be put on hold. He was hoping to reactivate the discussion with Morgan once he returned from England, allowing them to work jointly on this endeavor.[200]

Instead, upon his arrival in Philadelphia, Morgan jumped right into the plans, and made no attempts to share the undertaking with Shippen. Morgan's impressive accomplishments, memberships in various prestigious professional societies, and his polished presentation of himself and his plans for the medical school—all helped by a strong self-promoting style (at least according to Shippen)—knocked the socks off the decision-makers at the College of Philadelphia. The Board of Trustees was unanimous in its support, and appointed Morgan "Professor of the Theory and Practice of Physick" in the College. The colonies now had their first medical school.

Morgan was not slow in taking credit for the founding of America's first medical school. On the Commencement Day in May of 1765, Morgan sidelined Shippen and bragged about his own "qualifications without embarrassment."[201] To rub salt in Shippen's wound, Morgan claimed that although he and Shippen had discussed plans for an American medical school while they were both in England, they had not "recommended at all a collegiate undertaking of this kind." Although Morgan did recommend Shippen "as worthy of a professorship of anatomy," Shippen perceived this as a backhanded gesture.

Despite his bitterness, Shippen felt he had no choice but to accept the position as Professor of Anatomy and Surgery. In his acceptance letter of September 17, 1765, however, he gave the trustees an earful, explaining why he felt cheated:

> The instituting of medical schools in this country has been a favorite object of my attention for seven years past, and it is three years since I proposed the expediency and practicability of teaching medicine in all its branches in this city, in a public oration, read at the State House, introductory to my first course of Anatomy.
>
> I should have long since sought the patronage of the Trustees of the College, but waited to be joined by Dr Morgan, to whom I first communicated my plan in England, and who promised to unite with me in every scheme we might think necessary for the execution of so important a point.

Shippen then turned sarcastic and added, "I am pleased, however, to hear that you gentlemen on being applied to by Dr Morgan, have taken the plan under your protection, and have appointed that gentleman Professor of Medicine." Finally, he bit his tongue and accepted the appointment: "A professorship of Anatomy and Surgery will be gratefully accepted by, gentlemen, your most obedient and humble servant, William Shippen, Jr."[202]

In short time, the friendship between the two colleagues had been ruined, and replaced by bitterness and jealousy that would influence both during the rest of their lives.

Shippen, now thirty-three and newly appointed Professor of Anatomy and Surgery, had another decade ahead of him before the American Revolution broke out. It was ten years of relative calm, devoted to his clinical practice and what he probably enjoyed most in life: teaching anatomy and obstetrics to aspiring medical students. Shippen, who had started his own anatomical school three years earlier, had a head start in his teaching efforts at the medical school. He gave his first lecture in anatomy in November 1765. This marked an important milestone in what would become a forty-year career of teaching anatomy, surgery, and obstetrics. The influence of his time in London on his career as a lecturer was evident in a letter he wrote to William Hunter in 1765: "I am much pleased to hear you still continue to bless mankind by your very entertaining and improving lectures, to them I am indebted for the small attainments I have made in anatomy and the credit I gain in that way in the American world."

Despite disappointments and the conflict with Morgan, Shippen was an outgoing and jovial person who made friends easily (which he had already proven in London). He became a popular member of the Philadelphian socialites, enjoying good dinners, good wines, and good dancing. His open and cheerful demeanor made him a favorite doctor for many patients, and helped him build a robust and thriving practice of both surgery and obstetrics.

In the midst of continued bitterness and jealousy, Shippen and Morgan were able to develop respectful neutrality. This allowed them to be academic colleagues at the medical school and have joint appointments at the Pennsylvania Hospital. During this time, Shippen's path again crossed that of another person who would become one of his enemies. At the young age of twenty-four, Benjamin Rush was appointed Professor of Chemistry at the medical school in 1769. A decade later, he would join Morgan in the bitter quarrel between the colleagues.

The Feuds with Morgan and Rush and the Court Martial

With the start of the American Revolution, the relatively peaceful times were coming to an end. Shippen now entered a six-year period of personal upheaval. Accusations of malpractice, mismanagement of the army hospital, thefts, and corruption were flying back and forth between Shippen and Morgan. Morgan had been dismissed from the position as Surgeon-General of the Continental Army, and Shippen had replaced him. Shippen soon struggled with the same shortcomings of the Medical Department that Morgan had faced: "He had all the handicaps Morgan had to labor under—and one more, he did not like to work."[203] The feud between the colleagues exploded and ultimately led to Shippen's dismissal from the army, and his arrest and court martial in 1780. Morgan had opened his salvo in a letter to John Jay in Congress: "I do hereby charge Dr. William Shippen junr. in the service of the united States with Malpractices and Misconduct in Office."[204] By now, Morgan and Rush were expressing their disgust for Shippen together. Sensationally, Shippen was acquitted on most accounts despite strong evidence against him,[205] and he was reappointed as Surgeon-General. By now, however, Shippen was tired of the tumult and resigned from the army in 1781, only three months after his reappointment as Surgeon-General of the Army.

Rebuilding Reputation and Medical Practice

Shippen returned to his practice in Philadelphia and started to rebuild his reputation. He gradually eased back into his practice and the role as lecturer at the medical school. He reclaimed his spot in society, and again became a respected and admired member of his community.

It is amazing and almost miraculous that after what had transpired between them, the three antagonists were again able to coexist as fellow faculty members at the medical school, and as colleagues in the medical community of Philadelphia. They seemed to have been able to reach an agreement to live side-by-side without any further eruptions of animosity—although under the surface, the bitterness and jealousy most likely continued to smolder.

At this point, Shippen was again a favorite of the Philadelphian socialites. The Shippen house, where he and his family lived with parents and siblings, was known for its hospitality, lavish dinners, exclusive wines, and music with dancing that often followed dessert. With the Revolutionary War still going on, the Shippen home became a popular gathering place for such prominent Patriots as John Adams, Alexander Hamilton, and Thomas Jefferson. Washington himself was a night guest on several occasions. Being a proud member of the American Philosophical Society since 1767 helped Shippen build bridges in the society, and create important networks of support among the Philadelphian elite. Shippen was also a protégé of Washington, which may help explain why he had been exonerated at the court martial.

Shippen continued to successfully rebuild his surgical and obstetric practices. He became known as the most skillful obstetrician in Philadelphia. One reason for his success was his conservative approach. He avoided the use of forceps in deliveries unless absolutely necessary, and preached "against the dangerous and cruel use of instruments." He had learnt this conservative way to manage labors from two of his most influential teachers in London, William Hunter and Colin Mackenzie.

History has it that William Hunter used to show the students his forceps, "covered with rust from disuse." By showing the utmost restraints from using instruments during deliveries, many disastrous complications were probably avoided. On one occasion when Shippen thought he would have no chance to avoid using forceps, to his delight he found on his arrival that, "a very fine lusty fatt [*sic*] boy" had already seen the daylight. Both the mother and the doctor were relieved that the instruments had not been needed, but could remain in his pocket, "instruments, which…I have in my pocket, clapping his hands on his side, when I heard them rattle…."

Although Shippen did not leave much written material behind, there were many stories attesting to his skills as a male midwife. One of the better-known tales is that of Sally Drinker. Her mother, Elizabeth, has given us the account in her diary. When Sally was experiencing a difficult labor and could not be helped by two neighbor women, "probably experienced midwives," Shippen was sent for. He found Sally in severe pain, and that she was having "a footling labour."[206] With the two midwives still present, Sally's mother saw how the "doctor performed the safe delivery of the child by version." After a long and exhausting night, Shippen went home the next day and was pleased to note, "The little one seems hart whole…Sally sleeps sweetly this afternoon…the child put to the breast this evening."[207]

In addition to his social life and busy surgical and obstetric practices, Shippen had time for what he may have considered his favorite mission in life, teaching anatomy and obstetrics. He added to his lecture series in obstetrics "lectures on the diseases of women and children within the month and directions concerning the diet of each,"[208] subjects that were ahead of their time when Shippen introduced them.

Shippen's view on the importance of anatomical knowledge was strong. He argued that a thorough knowledge of the subject was "the foundation for all future medical training," and added, "Any medical surgical knowledge not built on this basis will be false and I would earnestly advise that no book on the theory and practice of medicine be ever put into the hands of a medical student till he be well acquainted with anatomy."[209]

The End

At the age of sixty-two, Shippen decided it was time to retire from his clinical practice.

His son had suffered ill health for several years and, tragically, died in 1798, an event that may have hastened Shippen's decision to give up his practice. When one of his favorite trainees, Casper Wistar (who later was to replace Shippen as Professor of Anatomy and Surgery), was able to take on more teaching obligations, it became possible for Shippen to fully retire, which he did in Germantown. The last decade of his life was spent in peace and tranquility, allowing him to reflect on some of his old passions in life, including religion, classic history, and Latin.

Shippen died in the summer of 1808, at the age of seventy-one. He had been sick for some time, possibly from diabetes and a skin infection reported as "anthrax." It is remarkable that he asked one of his old enemies, Dr. Rush, to attend to him on his deathbed. After returning home from seeing Shippen, Rush summarized some of his thoughts on his colleague and admitted that, although there were many traits in Shippen's character he did not like, "as a teacher of anatomy, he was eloquent, pleasing and luminous." Rush concluded, "Over his faults let charity cast a veil. He was my enemy from the time of my settlement in Philadelphia in 1769 until the day of his death July 11, 1808. He sent for me to attend him, notwithstanding, in his last illness, which I did with a sincere desire to prolong his life. Peace and joy to his soul for ever and ever."[210]

Although rivalry, jealousy, and perhaps even corruption and occasional misdeeds prevented Shippen from reaching the heights of prominence that he may have deserved, he is still remembered as one of the pioneers in American medical education and as a forerunner in the teaching of anatomy and obstetrics.

CHAPTER 6

BENJAMIN RUSH—
Healer or Killer?

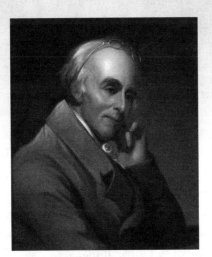

**Benjamin Rush (1745–1813). One of the best known
and highly respected physicians and surgeons
in America in the 1700s. (GL Archive)**

B enjamin Rush was born on Christmas Eve, 1745 (old style)[211] (January 4, 1746, new style[212]) into a well-to-do religious family farming a nine-acre property near Philadelphia. He was twenty-nine when the first shots of the Revolutionary War were fired at

Lexington and Concord. Although remembered for many nonsurgical achievements, Rush was also well trained in anatomy and surgery, and during his lifetime, his path crossed that of many accomplished surgeons.

The Early Years

Benjamin was the fourth of seven siblings. He became fatherless at the age of five when his father died at only thirty-nine years old. His widowed mother, Susanna, made certain that the importance of education was constantly imprinted on young Benjamin. He entered West Nottingham Academy in Maryland at age eight, and after five years he was ready for college. He had been so successful at the Academy that, upon starting college, he was admitted to the junior class. During his years in higher education, Rush developed a "love of knowledge" and excelled in his academic endeavors. He graduated from the College of New Jersey (the future Princeton University) in 1760 at the age of fourteen, making him the youngest individual to ever graduate from Princeton.

Medical and Surgical Training

Following college, Rush returned to Philadelphia and served an apprenticeship with Dr. John Redman from 1761 to 1766. The training provided a solid experience in medicine and surgery. John Morgan had completed a similar apprenticeship with Redman about a decade earlier. During his years with Redman, Rush also attended lectures in anatomy, surgery, and midwifery given by John Morgan and William Shippen Jr. at the newly founded Medical School in Philadelphia.

After completing the apprenticeship, Rush was encouraged by Redman to go to Europe for additional training. In 1766, he set sail for England and enrolled in the Medical School at the University of Edinburgh, which was considered the premier place for academic medical education in Europe at the time. During his time in Edinburgh, Rush continued to excel scholastically. Instead of participating in "the drunken orgies that marked Edinburgh night life," the Quaker Rush focused on his studies in anatomy, chemistry, mathematics, and Latin. His studiousness paid off with an MD degree in 1768. The subject of his thesis and its involved studies may sound repelling. He tested a theory about saliva, digestion, and fermentation by inducing his own vomiting. As though that was not enough, he then examined his vomits, as well as those of a friend who had participated as a "control."

In September of that year, Rush left Edinburgh for London, where he attended lectures in anatomy and human dissections. In London, Rush was introduced to many prominent members of English society who occupied medical and political positions. Benjamin Franklin supported him financially and, by letters of introduction, Rush also met with such high profile surgeons as Sir John Pringle, the court physician, and influential politicians such as John Wilkes, "an enthusiast for American liberty."

Before returning to the colonies, Rush made France the next stop of his European travel. While in Paris, he visited Versailles, and on one occasion he came close to King Louis XV. When standing in a large hall, Rush saw the king pass by on his way to mass, and Rush "stood within a few feet of him."[213] This reminded Rush of what he had heard about the corrupt life at the court and its appalling moral standards. Louis XV's appetite for women was legendary, and well accepted among the courtiers. The king had the royal privilege of picking and choosing among women, irrespective of their marital status or consent. John Wilkes told Rush "he had once dined with twelve gentlemen in Paris, eleven of whom declared it their duty to surrender their wives to the king if desired."

After the death of his mistress, Madame de Pompadour, in 1764 (four years before the death of his wife, Marie Leszczynska), the king had gone through a large number of women before ultimately casting his eyes on the twenty-year-old beauty Jeanne Bécu, who instantly bewitched him. Legend has it that when Louis XV first saw her, she was dining with one of the royal servants. Despite the servant's warnings that Jeanne was a prostitute and might have venereal diseases, the king, age fifty-eight at the time, swept her away and brought her to his chambers. In order to reduce the scandal, the king ordered Count du Barry to marry Bécu so that he could exercise his "legal" right to sleep with his vassal's bride on the wedding night. She would sleep with the king on many more nights, and in April 1769, he arranged what some critics called "a formal presentation at court of a whore from the streets of Paris and her elevation to the rank of Royal Mistress." Rush, a religious man, found this type of behavior deplorable.

Most important to Rush were his visits to the hospitals of Paris, including Hôtel de la Charité (which he found "remarkably neat and clean"), Hôtel Dieu ("crowded and offensive")[214], and his favorite hospital, the Foundling Hospital, to which abandoned babies were admitted every day. Rush commented in his journal that "the door of the hospital was always open, and a basket, made like a cradle, is placed near it into which the infant is placed. A bell is then rung to give notice to the keepers of the hospital…It is supposed that one-eighth of all children born in Paris are brought up by means of this institution."[215]

Before going back to the colonies, Rush also spent additional time in London where he bonded with Benjamin Franklin. They became lifelong friends and allies, and their relationship stimulated Rush in his development to becoming "a dedicated humanitarian."

When Rush returned to America in July 1769, almost three years after leaving the continent, he was still a young man of only twenty-three. With his prestigious degree from the University of Edinburgh, he quickly joined the ranks of the most accomplished physicians in the colonies. He seemed destined for an exceptional career. There was one problem, however. Rush had used all his funds during his tour of Europe, and was bankrupt when he again set foot on American soil.

Healing the Poor and Destitute in the Philadelphia Slums

The lack of money prevented Rush from buying a practice or establishing a partnership with other physicians. These circumstances, however, did not stop him from practicing his skills as a physician. Soon after his return to Philadelphia, Rush started making daily "rounds" in the poor quarters of the city. The poverty, filth, lack of sanitation, and destitution were appalling. They stood in stark contrast to the affluent Philadelphia with its beautiful brick houses, clean and elegant streets and squares, and well-fed, healthy-looking citizens wearing the latest fashion from London.

Early in the morning, Rush set out on his rounds and walked the streets and alleys of the poverty-stricken Philadelphia. He knocked the doors and shouted: "Doctor calling—Anyone need the doctor?"[216] What he saw stayed with him for the rest of his life. It strengthened Rush as a humanitarian to not only fight poverty, but to also fight other social injustices. When he entered homes of the poor, he was met by the stench of the filthy people. Most dwellings lacked water, and, even when water was available, people seldom bathed because they believed that bathing, particularly in warm water, caused illnesses to enter the body. Hungry, unhealthy-looking children with running noses peeked at Rush from behind their mothers. Multitudes lived with body lice and bed bugs. Contagious diseases were rampant, and outbreaks of infectious diseases were common. After long days, Rush usually came home late, exhausted and enraged by what he had seen.

Rush and the Abolition Movement

In addition to the poverty and degradation in the slums, other issues also upset Rush. Among those, slavery and slave trade were high on the list. Returning from Europe, where abolition was already getting strong support in many countries, Rush was distressed by the slavery in America.

On the way to his daily rounds in the slum, Rush often passed by the popular London Coffee House, where merchants carried out the business of slave trading over cups of coffee. This daily reminder of the institution of slavery enforced Rush's strong feelings against the subjugation of enslaved people. He joined the newly formed Pennsylvania Society for Promoting the Abolition of Slavery and the Relief of Free Negroes Unlawfully Held in Bondage. Members of the society encouraged Rush to write a pamphlet, "Address to the Inhabitants of the British Settlement in America on Slavekeeping," which was published in 1773. In it, Rush gave examples of the brutality of slavery, describing how one slave had lost "a foot as punishment for running away...another led to the gallows for eating a morsel of bread...."

Rush's pamphlet had a great impact in Pennsylvania, and resulted in a new law that imposed taxation on the sale of slaves. To Rush's happiness, the tax resulted in a sharp drop in slave trading. In some areas, including New York and Boston, the pamphlet created resentment and anger among slaveholders who thought Rush had "meddled with a controversy that was foreign to…[his] business."

Fighting Drunkenness

Poverty and drunkenness often went hand in hand, and together they were important factors in the misery and destitution of the poor. Due to his religious background, Rush despised alcoholism—but not its victims.[217] He became the first physician to label alcoholism a disease. He expanded on that theory in two publications, *Sermons to Gentlemen upon Temperance and Exercise* and *An Enquiry into the Effects of Spirituous Liquors upon the Human Body and Their Influence upon the Happiness of Society.* He argued that spirituous liquors were "the foundation of fevers, fluxes, jaundices, as well as dropsy, palsy, epilepsy, insanity, and other diseases." He continued that "spirituous liquors destroy more lives than the sword. War has in intervals of destruction—but spirits operate at all times and seasons upon human life…. Spirits…impair the memory, debilitate the understanding, and pervert the moral faculties…. They produce not only falsehood, but fraud, theft, uncleanliness, and murder…poverty and misery, crimes and infamy, diseases and death."

It is interesting that Rush limited his condemnation of "spirituous liquors" to hard liquor, and suggested that the alcohol in beer and wine was acceptable. Water, however, was first on his list of acceptable drinks, followed by "cider, malt liquor and wines," because they "inspired cheerfulness and good humor."

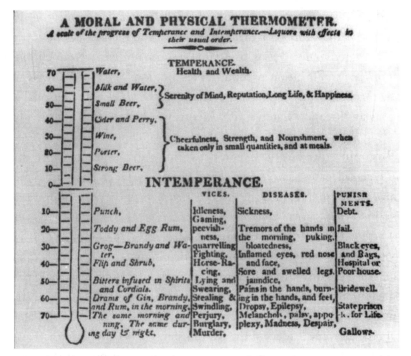

"A Moral and Physical Thermometer" from Benjamin Rush's
"An inquiry into the effects of ardent spirits upon the human
body and mind" published in 1785. (Public domain)

Cleanliness remained an important topic for Rush during his entire career. Along those lines, he became an opponent of tobacco and opined that "the use of tobacco in any way is uncleanly." As Rush explained in his essay "Observations upon the Influence of the Habitual use of Tobacco upon Health, Morals, and Property of Mankind," the risks for burn injuries and clothing and furniture stains were among the reasons he disapproved of tobacco.

Involvement in the American Revolution

As the British Parliament kept introducing new taxations on the colonies, Rush became a strong supporter of the resistance against the London government, and an early proponent of independence. When the First Continental Congress assembled in September 1774, Rush was among the

Philadelphians who eagerly welcomed the delegates. Upon meeting John Adams, he name-dropped Benjamin Franklin and mentioned their friendship. He shared many ideas with Adams, as both of them were abolitionists and opposed to "taxation without representation." His interactions with Adams resulted in a long-lasting friendship that had both personal and political significance. Later in life, Adams would turn to Rush for advice regarding the treatment of his daughter's breast cancer.

Rush proved to be effective in networking and connected with many prominent delegates to the Continental Congress. Later, he would remember how he "waited upon nearly all the members of the first Congress and entertained them at my table."

The First Continental Congress ended on October 26, 1774, with festivities and celebrations. Many Philadelphians at that time had tired of the delegates invading their city, in particular since the majority of Philadelphians were not in favor of America's potential separation from the motherland. Rush, however, continued to make friends with Patriots that would become leaders of the Revolution. He became more active and aggressive in his opinions about the British suppression of the colonies. Rush penned many of the ideas that were contained in Thomas Paine's pamphlet *Common Sense*.[218] He told Paine that he feared retribution from the Philadelphians, and suggested that Paine, who came from England, might face less criticism.

In early 1775, before the outbreak of the Revolutionary War, Rush encouraged Congress to stand up against England "with sword in hand." This was significant because, to many, it was not yet clear whether independence should be sought, in particular if it came at the price of violence. The events at Lexington and Concord on April 19, 1775, however, made it clear that war was inevitable.

On July 4, 1776, John Hancock, the President of Congress, signed the Declaration of Independence. Rush joined the Congress on July 20, and two weeks later, he added his name to what would grow to fifty-six signatures. In doing so, Rush became one of four physicians who signed the Declaration of Independence.[219] Like all signatories, he "pledged his life, fortune, and sacred honor to his province's independence from Britain." Like his fellow delegates, he understood he had committed treason against the king and would be hanged without trial if the British captured him. As a prominent physician in Congress, Rush became involved in important legislative work related to the Hospital Department, and was appointed a member of the medical committee created "to devise ways and means for supplying the continental Army with Medicines."[220]

Marriage

About a year before the Declaration of Independence was signed, Rush paid a visit to his alma mater, Princeton. There, he met with Reverend John Witherspoon, whom Rush had coaxed to leave Scotland and assume the presidency of the College of New Jersey. Rush was also invited to the home of the college trustee, Richard Stockton, and introduced to Stockton's daughter Julia.

Although Rush had met love earlier in life—his 1776 departure to England for medical and surgical training had almost been canceled because of Rush's involvement with his first love, Mary "Polly" Fisher—he was smitten by Julia. Julia was still a teenager, and known for her beauty, talents, and impressive education. Like her parents, she was a faithful Quaker. In a letter to a friend, Rush described her "brown hair, dark eyes, a complexion composed of white and red, a countenance at the same time soft and animated, a voice mild and musical, and a pronunciation accompanied with a little lisp."[221] He fell in love "from the moment [he] saw her" and was determined to pursue her heart.

His pursuits paid off. Reverend Witherspoon married them on January 11, 1776. Despite what would nowadays be considered an unacceptable view on the roles of husband and wife (Rush considered the marriage to be "the subordination of your sex to ours enforced by nature, by reason, and by revelation"), she remained his faithful wife till death parted them thirty-seven years later. Their marriage produced thirteen children, four of whom died as infants.

Military Surgeon

The battle at Trenton gave Rush his first exposure to the brutality of war and its devastating injuries. After the famous crossing of the Delaware River on the night of Christmas Day, 1776, Washington and his twenty-four hundred undisciplined and ragged men defeated fifteen hundred well-trained Hessian mercenaries, who were stationed at Trenton on the New Jersey side of the river. The attack caught the German soldiers by complete surprise. Legend has it that many of them were drunk after the Christmas celebrations, and were still in their nightclothes when the colonists awoke them. An officer in Washington's staff had written before the battle that "they make a great deal of Christmas in Germany, and no doubt the Hessians will drink a great deal of beer and have a dance tonight. They will be sleepy tomorrow morning." The hirelings rushed out in the snow to stop the Americans, but their attempts were to no avail. Although the description of the German soldiers as groggy and hungover has been questioned by some historians, Washington's victory was undoubtedly overwhelming, and badly needed after the disasters at New York. At the end of the battle, twenty-two Hessians were dead, eighty-three wounded, and more than eight hundred had been taken prisoners, including many in their underwear. The colonists suffered only two deaths from frostbite of uncovered feet, but several were wounded, including James Monroe, the future president.

When contemplating the horrific injuries at Trenton, Rush commented: "It was the first time war appeared to me in its awful plentitude of horrors. I want words to describe the anguish of my soul, excited by the cries and groans and convulsions of the men." The experience certainly differed from his rounds among the Philadelphia poor when, instead of war injuries, he had been fighting sores, infections, and running noses.

In his autobiography, Rush remembered "the first wounded man that came off the field was a New England soldier" with his right hand hanging from "above his wrist by nothing but a piece of skin. It had been broken by a cannon ball."[222] Rush started by cutting off the soldier's hand, and then performed an above-elbow amputation. He needed to amputate because both bones in the forearm, the radius and ulna, had been fractured by the projectile. When Rush used the bone saw to cut off the arm, the soldier mercifully passed out. When he woke up, the stump of his arm was wrapped with bandages torn from linen sheets and covered with a wood cap. Before the end of the day, Rush and his surgical colleagues had treated twenty additional soldiers; "... all the wounded – were dressed by

Dr. Cochran, myself, and several young surgeons who acted under our direction."[223]. True to his humanitarian philosophy, Rush rescued not only American soldiers, but cared for wounded enemy warriors as well.

Immediately following the victory at Trenton, Washington marched his soldiers to Princeton for another victory. Rush followed in the footsteps, and described in his autobiography how, when nearing Princeton, they "passed over a field of battle still red in many places with human blood. We found a number of wounded officers and soldiers belonging to both armies. Among the former...General Mercer...wounded by a bayonet in his belly in several places, but he received a stroke with a butt of a musket to the side of his head, which put an end to his life a week after the battle."

At Princeton, Rush was shocked and utterly distressed to find his father-in-law, Richard Stockton, walking along the road, distraught and in a bad condition. The British had ransacked his home and stolen his furniture, manuscripts, and all of his livestock. He was now a prisoner of war, and when Rush saw him, he was being marched up to New York City to be executed for treason. Frantically, Rush searched for someone who could help. Miraculously, Richard Henry Lee in the Continental Congress managed to get Stockton freed and returned to Princeton, thanks to connections with high-level British officials he had met while studying in England.

In April 1777, Rush was appointed Surgeon-General of the Middle Department Hospital of the Continental Army. In this capacity, Rush had a close look into the conditions of the Army Hospital—and was dismayed by what he saw. The lack of supplies, food, and the unsanitary conditions left wounded soldiers in horrific conditions. Men were dying from starvation. Infections and putrid fever (also known as "hospital fever") were rampant, killing both soldiers and surgeons. Like many others, Rush commented, "A greater proportion of men have perished with sickness in our army than have fallen by the sword."[224]

When Colonel Wayne encountered similar conditions, he described the hospitals as "a house of carnage." The hospitals were overcrowded (often with multiple wounded men in the same bed), the hygiene was inadequate (or nonexistent), and the patients and beds were infested with lice and bed bugs. Epidemics, including smallpox, were spreading like wildfires.

In order to increase the awareness of the deplorable conditions in the hospitals, Rush pleaded with influential members of Congress, and also turned directly to Washington for support, but his cries for help fell on deaf ears. To increase the pressure, Rush published a provoking pamphlet, "Directions for Preserving the Health of Soldiers" in September 1777. He described how "the gallant youth…who had plighted his life to this country in the field and…courted death from a musket or cannon ball was often forced from the scene of action and glory by the attack of fever and obliged to languish for days or weeks in a hospital."

Rush requested changes in several areas and was quite specific in his demands. He requested that the soldiers dress in thick flannel rather than linen. Not only would it provide warmth, but it would also prevent mosquito bites. He wanted soldiers to wash their hands and faces daily, and their bodies at least three times every week. He requested that soldiers keep their hair short, and comb their hair on a regular basis to get rid of lice. He talked about the risks of establishing encampments in damp surroundings, such as near swamps and marshes. He also requested that soldiers dig privies at a distance from the tents, and that they use them instead of relieving themselves around the camp.

The Feud with Shippen Jr. and the Opposition to Washington

The appointment of Shippen as Director-General of the Continental Army (succeeding John Morgan) did not make life easier for Rush. Although Shippen had been Rush's teacher in anatomy during the apprenticeship with Redman, Rush soon became an outspoken enemy of Shippen. In 1777, Rush was attacking Shippen, accusing him of "want of checks upon the lower officers of the hospital," which he implied was a reason why the patients had to suffer deplorable conditions.[225]

Shippen was a formidable enemy to take on, as he was well connected with influential members of society. Shippen's sister had married General Benedict Arnold (still considered a faithful Patriot and very much involved in the Revolution), and his wife was the sister of two powerful congressmen from Virginia, Richard Henry Lee and Francis Lightfoot Lee. Shippen's circle of acquaintances also counted other prominent leaders, including Washington himself. Despite the risks, Rush became an open and vigorous opponent of Shippen. Along with Morgan, Rush ended up playing an important role at Shippen's court martial.[226]

Because Washington had ignored Rush's complaints about Shippen's mismanagement of the Army Hospital, and Rush was disappointed in Washington's war conduct, he became involved in what is sometimes referred to as "Conway Cabal," (although some historians have expressed doubt that Rush realized that the ultimate goal of Conway and his accomplice General Horatio Gates, the "hero of Saratoga," was to have Washington overthrown as Commander-in-Chief and replaced by Gates). Washington became aware of Rush's critical view of him when he saw an unsigned letter sent to Patrick Henry and recognized Rush's handwriting. In the letter, Rush opined that "the Northern Army has shown us what Americans are cable of doing with a general at their head. The spirit of the southern army is in no ways inferior to the spirit of the northern. A Gates, a Lee, or a Conway would, in a few weeks, render them an irresistible body of men." As soon as Henry received the letter from "one of your Philadelphia friends," he handed it over to Washington. They quickly realized who "the friend in Philadelphia" was.

This was a dramatic departure from Rush's earlier assessment that Washington "has so much martial dignity in his department that you would distinguish him to be a general and a soldier from among ten thousand people. There is not a king in Europe but would not look like a valet-de-chambre by his side."[227]

When Henry forwarded the letter to Washington, he warned him that "there may possibly be some scheme or party forming to your prejudice" and pledged his allegiance to Washington: "I will not conceal anything from you by which you may be affected." Washington was grateful to Henry for informing him and replied, "I can only thank you again, in language of the most undissembled gratitude, for your friendship."

Other officials who had also become critical of Washington, and his lack of military successes, included Richard Henry Lee in the Continental Congress and General Thomas Mifflin, the quartermaster of the army. Even John Adams was concerned about Washington's ability to lead the army, but was not as active and outspoken in his judgment of Washington as others.

More Battles and Wounded Soldiers

Before the end of 1777, Rush would be exposed to more military surgery. The Battle of Brandywine resulted in 250 killed and 600 wounded on the American side, and 93 dead and 488 injured among the Redcoats. About only three weeks later, the Battle of Germantown resulted in 152 killed and 521 wounded rebels, and the British seeing 71 killed and 448 wounded. The massacre at Paoli on September 20 also took place between the two battles. More than 200 Americans were slaughtered or wounded in a surprise attack during the dark of the night (with only nine being killed or wounded on the British side).

The disastrous losses resulted in overcrowded hospitals and significant stress on Rush and other military surgeons. At Brandywine, Rush was left on the battlefield with wounded and dying soldiers all around him. He felt powerless. Once the smoke cleared, Rush saw young boys "soaked in blood, sweat and dirt" and heard combatants from both sides screaming in pain. Rush described how he "a few days later went with several surgeons into the British camp with a flag from General Washington to dress the wounded" who had been left on the field of battle: "I was introduced to a number of British officers [who]...treated me with great politeness."[228] One of the British officers expressed his gratitude to Rush for treating both American and enemy victims at Trenton.

The experience made the differences between the undisciplined, ragged, and dirty colonists, and the professional, disciplined British soldiers in their imposing red uniforms, even more obvious. Rush was again outraged. He felt the American soldiers were the same quality as the British, and blamed the lack of equipment, cleanliness, and clothing on Shippen, who had been appointed Surgeon Director–General of the Continental Army on the very same day that saw the Battle of Brandywine. In a letter to John Adams, Rush vented his frustration: "The waste, the peculation... are enough to sink our country. It is now universally said that the system was formed for the Director-General and not for the benefit of the sick and wounded.... The sick suffer, but no redress can be had for them. Upwards of one hundred of them were drunk last night. We have no guards to prevent this evil." In a second salvo to Adams, Rush wrote, "The fashion of blaming our soldiers and officers for all the disorders of our army was introduced in order to shelter the ignorance, cowardice, the idleness, and the drunkenness of our major generals."

At this point, Rush's disdain for Shippen was well cemented, and he did not spare his words or hide his opinion. Along with John Morgan, he managed to get Shippen court-martialed. However, as we have seen, Shippen was acquitted on most points, which probably reflected his connections with many powerful men.

Rush at Valley Forge

Rush was one of many surgeons and physicians who followed Washington and his army into winter camp at Valley Forge in December 1777. During the encampment, Rush continued his fight against the unclean and unsanitary conditions that wounded soldiers had to endure in the flying and general hospitals. It was also during the six months at Valley Forge that Rush got involved in the Conway Cabal.

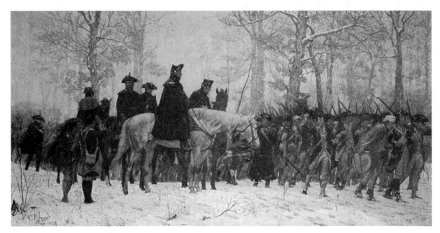

George Washington marching his troops to winter camp at Valley Forge, December, 1777. Benjamin Rush joined Washington at Valley Forge together with dozens of other Revolutionary Surgeons. (Asar Studios)

Rush, like many of his fellow Patriots, was enraged by the lack of food, clothes, and other supplies at Valley Forge. The anger grew even more intense when he realized that much of the suffering was caused by the actions of quartermaster Mifflin. Thomas Mifflin, who was a wealthy and influential merchant in Philadelphia, had reluctantly accepted the position of quartermaster for the Continental Army. He, instead, would have preferred a more active role in the army with the opportunity to gain fame and glory on the battlefield. As the quartermaster, he was charged with securing supplies to the army, a challenge that became particularly difficult at Valley Forge. Because of his inadequate—and sometimes even criminal—behavior, his performance became a fiasco and an important factor for the horrible conditions at Valley Forge.

Responding to the lack of clothing, housing material, and food as well as the real threat of starvation, Patrick Henry in Virginia confiscated wagonloads of food, clothing, and blankets from the British and directed them to Valley Forge. However, the material which had been sent to him for distribution, was stolen by the Mifflin, who put it in his own warehouses and sold the goods in surrounding towns. Like Rush, Henry was enraged and wrote about Mifflin to Richard Henry Lee at the Continental Congress: "I am really shocked at the management of Congress. Good God! Our fate committed to a man utterly unable to perform the task assigned to him!....I grieve at it."

A congressional investigation of Mifflin was conducted. When Washington confronted him with the findings, Mifflin confessed not only to the theft of supplies, but also to his role in the Conway Cabal. The revelations ultimately led to the resignations of both Mifflin and Conway.

Although Rush might not have understood the ultimate purpose of the Conway Cabal, he was found guilty in the eyes of public opinion—and importantly, in the eyes of Washington. Rush—one of the Founding Fathers!—was summoned to appear before Congress. He resigned from the army shortly thereafter.

Back in Philadelphia

In early 1778, Rush found himself out of work. He had resigned from the medical service in the army, and his medical practice in Philadelphia was not available, because the city was still occupied by the British. Rush went to live with his wife, Julia, and their young son, John, at the home of Julia's family in Princeton. He was encouraged by his father-in-law Richard Stockton (who had also signed the Declaration of Independence), to start studying law. However, when the British evacuated Philadelphia on June 18, 1778, Rush hurried back to his hometown, where he ended up spending the remaining thirty-five years of his life and career.

Back in Philadelphia, Rush found a devastated city, with filth and trash that the British army had left behind. He resumed his medical practice and again started making daily rounds in the slums of Philadelphia. His private practice started to thrive, and during the first two months of reopening his practice, he saw his patient population more than quadruple. In his autobiography, he commented that he "quickly recovered [his] business, with a large accession of new patients."

Like before the war, Rush remained upset by the horrific conditions the poor had to endure. He kept advocating for cleanliness to prevent diseases. He remarked, "The filth left by the British army in the streets created a good deal of sickness."[229]

Along with his medical practice, Rush involved himself in many other aspects of society. Although the common denominators for most of his endeavors were his humanism and religious background, winning him huge admiration among the Philadelphians, the positive opinion of Rush was not universal. One of his colleagues, Dr. Thomas Bond, felt otherwise and wrote that Rush was "capable of LYING in the WORST SENSE of that approbrious [*sic*] word" and called him "an unprincipled man."[230]

Continued Fight against Shippen

Like Morgan, Rush was infuriated by Shippen's acquittal at the court martial in 1780. In a letter to John Adams, who at this point served as an envoy in Paris, Rush wrote, "Would you have winked at…the Director General having bought six pipes of wine at £150 a pipe…and selling them upon his *own* account for £500 a piece?…. Would you have winked at the Director General being unable to produce a single voucher from the surgeons of the hospital of the expenditure of his stores and medicines? Would you have winked at bills for poultry and other delicate articles bought for the hospital which no sick man ever tasted? Would you finally have winked at false returns of…the mortality in the hospitals? No, you would not." He also vented his frustration to Adams by writing, "Our hospital affairs grow worse and worse…. The fault is both in the establishment and in the Director General. He is both ignorant and negligent of his duty."[231] To another congressman, Rush complained: "For God's sake, do not forget to take the medical system under your consideration. It is a mass of corruption and tyranny."[232]

Rush then wrote Shippen an open letter for publication in *Pennsylvania Packet*. In it, Rush did not spare his angry words: "Your reappointment, after the crimes you have committed, is a new phenomenon in the history of mankind. It will serve like a high-water mark to show posterity the degrees of corruption that marked the present stage of the American Revolution." Rush also reminded newspaper readers that Shippen's brother-in-law, Benedict Arnold, had recently committed treason and defected to the British. He accused Shippen of "selling large quantities" of wine and sugar from the hospital stores and pocketing the proceeds for himself.

The pressure ultimately became too strong even for the well-connected Shippen. He resigned from his position as Surgeon-General of the Army on January 3, 1781.

Rush the Do-Gooder

After taking care of the Shippen issue, Rush carried on with many of the humanistic causes he had supported before the revolution. He continued to be a strong spokesman against slavery, and was elected president of the Abolition Society in 1803. His contempt for slavery, however, had been expressed much earlier. In as early as 1773, he published *An Address to the Inhabitants of the British Settlements in America upon Slave-Keeping.*

Rush kept preaching against the evils of drunkenness, and proclaimed "spirituous liquors destroy more lives than the sword."[233] In 1790, he published *An Inquiry into the Effects of Spirituous Liquors on the Human Body and the Mind*, which became a bestseller, with more than 170,000 copies sold among the Quakers alone.

Rush continued to be appalled by the cruel treatment of prisoners, and wanted to put an end to death penalty for noncapital crimes. He was against public punishments that he considered demeaning and nonproductive. He proposed establishing houses of worship in each prison, and also advocated for gardens and workshops to give the prisoners a chance to learn vocations before they were released. He argued that the purpose of jail time was not only punishment, but should also provide a chance for repentance and rehabilitation.

In his outrage over the conditions in the prisons, Rush reported that "boys and girls, men and women [were] crowded together in dark, filthy, unlit, unheated cells, without means to avoid fouling themselves and their surroundings."[234] Rush described how jailers often robbed the inmates of their clothes and other belongings, and abused them mentally, physically, and sexually. To further his fight for better conditions in the prisons, Rush joined the Philadelphia Society for Alleviating the Miseries of Public Prisons.

Rush's fight for society's poor and sick was constant. With the financial support of Benjamin Franklin, Rush opened the Philadelphia Dispensary for the Poor, the first free clinic in America, where he and a colleague saw patients for a couple of hours, three days a week. More than 7,000 patients were treated free of charge during the first five years at the clinic. Medicine was provided to patients at Rush's own expense.

At a time when public free schooling was only legislated in Massachusetts and Connecticut, Rush also called for the establishment of "free schools in every township or district consisting of one hundred families…. Let children be taught to read and write!"[235] Rush's call for free public schools was radical for the time, and was met with skepticism and even open resistance by some segments of society. The controversy grew even greater when Rush had the audacity to propose that the schools should not only be open for boys, but for girls as well.

Higher education was also close to Rush's heart. He helped found the Dickinson College in Carlisle, Pennsylvania, and the Franklin College (named in honor of Benjamin Franklin) in Lancaster, outside Philadelphia.

Rush, the Medical Educator

Six years after returning to Philadelphia, Rush was appointed surgeon at the Pennsylvania Hospital, a position he occupied until his death. During more than three decades of faithful devotion to academia and the care of his patients, Rush gained increasing admiration, and became one of the best-known physicians on the continent. He also gained international fame, and was elected to membership in many prestigious societies, including the Royal Swedish Academy of Sciences in 1794.

In 1789, Rush was appointed Professor of Medicine at the College of Philadelphia. Two years later, the college merged with the University of the State of Pennsylvania to become the University of Pennsylvania, and in 1792, Rush was named Professor of Medicine at the Medical School of the University of Pennsylvania. Rush's academic endeavors were extensive and included lectures, publications of scientific reports, and, importantly, textbooks that would become enormously influential in years to come. Particularly important were the four-volume *Medical Inquiries and Observations* that became part of the curriculum for thousands of medical students and young physicians-in-training for decades to come.

In his teaching, Rush emphasized the importance of combining book studies and bedside training. He insisted that "diseases are much more instructing than books; as well might a man attempt to swim by reading as practice medicine from books…. The good physician…combines observation and reasoning."

Rush was a popular lecturer and taught and trained more than three thousand students and young physicians over the next two decades. His academic achievements and large medical practice helped his reputation grow. At the time, it was generally agreed that he was the "greatest physician" in the land.

True to his values, Rush emphasized many moral aspects of the physician's profession in his teaching. He counseled future doctors to "never give up hope" and pointed out that "many patients have recovered, who have been pronounced incurable, to the great disgrace of our profession." He also emphasized the importance of continued study and research throughout one's medical career. Rush lectured on the importance of always putting the patients' interests first. He taught future doctors not to become greedy, or demand excessive fees. He instead encouraged humility and simplicity "in your manners, dress and general conduct." Rush detested a haughty attitude and called the pompous manners of some physicians, evidence of "little minds."

Astonishingly, Rush had to tell his students to avoid drinking while on duty. In a February 7, 1789 lecture at the University of Pennsylvania, entitled "Observations on the Duties of a Physician and the Methods of Improving Medicine, Accommodated to the Present State of Society and Manners in the United States," he said, "Let me charge you to lay an early restraint upon yourselves.... Many physicians have been innocently led by it into drunkenness. You will be in the more danger of falling into this vice from the great fatigue...to which you will be exposed.... But...strong drink affords only a temporary relief from those evils."

During his further career, Rush had several interactions with friends in the American Revolution. We have already seen how Rush became an important advisor to Nabby Adams, and her parents John and Abigail, when she developed breast cancer. It was mainly Rush's advice that convinced Nabby to consent to her mastectomy.[236]

Even before Nabby's illness, Rush was involved in the health care of the Adams's family. In 1792, while residing in Philadelphia with her Vice President husband, Abigail fell ill with "fever and rheumatism." Rush applied the remedy that he trusted the most, and bled Abigail of large volumes, a treatment that probably felt worse than the underlying illness. She grumbled, "I have scarcely any flesh left in comparison to what I was." It was not until she was able to move back to her house in Braintree, Massachusetts, and avoid Rush's bleedings, that she started to feel well again.

When the "Hero of Saratoga," Horatio Gates, complained at one point to Rush about aches and pain that caused him agony at a high age, Rush told Gates that "old age has no cure." Rush advised Gates to improve his symptoms by taking "a warm bath three times a week or daily…a clove of garlic every morning and evening" and "go to bed early."

Rush's old friend, Thomas Jefferson, also had a great interest in medicine throughout his life. Although he was a lawyer by profession and became engulfed in politics later in life, he read medical books throughout his days and was often involved in discussions and exchanges of opinions with physicians. He was a driving force behind the Schools of Medicine at the College of William and Mary and at the University of Virginia. So when he opined to Rush on several occasions that he did not always believe in doctors and their medicine, Jefferson had some credentials. He used strong words and expressed the opinion that doctors "destroy more of human life in one year than all the Robin Hoods…do in a century" and argued that "the patients…sometimes gets well in spite of the medicine."[237] Jefferson argued that scientists would one day find cures to many diseases, but until then the physicians should stop their "experiments on those who put their lives into hands [of the doctors]."[238] Such strong words about physicians!

One type of treatment that supported Jefferson's view of the medical profession was related to the old theory that diseases were caused by an imbalance between the fluids of the body. This theory was still prevailing in the medical community, and would continue to do so for another century. For thousands of years, physicians had observed that inflammation was associated with redness as a sign of increased blood flow. With those observations in mind, it is not surprising that bloodletting was used as a remedy for many (if not most) illnesses. Purging induced by drugs that also caused diarrhea and vomiting was believed to help further restore the fluid balance in the body. This was part of the armamentarium used by physicians since ancient times, and it certainly remained popular during the 1700s. Although Jefferson seemed to believe that an imbalance between body fluids did play a role in illnesses, he felt that nature should be allowed to restore the balance, rather than having physicians give medicines that accomplished the same effect. Jefferson explained "nature… was the controlling force in human maladies" that could reestablish a balance "by exciting some salutary evacuation of the morbific matter." He further argued that nature "brings on a crisis, by stools, vomiting, sweat, urine, expectoration, bleeding, &c., which, for the most part, ends in the restoration of healthy action." What Jefferson did not agree with was physicians intervening and causing diarrhea, vomiting, sweating, and blood loss.

Rush, on the other hand, was a strong believer in all those treatments, particularly purging and bleeding. He was particularly aggressive in the use of bloodletting, something that caused him to lose popularity and respect among the Philadelphians during the Yellow Fever Epidemic of 1793. Because of his aggressive purging and bloodletting, some, including his own colleagues, started to wonder whether Rush was a healer or a killer.

The 1793 Yellow Fever Epidemic

Had yellow fever not struck the continent in the late summer of 1793, America may have been a French-speaking country today.

1789 saw the eruption of the French Revolution. The upheaval in France caused a rift in Europe with hostilities between France and England, and it also caused a divide in America. Thomas Jefferson and Benjamin Rush were among influential individuals who embraced the developments in France, whereas others, including John Adams, Alexander Hamilton, and Henry Knox, were strong opponents of the philosophy and deeds seen in Paris. Hamilton and Knox even argued for US military intervention on Britain's side. Washington wanted to stay out of the debacle, taking a stance for neutrality.

Louis XVI's execution by guillotine in January 1793, followed by the beheading of his spouse, Marie Antoinette, in October of the same year, outraged many in America and strengthened the pro-British sentiment in some quarters. In contrast, the anti-British side was bolstered when the British Navy blockaded ports in France, and captured American ships that tried to break the blockade. In the process, the British impressed large numbers of American seamen and passengers into the British Navy. Of course, the memory of France's intervention in the American Revolution, which had made it possible to defeat the British, was still fresh in the memory of the Americans, and this helped to generate support for France.

In the midst of these tensions, France appointed a new ambassador to the United States, Edmond-Charles Genêt, also called "Citizen Genêt." He arrived in America in April 1793 with the official charge of getting the United States to intervene in the war between Britain and France.[239] Some historians claim that Genêt also had a secret agenda to try to get Washington's government overthrown. When Genêt met with Washington, he pleaded with the president to support France, but Washington remained faithful to the Neutrality Proclamation issued the same month that Genêt had had set foot on the American continent. Genêt, however, did not take no for an answer and continued to aggressively stir up strong sentiments among American Francophiles.

Considering the pivotal role France had played in the American Revolution, it was not surprising that large segments of the society, including members of the government, were outspoken Francophiles. Thomas Jefferson, secretary of state at the time, proclaimed, "The liberty of the earth depends on the success of the French Revolution…. I would have seen half the earth devastated rather than it should have failed." His view on the tumultuous events in Paris reflected his philosophy that "the tree of liberty must be refreshed from time to time with the blood of patriots and tyrants."

When Genêt arrived in Charleston, South Carolina, in April 1793, he was met by crowds of cheering citizens, waving French flags in support of the French Revolution. The Francophilia was spreading like a wildfire along the east coast, and soon, throngs of people were marching the streets of Philadelphia, New York, and Boston. Despite Washington's refusal to get involved in the conflict between France and England, Genêt continued to press on.

While in Philadelphia, Genêt carried on, creating commotion. Thousands of Philadelphians were in the streets, causing tumults and spreading fear. John Adams later reflected about "the terrorism excited by Genêt in 1793, when 10,000 people in the streets of Philadelphia, day after day, threatened to drag Washington out of his house and effect a revolution in the government or compel it to declare war in favor of the French Revolution and against England." Adams was concerned about the safety of his family and "judged it prudent and necessary to order chests of arms from the war office" to protect his own home. Washington thought it would be necessary to send his wife and the rest of his family to Mount Vernon, out of harm's way.

The British Counsel also feared for his safety and wrote to London, "The town is one continuous scene of riot," adding, "The French seamen range the streets by night and by day armed with cutlasses and commit the most daring outrages. Genêt seems ready to raise the tricolor and proclaim himself proconsul. President Washington is unable to enforce any measures in opposition."

When Genêt continued to defy the decisions of the United States government, Washington requested that France recall Genêt as its ambassador. Instead, Genêt embarked the flagship of the French warships assembled in Philadelphia and sailed to New York, where he created similar tumultuous scenes as in Philadelphia. Thousands of French sailors and marines joined cheering and drunk New Yorkers shouting "Down with Washington!" and "Genêt to power!" Genêt felt that the moment had arrived to oust Washington, reclaim Canada (New France), and reestablish the glory of France on the American continent.

However, a couple of days into the events, Genêt had a rude awakening. When entering an inn to enjoy his breakfast, he found a city being deserted by hordes of citizens, leaving empty streets behind. When he asked one of the few remaining servers at the inn what was going on, the servant replied: "Yellow fever, Monsieur."[240]

So died the French dreams of a takeover of America. John Adams commented that "nothing but the yellow fever…could have saved the United States from a fatal revolution of government." He was convinced that if the yellow fever had arrived only a month later, Genêt's supporters would have taken control of New York, Philadelphia, and Boston.

In Philadelphia, the first victims of the epidemic were reported in late July. Yellow fever was a feared disease, and rightfully so. The suffering was severe, and the death rate was extremely high, about 30–40 percent. Philadelphia, like other communities on the continent, was afflicted by recurrent epidemics of yellow fever in the 1700s. The epidemic that hit Philadelphia in 1793 was particularly serious.

There was no understanding of how the disease was spread. The theories that were most prevailing was proliferation by direct contact between individuals, or by environmental factors, such as filthy conditions in the streets and elsewhere. Rush was a subscriber to the idea that yellow fever was caused by "noxious miasma." At the time, there was a heated debate about whether the cause was "dirty streets or dirty foreigners." In Philadelphia, the summer of 1793 saw a major influx of people fleeing slave revolts, as well as epidemic diseases in the West Indies. In particular, French settlers came in droves. Thousands of refugees were quartered under poor and unsanitary conditions. They became scapegoats, and were suspected of being the source of the ongoing epidemic. Thomas Jefferson was appalled by the trash and raw sewage in the waterfront streets, and accused refugees from Haiti, and French soldiers, of creating the unhealthy conditions.

The 1793 yellow fever epidemic was preceded by an unusually mild and wet winter, which explains why the mosquito population was large during the spring and summer. Nowadays, we know that yellow fever is caused by a virus carried by mosquitos, but in those days, the connection between mosquitos and yellow fever was not understood. In hindsight, the fact that yellow fever epidemics typically subsided after the first days of fall frost could have given people an important clue.

Thomas Jefferson elaborated on the signs and symptoms of yellow fever in a letter to James Madison in September 1793: "It comes on with a pain in the neck, sick stomach, then a little chill, black vomiting and stools, and death from the second to the eighth day."[241] In an equally vivid description, Rush wrote about the patients' suffering in an August letter to his wife:

> The disease has raged with great virulence this day.... Its symptoms are very different in different people. Sometimes it comes on with a chilly fit and a high fever, but more frequently it steals on with headache, languor, and sick stomach. These symptoms are followed by stupor, delirium, vomiting, a dry skin, cool or cold hands and feet, a feeble slow pulse.... The eyes are first suffused with blood, they afterwards become yellow, and in most cases a yellowness covers the whole skin on the 3rd or 4th day. Few survive the 5th day, but more die on the 2nd or 3rd days.

Rush went on to report the disease among his patients who were felled by the disease in less than a day: "One of my patients stood up and shaved himself on the morning of the day he died. Livid spots on the body, a bleeding at the nose, from the gums, and from the bowels, and a vomiting of black matter...closed the scenes of life."

The epidemic of 1793 lasted more than three months. Over four thousand Philadelphians lost their lives, making almost 15 percent of the population. Individuals who could afford it fled the city for the surrounding countryside, and did not return until the epidemic had subsided. Many doctors also left. Among physicians who stayed, ten died in the epidemic. Rush was one of the brave and compassionate doctors who remained in the city. He reported that at one point, only three physicians were available to treat thousands of patients. One of the remaining physicians was Philip Syng Physick who, like Rush, had studied surgery in London, and obtained his MD degree at the University of Edinburgh. Physic was mentored by Rush, and adopted Rush's bleed-and-purge treatment for yellow fever. When Rush himself was hit by the disease, he was treated by Physic—and survived.

People avoided contact with each other to prevent spread of the disease: "The old custom of shaking hands fell into disuse." People walked in the middle of the street to keep their distances from houses that had been stricken by yellow fever. Tobacco smoke was believed to be a preventive by many. As a result, "many persons—even women and small boys—had cigars constantly in their mouths." Garlic was also believed to keep yellow fever away, and some individuals placed "full confidence in garlic, chewed it almost the whole day; some kept it in their pockets and shoes."

Throughout the epidemic, Rush continued to manifest a remarkable compassion for the sick and poor. He had the courage to enter the filthy slum neighborhoods, where he saw dead bodies rotting in the midst of garbage, and chamber pot contents dumped into the streets.

Although initially Rush was much admired for his bravery and compassion, Philadelphians started to suspect that his treatments were causing more harm than good. The pendulum had begun to swing away from depletion therapy (bloodletting and purging). Rush, however, was headstrong in his practice. He became overzealous and probably "treated" some patients to their death by his extreme measures. Indeed, both colleagues and nonmedical members of the society became upset and quite critical towards Rush. Some even accused him of murdering people. The sentiments against him grew even stronger when Rush continued the extreme depletions during the subsequent yellow fever epidemics in 1794 and 1797. Some of the members of the College of Physicians called the cures provided by Rush "murderous," or described them as "doses fit for a horse" (referring to extremely high doses of calomel, a mercury compound commonly used as a purgative). Medical historians have commented that Rush's treatments became "the most popular and also the most dangerous 'system' in America."[242]

At the height of the epidemic, Rush and his assistants bled hundreds of patients on a daily basis. As a result, pale, exhausted, and dizzy individuals stumbling around in the streets of Philadelphia became a common sight. Many of the treatments took place in Rush's home, where many were housed on a frequent basis. The front yard was soaked with so much blood that it gave off a stench that attracted large swarms of flies.

It may seem surprising that learned men like Rush (and many other members of the medical profession at the time) advocated treatments that actually made patients sicker, and sometimes even resulted in their demise. Rush's view of the disease process partly explains this. He believed that fever was a "unitary principle of disease" and fighting the fever, regardless of its cause, was the primary objective of the cure. The direct cause of the fever, Rush argued, was an "irregular convulsive action of the blood vessels," and the treatment should be directed at "calming the excited vessels." The purging and bloodletting (the depletion therapy) were supposed to do just that.

The stories about Rush and the yellow fever epidemics are thought provoking for several reasons. Rush actually made several observations and recommendations that were sound, although he did not understand why he was on the right track. In his research of early literature on the subject, he discovered a recurring theme. Many previous writers had come to the conclusion that bad air from stagnant water was a cause of yellow fever. Rush therefore encouraged the citizens of Philadelphia to get rid of bad-smelling water from wherever they could find it, such as puddles in the streets, gutters, sewers, and privies. By recommending removal of breeding grounds for mosquitos, Rush was close to discovering the source of yellow fever without realizing it. So, it can be said that Rush was both right (advocating the removal of stagnant water), and wrong (believing that yellow fever was caused by bad air emanating from stagnant water).

Unfortunately, Rush's stubborn embracement of aggressive bleeding and purging of sick people led him down the wrong path, although at the time, Rush justified his treatments with theories that were supported by many others in the scientific and medical fields, including the prominent surgeon Physick. Belief in depletion, however, was not universal, and Rush started to experience venom from both colleagues and other members of the society. As the death tolls continued to rise, many began to suspect that his methods were not effective but were even harmful and could hasten the demise of patients.

Rush Losing Ground

The propaganda against Rush led patients to leave his practice, and his finances started to suffer. He was no longer respected in Philadelphia, and multitudes wanted him to leave town. He lamented, "Such has been the clamor against me that a proposal has been made in a company of citizens to drum me out of the city."[243] The criticism, however, strengthened Rush's resolve: "I am not moved by insults, but persist in asserting and defending all my opinions respecting the disease." Some of the harshest criticism originated from Rush's colleagues. Dr. Hugh Hodge, whose daughter had been one of the first victims when the 1793 epidemic erupted, was particularly intolerant in his critique, something that was painful for Rush. In a letter to his wife, Rush wrote, "Dr. Hodge leads the list of my calumniators. I give him no offense. I never intended to begin a controversy with him."

Even more ruthless nemeses were found among nonmedical individuals, especially journalists. John Fenno, the editor of the *Gazette of the United States,* assaulted Rush in "Letters to the Editor" (written by Fenno himself), comparing Rush's bloodletting to the guillotines of the French Revolution. Fenno's assaults had a political undertone. He was an ardent Federalist who despised the Republican Thomas Jefferson. Fenno thought Rush was a weak member of Jefferson's inner circle, and used him in his attacks on Jefferson. Fenno's attacks on Rush became so toxic that Rush sued for libel. Ironically, Fenno and his family ended up being wiped out by yellow fever before the trial even started.

The Cobbett Affair

The cruelest antagonist of Rush was William Cobbett, owner and publisher of the *Porcupine's Gazette.* Cobbett, an Englishman, had arrived in Philadelphia in 1793 at the age of thirty. He used his newspaper to spew vitriol at Rush for the bleed-and-purge treatment. He used language that makes even today's rhetoric look tame. He relentlessly affronted Rush and other physicians who had adopted Rush's methods. His disdain for the compassionate Dr. Rush saw no boundaries: "The remorseless Dr. Rush shall bleed me till I am white as this paper before I'll allow that [he] was doing good to mankind."[244] He went on to compare Rush to a mosquito, a horse leach, a ferret, a polecat, and a weasel: "for these are all bleeders, and understand their business full as well as Dr. Rush." He even accused Rush of murder, claiming that the bleedings had "slain tens of thousands."

Still more insulting was the accusation that Rush was knowingly killing his patients for profit. In a fictitious advertisement inserted into one of his poisonous articles, Cobbett wrote, "Wanted, by a physician [meaning Rush], an entire new set of patients, his old ones having given him the slip; also a slower method of dispatching them than phlebotomy, the celerity of which does not give time for making out a bill."

When Cobbett's hatred ultimately began to concern Rush about the safety of his family, Rush sued Cobbett for libel and demanded $5,000 in compensation (more than $100,000 in today's money). When the day for the trial finally arrived on December 13, 1799, Philadelphia was all but consumed by the event. After Rush and his family had arrived, the court waited for the defendant to show up. After a long wait, a messenger arrived with the information that Cobbett had taken refuge in New York, and the court proceedings had to be carried out without Cobbett.

Despite the fact that the judge, Chief Justice Edward Shippen, was the brother of Dr. William Shippen, whom Rush had brought before the infamous court martial in 1780, Rush won the case and was awarded the full amount he had demanded. In addition, Cobbett was ordered to pay an additional $3,000 for the cost of the trial.

Rush, of course, was happy with the verdict, but his happiness only lasted for a short time. On the day after the trial, the nation was reached by the news that its first president had died. One of the physicians that Rush had trained had been at the bedside of Washington during his illness (epiglottitis), and had directed repeated bleedings. Even during this time of national grieving, Cobbett continued his hateful attacks on Rush and his treatment, claiming that the bleeding had been a factor contributing to, if not even causing, Washington's death—[245] which may, of course, have been true.

The verdict against Cobbett in Philadelphia stood. It bankrupted Cobbett, who sailed back to England the following year. Before leaving New York, however, Cobbett could not restrain himself from further insulting Rush. In the pamphlet *The American Rush-Light*, he called Rush a "quack" and repeated his accusation that Rush "slew his patients." Sarcastically, he added that Rush's bleed-and-purge methods were one of "the great discoveries...which have contributed to the depopulation of the earth." He also claimed that Rush had won the lawsuit in Philadelphia by corrupting the judge and jury.

Retirement

Exhausted from the Cobbett controversy and starting to feel a threat to his life, Rush retired from his medical practice and settled at his farm at Sydenham. Rush devoted the remaining twelve years of his life to his family, trying to be a more present figure than he had been before. He also spent time writing and editing the book that would become an important part of his legacy, the four-volume *Medical Inquiries and Observations* (the last edition, published two years after his death, had five volumes). Despite his continued belief in and defense of bloodletting as an effective treatment for most diseases, the work came to influence the teaching of medical students for generations.

Rush allocated one of the last chapters in Volume 4 to his method of bloodletting, "A Defense of Bloodletting as a Remedy for Certain

Diseases." He justified his belief in bleeding by quoting his theory of disease unity. This "unitary system" argued that all fevers and diseases were caused by a disturbance of the bloodstream, mainly in the arteries. According to the theory, all types of inflammation, regardless of where they occurred in the body, were the result of one disease, namely the disturbance of the arteries and other components of the bloodstream. It is interesting that today we favor another theory that comes close to a "unitary system." In our modern thinking, inflammation is thought to be involved in a wide variety of diseases, including arteriosclerosis, diabetes, obesity, hypertension, arthritis, and cancer. It may be interesting to contemplate that one of the hallmarks of inflammation is increased blood flow.

The *Medical Inquiries and Observations* was based on lectures given to medical students at the University of Pennsylvania. In his lectures, Rush covered many topics that are even relevant today. He emphasized the importance of listening to the patients ("taking a good history"), performing thorough examinations, and considering all symptoms that the patient reports. Rush also discussed moral and ethical issues, encouraging the students to be charitable and act as humanitarians. He expressed disdain for colleagues who thought more about money than helping the poor and sick. Rush considered living up to moral and ethical standards to be "the duties of the physician." In many of the lectures, Rush also described the symptoms and treatments of many diseases that were common, such as hemoptysis (coughing up blood), consumption (tuberculosis), smallpox, gout, rabies, cholera, scarlet fever, measles, and the flu.

Rush was also early to use the vaccination against smallpox, and described it as "the most important discovery of the 18th century." By 1800, vaccination had replaced inoculation in most of Europe. Edward Jenner reported the method in 1796, and the Harvard professor, Benjamin Waterhouse, introduced it in America and was soon followed by Rush.

In addition to spending time with his family, reading, writing, and following new developments in the medical field, Rush also served as a consultant, and provided medical advice to many in need during his retirement years. In 1802, Thomas Jefferson, then the president of the United States, wrote to Rush about his health that "has always been so uniformly firm that I have for some years dreaded nothing so much as living too long. I think, however, that a flaw has appeared that ensures me against that...."[246]

The "flaw" that Jefferson talked about turned out to be chronic diarrhea. In the reply to his old friend, Rush wrote, "I have the great pleasure to tell you that complaints of the bowels such as yours have very generally yielded to medicine under my care," such as small meals of bland foods with a bit of sherry, or Madeira, and water. "When your bowels are much excited, rest should be indulged.... Carefully avoid fatigue of body and mind from all its causes. Late hours and midnight studies and business should likewise be avoided.... To relieve the diarrhea when troublesome, laudanum should be taken in small doses during the day and in larger doses at bedtime to prevent your being obliged to rise during the night."

Because Rush knew that the president was skeptical towards doctors and their treatments, he was surprised to learn that Jefferson had, in fact, followed his orders, and that the "flaw" had indeed disappeared. Rush replied, "I was made very happy by learning...that your disease is less troublesome than formerly. As I know you have no faith in the principles of our science, I shall from time to time combat your prejudices (and your disease, should it continue) with facts."

During his retirement, Rush continued his humanitarian endeavors, although at a slower pace. His sentiments against slavery, cruel treatment of prisoners, and the barbaric treatment of mentally ill, remained unmoved. In particular, his fight for better treatment of the mentally ill helped support his reputation as the best known and respected physician all over the continent. In 1812, when he published the groundbreaking work, *Medical Inquiries and Observations upon the Diseases of the Mind,* it resulted in both national and international accolade. In the book, Rush emphasized the necessity of providing important and meaningful activities to patients in mental hospitals, recommendations that were considered groundbreaking in the field of occupational therapy. He wrote: "It has been remarked that the maniacs of the male sex in all hospitals, who assist in cutting wood, making fires, and digging in a garden, and the females who are employed in washing, ironing, and scrubbing floors, often recover, while persons, whose rank exempts them from performing such services, languish away their lives within the walls of the hospital." For his work,

Rush was awarded a gold medal by the king of Prussia, a diamond ring by the czar of Russia, and special thanks from the king of Spain.

Early in his career, Rush saw mentally ill patients housed in the basement of the Pennsylvania Hospital under the most deplorable conditions. The "maniacs" were housed in locked cells, and were often chained to the floor. People were allowed to take tours to look at the patients, as though they were animals in cages. Visitors found "some of them…extremely fierce and raving, nearly or quite naked; some singing and dancing; some in despair." They were "entertained" by finding that "some were dumb and would not open their mouths; others incessantly talking." Rush was outraged by the way the mentally ill were treated, and for many years he fought with the hospital to allocate resources allowing for the creation of more humane conditions. Finally, a special building was created where psychiatric patients could be housed, which provided a clean and respectful treatment. In addition to allowing the patients to go outdoors for fresh air, and instructing the caregivers to talk to the patients to try to understand their diseases, Rush also introduced some treatments that may seem odd today. The centrifugal spinning board was used to improve circulation to the brain and the "tranquilizer chair" was believed to improve the condition by sensory deprivation, achieved by having the head enclosed and the eyes blocked. Rush's interest was personal because, sadly, Rush's son John was afflicted by mental illness and became a patient of his father for several years. This was a tragedy that impacted Rush till the end of his life.

Ultimately, Rush's contributions to the field of the mental illness earned him the epithet "the Father of American Psychiatry."

Reconciling John Adams and Thomas Jefferson

From a political standpoint, perhaps the most remarkable achievement toward the end of Rush's life was his ability to reconnect two giants in American history, John Adams and Thomas Jefferson.[247] They had been best friends during the early years of the Revolution but had later turned on each other. The unfortunate development of their personal relationship was multifactorial and has been well documented by historians. An important factor in the disruption of their friendship was Jefferson defeating

Adams in what would have been Adams's second presidential term. So upset was Adams about his loss that he did not even attend Jefferson's inauguration. Adams was a strong believer in the Federalist system, which continued to put him in a collision course with the Republican Jefferson.

Rush was in the unique position of being a friend to both Adams and Jefferson, and carried on a proliferative correspondence with both. He urged the two gentlemen to reconcile, realizing the benefits it would have for the country. Once Adams and Jefferson were convinced they did not actually hate each other, but instead loved and respected each other (Adams wrote "I always loved Jefferson, and I still love him"), letters started to be exchanged between the two, letters that addressed both the political situation in the country and personal affairs. Between 1812 and 1826, more than 150 letters were exchanged between the two men, letters that historians consider some of the most historically significant documents in American history.

Rush was exhilarated by seeing the reconciliation between the two ex-presidents, and understanding that he had indeed made this happen. In a letter to Jefferson, Rush wrote, "Few of the acts of my life have given me more pleasure than to hear of a frequent exchange of letters between you and Mr. Adams."

The End

Only a year after this accomplishment, Rush left this world. In April 1813, he became ill with fever and other symptoms that suggest pneumonia. In a letter to Adams on April 10, Rush wrote, "my time is short and…death is fast approaching." Despite (or maybe because of) vigorous bleeding performed by Rush's trainee and colleague, Dr. Physick, Rush died on April 19, aged sixty-seven seven years old. Rush was survived by Julia, his wife for thirty-five years.

After Rush's death, Adams and Jefferson continued their correspondence for thirteen more years, until their deaths in 1826. Amazingly, they died only five hours apart on the same day. The day was the 4th July, exactly fifty years after the signing of the Declaration of Independence.

CHAPTER 7

JOHN AND SAMUEL BARD—
Father and Son Surgeons

John Bard (1716–1799)

J ohn Bard initially practiced medicine and surgery in Philadelphia, but
moved to New York City in 1746. He counted Benjamin Franklin
among his friends, and it was Franklin who had advised John to move
to New York to take over the practice of a colleague who had died from
yellow fever. John would become highly respected and revered, and generate statements such as, "Dr. John Bard, a man who will not be quickly
forgotten where he was once known."[248]

Throughout his career, John's reputation as an excellent physician and
surgeon was solid. Despite growing a large and successful practice, however, he had persistent financial difficulties, some of which were caused
by expenses incurred by supporting his son's medical training in England.

Many physicians in the 1700s had a great interest in botany and horticulture, reflecting the role of herb-based medicines in those days. In 1763,
John Bard acquired Hyde Park, an estate of approximately 3,600 acres on
the east side of the Hudson River, about seventy-five miles north of New

York City. While designing his property at Hyde Park, he applied new European ideas in garden architecture, many of which had been provided in letters from his son Samuel who, at the time, was in England for medical and surgical training. Gardening also gave John the opportunity to explore and learn more about botany. He developed a large orchard, and after Samuel returned from Europe, he also grew plants for his son's medical practice in the city down the river. John retired to his beloved Hyde Park in 1778, but returned to New York to resume his practice after the end of the Revolutionary War in order to recover some of the economic losses he sustained while improving Hyde Park.

John and Samuel had a close relationship. Samuel's choice of career was, of course, influenced by his father. When studying in England, Samuel kept up an active correspondence with his father, not only related to his medical and surgical training in London and Edinburgh, but also related to his father's plans for developing and expanding Hyde Park. In particular, ideas were exchanged between father and son regarding landscape gardening, and what Samuel had learned about European horticulture in Edinburgh. He frequently expressed the desire to be with his father "in laying out your grounds."

Hyde Park would play an important role in the lives of both John and his son. Due to economic restraints, John had to give up some of the ideas he had for expanding the property, and even had to sell parts of the estate to make ends meet. Despite that, Hyde Park remained a beautiful place with magnificent views over the Hudson River. Despite returning to his medical practice in 1783, John was able to spend time farming, growing apples, and practicing botany and horticulture at Hyde Park towards the end of his life. Being close to his wife and the rest of his growing family was also important to him.

Although spending time as often as possible at Hyde Park, John remained involved in the medical and academic world of New York. When the Medical Society of the State of New York was established, John Bard was elected its first president. He did not leave many publications behind, but papers on yellow fever and pleurisy belong to his legacy. The most important report, however, is that of what may have been the first successful laparotomy in America.[249]

John Bard's 1759 Laparotomy

In the surgical annals, John Bard is most remembered for a heroic procedure he performed in 1759. In a letter to the well-known London physician John Fothergill, dated December 25, 1759, John described how he had performed a successful laparotomy to remove a nonviable fetus in a twenty-eight-year-old woman with ectopic pregnancy. Fothergill reported this case of an "extra-uterine foetus" to the *Society of Physicians of London* on March 24, 1760. He subsequently published John's letter in its entirety in 1764 in Volume 2 of *Medical Observations and Inquiries by a Society of Physicians in London.*[250] The letter provides fascinating details about the case:

SIR,

Dr. Colding, some time ago, showed me a letter he was favoured with from you; wherein you acquaint him with the design of publishing the London Medical Essays; and invite him to encourage that work, by communicating any useful or curious observations, which might fall under his notice in this part of the world. Encouraged by this invitation to the Doctor, whom I have the honour to be intimate with, I have taken the freedom, though a stranger, to send you the history of a case, which was lately fallen under my care.

Mrs. Stagg, the wife of a mason, about 28 years of age, having had one child without any uncommon symptom, either during her pregnancy or labour, became, as she imagined, a second time pregnant. She was more disordered in this, than in her former pregnancy, frequently feverish, the swelling of her belly not so equal, not the motion of the child so strong and lively. At the end of nine months, when she expected her delivery, she had some labour pains, but without a flow of waters, or any other discharge. The pains soon went off, and the swelling of her belly grew gradually less; but there still remained a large, hard, indolent, movable tumour, inclining a little to the right side. She had a return of her menses, continued regular five months, conceived again, and enjoyed better health: the swelling of her belly became more equal and uniform, and, at the end of nine months, after a short and easy labour, she was delivered of a healthy child. The tumour on the right side had again the same appearances as before her last pregnancy. Five days after delivery, she was seized with a violent fever, a purging, suppression of the lochia, pain in the tumour, and profuse fetid sweats. By careful treatment, these threatening symptoms were, in some measure, removed; but there still remained a loss of appetite, slow hectic fever, night sweats, and diarrhea. To the tumour, which continued painful, and gradually increased, were applied fomentations, and emollient pultices; and, at the end of nine weeks, I perceived so evident a fluctuation of matter in it, that I desired Dr. Huck, physician to the army, to visit this patient with me, and be present at the opening it. From the whole history, we concluded, that we should find an extra-uterine foetus. I made an opening in the most prominent part of the tumour, about the middle of the right rectus muscle, beginning as high as the navel, and carrying it downwards. There issued a vast quantity of extremely fetid matter, together with the third phalanx of a finger of a child. Introducing my finger into the abscess, I found an opening into the cavity of the abdomen by the side of the rectus muscle, through which I felt the child's elbow. I then directed my incision obliquely downwards to the right ilium, and extracted a foetus of the common size, at the ordinary time of delivery. The frontal, parietal, and occipital bones, as also the third phalanges of the fingers of one hand, separated by putrefaction, remained behind; which I also took out. We imagined the placenta and funis umbilicalis were dissolved into pus, of which there was a great quantity. By the use of fomentations and detersive injections, while the discharge was copious, fetid, and offensive; and by the application of proper bandages, and dressing with dry lint only, when the pus became laudable, the cavity contracted, filled up, and was cicatrized in ten weeks. The source of the hectic being removed, with the help of the bark, elix. of vitriol, and a proper diet, she quickly recovered good health. Her milk, which had left her from the time she was first seized with the fever, returned in great plenty after the abscess was healed; and she now suckles a healthy infant.

I am,
SIR,
With great respect,
Your most humble servant,
JOHN BARD.
New York,
Dec. 25, 1759.

Although John did not give the date for his operation in the letter, it was obviously performed during or before 1759, at least fifty years before McDowell's laparotomy, which many textbooks and articles incorrectly credit as the first laparotomy on the American continent. McDowell's laparotomy was probably the fifth successful laparotomy performed in America. We have already seen how John Warren performed a laparotomy in 1785. In the 1790s, William Baynham, a surgeon in Virginia with a nationwide reputation, performed two laparotomies for ectopic pregnancy.[251] It is interesting that the first laparotomies were performed for gynecological conditions. One reason for this is that tumors of the female organs often become both visible and palpable, whereas other intra-abdominal tumors, such as tumors of the bowels and stomach, were not easily detectable.

Although John Bard and John Warren preceded McDowell by fifty and almost twenty-five years, respectively, and McDowell performed his laparotomy almost thirty years after the end of the American Revolution, it is worth describing McDowell's procedure here because of the detailed description of the surgery that has been preserved for history. In addition, the patient subjected to the operation was an amazing woman with a remarkable history.

McDowell's Laparotomy in 1809

One reason why the December 1809 laparotomy performed is often credited as the first successful laparotomy undertaken in America—and perhaps in the world—is that many details surrounding the procedure have been preserved for posterity. Although the surgery took place twenty-six years after the end of the Revolutionary War, the country was still young, and the memories from the revolution were fresh. In addition, surgery at the time was not much different from earlier surgeries the 1700s.

The surgeon, Dr. Ephraim McDowell, had moved from Virginia to Kentucky when his father was appointed a judge in Danville. After completing a surgical apprenticeship in America, McDowell journeyed to Edinburgh in 1793, and stayed there for two years of additional training in anatomy and surgery.

Upon returning to the country that was now the United States, McDowell went back to Danville and quickly built a busy surgical practice serving a large area of Kentucky. When making house calls, he had to get to the patients by long rides on horseback through the wilderness, where Natives and wild animals remained a danger.

The patient undergoing the 1809 laparotomy was a forty-four-year-old woman, Mrs. Jane Todd-Crawford, who resided with her family in a simple log cabin sixty miles from Danville. McDowell was called to help her deliver at the end of a presumed pregnancy. When McDowell examined Mrs. Crawford, he saw she did indeed have an enlarged abdomen, which had made her and her family believe she was at the end of a regular pregnancy. When he examined her more carefully, however, McDowell realized that the patient was not pregnant, but instead had a large abdominal tumor, most likely "an enlarged ovarium." He offered to try to remove the tumor if the patient was able to make it to Danville. To McDowell's surprise, the remarkable woman appeared on his doorstep a couple of days later after a long—and probably painful—horseback ride. She asked to undergo the surgery McDowell had promised her.

McDowell took her in and started to make preparations for a laparotomy. At the time, McDowell had been joined in his practice by his young nephew, Dr. James McDowell, who was fresh out of medical school in Philadelphia. He was appalled by his uncle's proposition and tried to talk him out of it, but together, McDowell and Mrs. Crawford decided to proceed.

The front room of McDowell's' house was converted into an "operating room." The kitchen table was moved into the room to serve as the operating table. Once the operation had commenced, Mrs. Crawford was able to endure the pain by reciting and singing psalms and hymns. McDowell described the operation in vivid terms:[252]

> Having placed her on a table of ordinary height, on her back, and removed all her dressing which might in any way impede the operation, I made an incision about three inches from the musculus rectus abdominis, on the left side, continuing the same nine inches in length, parallel with the fibres of the above-mentioned muscle, extending into the cavity of the abdomen.... The tumour then appeared full in view, but was so large that we could not take it away entire. We put a strong ligature around the Fallopian tube near the uterus, and then cut open the tumour, which was the ovarium and fimbrious part of the Fallopian tube very much enlarged. We took out 15 lbs of a dirty gelatinous-looking substance, after which we cut through the Fallopian tube and extracted the sack, which weighed 7 lbs and one-half. As soon as the external opening was made the intestines rushed out upon the table and so completely was the abdomen filled by the tumour that they could not be replaced during the operation, which was terminated in about 25 minutes. We then turned her upon her left side, so as to permit the blood to escape, after which we closed the external opening with the interrupted

suture, leaving out at the lower end of the incision the ligature which surrounded the Fallopian tube.

Mrs. Crawford was indeed an exceptional woman. After only five days, she was up and about, able to take care of herself, and even participated in the housekeeping of her sickroom. Less than four weeks later, she mounted the horse and rode back to her home the same way she had come. Together with her husband, she later moved to Indiana, became a wealthy landowner, and got involved in politics as a representative in the Indiana legislature. She survived her laparotomy by more than thirty years and died in 1842, seventy-eight years old.

Dr. McDowell was a humble man not eager to blow his own horn. He did not publish his case until 1817, by which time he had performed two additional laparotomies (in 1813 and 1816, respectively). His report appeared in *Eclectic Repertory and Analytical Review* and was published in Philadelphia. McDowell's report was initially met with skepticism, particularly by the English medical establishment. In an article published in *The London Medical and Chirurgical Review*, it was stated, "We candidly confess that we are rather sceptical respecting these things...." After publishing a new report, describing two additional laparotomies, McDowell was vindicated by an article published in the same journal that had initially expressed skepticism: "A back-settlement of America—Kentucky—has beaten the mother country, nay, Europe itself, with all the boasted surgeons thereof in the fearful and formidable operation of gastrotomy, with extraction of diseased ovaria...there was circumstances in the narrative of some of the first three cases that raised misgivings in our minds, for which uncharitableness we ask pardon of God and of Dr. McDowell of Danville. Two additional cases now published...are equally wonderful as those with which our readers are already acquainted."

Even after McDowell was credited and honored for what was believed to be the first successful oophorectomies, he remained low-key. He has been quoted as saying, "How is it that I have been so peculiarly fortunate with my patients of this description? I know not; for, from all the information I can obtain, there has not one individual survived who has been operated on elsewhere for diseased ovaria. I can only say that the blessing of God has rested on my efforts." In retrospect, of course, McDowell was wrong in his statement that "not one individual survived who has been operated on elsewhere for diseased ovaria." As we have seen, at least two women had undergone successful laparotomies during the preceding century, and in one of those patients the ovary was indeed diseased.

Nevertheless, today McDowell is considered one of the fathers of oophorectomy and abdominal surgery. He continued to have a successful surgical practice, and performed many groundbreaking procedures in the area where he lived and practiced. He also attracted some very prominent patients. Perhaps his most famous patient was James K. Polk, who would become the eleventh president of the United States and for whom McDowell removed a bladder stone and repaired a hernia.

It is somewhat ironic that McDowell seemed to have died from a "surgical disease." In June 1830, he experienced acute abdominal pain and developed nausea and fever. He died on June 25 from what was most likely acute appendicitis.

McDowell is remembered with a granite monument at his grave in Danville with an inscription reading, "Beneath this shaft rests Ephraim McDowell MD, the father of ovariotomy who by originating a great surgical operation became a benefactor of his race, known and honored throughout the civilized world."

McDowell's home in Danville has been carefully preserved and now serves as a museum.

John Bard's Last Year

John Bard and his son Samuel remained close until John's death. After Samuel retired in 1798, they still had another year of nearness and fond respect. Samuel had built his own dwelling at Hyde Park only walking distance from his father's house. In several letters to family and friends, he described some of the circumstances surrounding his father's passing. Samuel's recognition of how much his father had done for him during his training in London and Edinburgh, and during the time they shared a New York practice, made his heart tender.

John Bard died in early April 1799 at the age of eighty-three. He was in good health up until one night, when a stroke befell him; in the afternoon preceding his death, John had visited his son's home. As was his routine, he came knocking on the door, accompanied by his servant who carried his master's obligatory two bottles of water "from his own favourite spring." As always, he took the "high backed elbow-chair, and was more than usual the delight and admiration of the family circle." Upon seeing his family and looking out the window at "the brilliancy of the setting sun" across the Hudson River, he exclaimed, "I think I am the happiest old man living."

The following morning, Bard's servant found his employer speaking incoherently. When Samuel rushed to his father's house, he found him "with symptoms that indicated an approaching palsy, his ideas incoherent, and his articulation very bad...[and] for the most part in a sweet sleep." A short time later, John Bard left this world.

Great respect for Bard is expressed on a plaque close to his grave: "A prominent physician, Bard investigated and helped prevent a malignant fever outbreak. He was the first president of the New York Medical Society. The town of Hyde Park derives its name from his estate, which he named "Hyde Park" in honor of Edward Hyde, the governor of New York and New Jersey during colonial times. His grave is the first in this churchyard."

Samuel Bard (1742–1821)

When he moved with his family from Philadelphia to New York, four-year-old Samuel saw the place where he would spend most of his future professional career. During his lifetime, he would leave his stamp on the city, not only in regard to medical care and education but also with regards to the overall cultural environment.

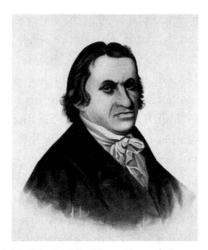

Samuel Bard (1742–1821). Founder of the second Medical School on the American continent. He was the private surgeon of George Washington and saved the President's life by cutting open and draining a large abscess on his left thigh. (History and Art Collection)

Samuel's Early Years

John Bard and his wife, Suzanne Valleau Bard, were keen on providing their children with a solid Christian upbringing that emphasized the importance of truth. In the 1822 book, *The Life of Samuel Bard, M. D.—A Domestic Narrative,* John McVickar (an Episcopalian clergyman from New York and a Professor of Political Economy and Moral Philosophy at Columbia College) tells the story of Samuel's father rebuking him for lying, even though Samuel had performed a generous and goodhearted deed. A young servant boy accidentally broke John Bard's cane. Samuel felt bad for the perpetrator and took the blame himself. When his father found out, he praised Samuel for his kind act but in the same breath scolded him for his "falsehood."[253] This lesson greatly impacted Samuel, and he remembered it through the rest of his life. He later passed on the same moral value to his own children, emphasizing that "any fault may be excused, but want for truth."

Samuel's parents did not only emphasize the moral values in life but also understood the importance of a good education. Samuel was sent to the grammar school of Mr. Smith, "a teacher of considerable merit." Samuel seems to have been an exemplary student, and was described "as a quick, industrious, and amiable child."[254] His parents considered Samuel smarter than his brother, Peter. Their mother wrote a note with instructions to their teacher: "If Peter does not know his lesson, excuse him—if Sam, punish him for he can learn at will."

Samuel entered King's College in New York at the age of fourteen. To improve their son's education, John and Suzanne made financial sacrifices and paid for board and private tutoring in the home of the classical scholar Dr. Leonard Cutting. The college years and Dr. Cutting's tutelage were formative experiences, and Samuel always remembered pearls of wisdom from those years. He adopted what was considered in those days the "great instrument of learning, repetition...line upon line."[255] Samuel also absorbed many other qualities during his years at King's College and with Dr. Cutting, such as "refined taste and critical acuteness," and he always remembered his professors with "affection and respect."

There is no doubt that during these years Samuel was influenced by his father as well. That Samuel would follow in the footsteps of the senior Bard seemed to have been a given. After college, he was apprenticed by his father and received a robust training in medicine and surgery. During these years, Samuel proved to himself and his surroundings that he had the stamina that was needed for a successful surgical career. He "laid the foundation of that habit of early rising which doubles the powers both of body and mind; a practice from which, in the remainder of his life, he never swerved." His biographer explained, "Daylight in summer, and an hour previous to it in winter, seldom found him in bed."[256]

Understanding the importance of schooling abroad, Samuel went to Europe for additional medical training. In October 1761, he set sail for the motherland. In a farewell letter, an anxious father gave Samuel many words of advice. Reflecting on the Christian and moral upbringing that Samuel had been given, John assured his son that "I have the greatest confidence in your piety, prudence, and honour." But, he warned, "you are going to a part of the world where you will be surrounded with allurements."[257]

Samuel was advised to choose friends carefully and to avoid people of lesser character, because "should you suffer yourself to be captivated with the idle of the gay, so far as to give into their schemes of dissipation...your mind may become enervated." Instead, "I do recommend to you...to attend upon the public worship of God constantly...."

As it turned out, Samuel did not have to wait until his arrival in England to learn that the world was full of dangers. The voyage itself would offer more excitement (and dangers) than Samuel could have imagined.

Voyage to England and Imprisonment in France

When Samuel left for England, the Seven Years' War was raging and England and France were the major foes. Anybody sailing the seas ran the risk of enemy ships apprehending them. In a letter to his father, Samuel described how "three weeks after I left you, being the 2d of November, we unfortunately fell into the hands of the enemy, and on the 24th arrived at St. Jean De Luz, a small town on the coast, in the South of France, from where I was carried to Bayonne Castle."[258] In the initial letter sent from Bayonne Castle, Samuel sugarcoated the situation to not worry his parents or anger the guards. Samuel knew that letters sent from the prison were censored. In subsequent communications, however, he was more forthcoming about what was really happening.

In his biography of Samuel Bard, John McVickar described how Samuel was "pillaged at the time of his capture, robbed of what little remained to him on landing, by the military police, defrauded by the commandant... he was literally starving upon two and a half pence a day."[259] His situation was desperate, and it even pushed him to "attempt an escape by the connivance of one of the guard." Finally, Benjamin Franklin, who was in London as an agent for several of the colonies, intervened, and Samuel was freed. After five months under French imprisonment, he could jubilantly write to his parents that "it is with the greatest joy I acquaint you with my deliverance from the French prison, and safe arrival at London."[260]

It was now time to get down to the business of learning medical and surgical skills in the metropolis.

London

We have learned a lot about Samuel Bard's time in London from letters penned by the young medical student. He kept updating his father about his activities, and frequently asked for advice. Bard Sr. was generous in his advice, and also complimented his son for his honorable, industrious, and successful life on the other side of the ocean.

Bard arrived at London in April 1762 and spent almost six months in the capital. Like many other American medical students, Bard connected with Dr. John Fothergill, one of the most revered physicians in London at the time, and asked for guidance regarding his education. He also sought the advice of Dr. Colin Mackenzie, the famous surgeon specializing in male midwifery. Both Fothergill and Mackenzie recommended that Bard spend time in London before going to Edinburgh for an MD. Bard explained in a letter to his father that "their reasons were, that they thought it best to lay a foundation by practice before I entered upon theory."

During his stay in London, Bard was admitted to St. Thomas' Hospital "as a physician's pupil, ... and constantly attended all the operations at both St. Thomas's and Guy's hospital." He also attended Mackenzie's lectures. He was lucky to be taken under the wings of many "able and amiable" men. Between the two Hunter brothers, Bard favored the older William with his "suavity of manners" rather than the younger John, "with the morbid irritability of temper which both embittered and shortened [his] life."[261]

Three months into his stay in the British capital, he reported in a letter to his father: "I never found one so unsocial [place] as London. Nothing is minded here but business; every one you meet is in a hurry, and if you do not walk with circumspection, you run the risk of being shoved into the gutter. I assure you I am most heartily tired of it...."[262]

It was with great anticipations, and probably a sigh of relief, that Bard, on September 1, 1762, climbed onto a stagecoach to Edinburgh.

Edinburgh

When arriving in Edinburgh, Bard quickly discovered the richness of its academic world. He got to attend lectures by scholars who were world leaders in the medical field. In a letter sent home to New York on December 5, 1762, Bard described his favorite lecturers: "I attend three classes, Drs. Cullen, Monro, and Ferguson. Cullen, professor of chemistry, at first gave us the history of his art...next proceeded to give an account of its objects... he is a very good speaker...lectures in English, in a clear, nervous style, and with a natural strong tone of voice."[263]

Although Cullen was probably Bard's favorite professor, he had some very good words to say about the other scholars as well: "Monro [secundus], professor of anatomy...is a very good demonstrator, and a pretty orator. I have procured a skull and a few old bones, in order to ground myself well in this fundamental part of anatomy [osteology]." Another favorite, Professor Ferguson was occupied by the science of magnetism and the "doctrine of attraction and repulsion.... He illustrates his lectures with a variety of very entertaining experiments; they are very agreeable, and with him we read the Newtonian philosophy."

During the beginning of the courses, Bard was overwhelmed and had a hard time writing down all the new knowledge he was exposed to: "When I first began to attend these gentlemen, I found much difficulty in taking notes." He soon, however, got acclimated and commented, "I have now by practice conquered it, and can carry off near the whole substance of the lecture." He was happy about the acquired skill because, when he returned to New York, he would "have a system of the different parts of the course in my own writing" that he would be able to share with his father and other colleagues.

That Bard was studying diligently and putting in long days is obvious from many of his letters. He wanted to make sure that his parents—his father in particular—were aware of his tough schedule. Bard knew his father was making financial sacrifices so he could study abroad. As Bard's biographer, McVickar, pointed out: "The application of his time, as given by himself, affords no weak proof of firmness of mind." In support of that statement, McVickar provided a quote by Bard in which the surgeon in training described his schedule:

My day, in general, is thus spent: from seven to half after ten I am at present employed in…professional reading and the examination of my notes; I then dress, and by eleven at college, attending professor Ferguson until twelve; from that hour until one, at the hospital; from one till two, with Dr. Cullen; from two to three, I allow to dinner; from three to four, with Monro in anatomy; from four to five, or half an hour after, I generally spend at my flute and taking tea…after this I retire to my study, and spend from that time until eleven o'clock, in connecting my notes and in general reading.

On several occasions, Bard expressed a desire to establish a medical school in New York. He was aware that the Philadelphians were ahead of him in this endeavor. In December 1762, Bard wrote to his father, "You no doubt have heard that Dr. Shippen [who had recently returned to Philadelphia from England] has opened an anatomical class in Philadelphia." Bard met with John Morgan in Edinburgh. They bonded, and developed a close relationship: "I have taken a small room, find my own breakfast and supper, and dine at an ordinary, with several agreeable young men; all students, among whom is…a Mr. Morgan, from Philadelphia, a person of distinguished merit, who knew our family and has taken particular notice of me."[264] Bard then continued by describing why he appreciated Morgan's friendship: "I can with more freedom apply to him in any trivial matter than to a professor, I promise myself much advantage from his friendship."

In the December 1762 letter to his father, Bard continued to think about Shippen's anatomical school in Philadelphia and commented, "The whole of that scheme…is not to stop with anatomy, but to found, under the patronage of Dr. Fothergill, a medical college in that place: Mr. Morgan, who is to graduate next spring, and will be over in the fall, intends to lecture upon the theory and practice of physic, and is equal to the undertaking." This statement lends credence to Shippen's claim that he and Morgan had together planned to establish the medical school as a joint endeavor, once Morgan returned to Philadelphia. As we have already seen, Morgan's supposed betrayal with regards to the Philadelphia medical school became the source of a lifelong bitterness and conflict between the two men.

Bard regretted that he would not be able to participate in the milestone event that would soon take place in Philadelphia. He wrote, "I wish with all my heart, they [Shippen and Morgan] were at New-York that I might have a share amongst them, and assist in founding the first medical college in America."[265] In the rest of the letter, Bard continued to lament the fact that he would not be the first: "I am afraid that the Philadelphians…will have the start of us by several years." He continued, "I own I feel a little jealous of the Philadelphians."

It would be another six years before Bard saw his dream fulfilled. He was one of the driving forces (and probably the most important) behind the establishment of the King's College medical school in 1768. Although by then the Philadelphia medical school was already three years old, the establishment of New York's first medical school was still an honorable achievement.

Bard spent almost three years in Edinburgh. During this time, he continued his studies with Cullen and Monro. He also built close relationships with other American students in Edinburgh and helped them advance their knowledge.

With pride, Bard reported to his father that he had been elected a member of the Royal Medical Society of Edinburgh. The society had been initiated in 1737 after beginning as a series of informal meetings among medical students. The gatherings initially took place at local taverns, which may be one reason membership was highly sought after. When Bard joined the society, it consisted of twenty to thirty members, who were now meeting at a more legitimate location. Bard stated that the members "meet every Saturday evening, in a room in the infirmary" discussing "medical subjects." The students exchanged opinions about recent medical publications, and discussed what they had learned during cadaver dissections.

Towards the end of his time in Edinburgh, Bard and his father exchanged multiple letters discussing what he still needed to accomplish before returning to the colonies. The plan included travels to Leyden and Paris, followed by a second stay in London. For unclear reasons, the travels to Leyden and Paris never took place. Instead, Bard spent the last ten months of his European sojourn in London. During this time, Bard spent most days at Guy's and St. Thomas' hospitals. He tried to focus on surgery but found that his "natural sensibility was too keen for a calm and scientific operator." He probably found that cutting into awake, screaming, and kicking patients was more than he could stomach at the time.

Bard's father was concerned that the English and Scottish education might change his son's manners. He repeatedly told Samuel to keep his humble and down-to-earth demeanor, both in his interactions with patients and with the public: "A physician should never assure...at his patient's bedside...formality." Upon his return to New York, Bard was also advised to keep a plain style of dressing: "In your taste of clothes preserve a plain and manly fashion, as well as in your manners." He went on asking his son to consider "that New-York is to be the place of your residence, where plainness in dress has been long the taste of men of the greatest fortune, and much respect is due to the fashion and custom of the country where you live."

Bard Receiving his MD Degree

In what may have been the last letter sent to his father from Edinburgh, Bard wrote on May 15, 1765, "My work being now over...and communicating to you a little of the satisfaction I myself feel." He mentioned "the day before yesterday, I received my degree." (He would have had to wait until September 6 to get his official printed diploma.)

Bard's thesis and defense are interesting. The subject of his dissertation, "*de viribus opii*," was the effect of opium on the human body. When he started the project, Bard regarded opium as a stimulant, an opinion that was shared by many at the time. To test his hypothesis, Bard performed experiments on himself and a fellow student (making the number of subjects in the study two). After administering the drug to himself and the fellow student, Bard had to admit that he had been wrong. The experiments, which were "frequently and carefully repeated," proved, based on the "debility which succeeds [the administration of the drug]...to all practical purposes [opium] may be ranked as a sedative, though it must be acknowledged that its powers of nervous excitement [becoming high] before falling into a stupor are often at variance with this opinion."[266]

The experiments, of course, were dangerous—and crazy! In an earlier letter, Bard's father commented, "We think you went too far in the experiments you made upon yourself."[267]

Publicly defending the thesis was the most important component of the MD examination. This examination stretched over several days, and also covered topics not directly related to the thesis. The committee examining Bard consisted of the two Monros ("primus" and "secundus"), Cullen (the Professor of Chemistry), and "my good friend Dr. Hope" (a botanist) who "publicly impugned my Thesis."

On the first day of the examination, Bard did not have "the most distant hint what was to be the subject of my trial," and he had to confess that he "went in…trembling." Cullen started the interrogation with some general questions, and then proceeded by inquiring about "the structure of the stomach and alimentary canal…and their diseases, with their diagnosis and method of cure." Then, Monro secundus continued the trial with "similar topics," and Bard concluded, "This ended my first examination, which lasted near an hour."[268]

The next day, Bard was asked to write "commentaries upon two aphorisms of Hippocrates, and defend them against Monro primus and Dr. Cullen." That exercise also lasted about an hour.

On the third day, Bard was charged with "writing commentaries upon two cases in practice," and had to defend the script against Monro secundus and Cullen for an hour and a half. The last component of the examination was the public defense of the doctoral thesis.

All examinations were conducted in Latin: "During all these trials, my exercises were not only written in Latin, but I was obliged to defend them in the same language; not even…being allowed to speak a word of English."

So, to obtain his MD degree from the University of Edinburgh, Bard had to go through a process characterized by impressive academic rigor, on top of three years of medical and surgical training, and daily lectures. No wonder he happily reported to his father about his "work being now over, and my mind at ease."

Returning to New York

After his second stay in London, it was time to return to New York. Five years prior, the voyage from New York to England had had its perils and risks. Now, his departure from London would attract new dangers and even renewed imprisonment, this time by local thugs.

On the way to the merchant ship on which Bard and a friend had booked accommodations for the return voyage, they got lost in the darkness of the night and ended up in a "lone house upon the heath," where they tried to get rest and sleep. When waking up, they found to their horror that they had been locked in with no way to escape. Convinced they were under the threat of criminals, they panicked. They also feared they were going to miss the boat. At last, they found a "narrow and concealed door...that yielded to their cautious efforts to open it." The rest of the account reads like a suspense novel: the door they had managed to open "was connected to a descending step-ladder, at the bottom of which lay a cloak and a sword, with a dark lanthorn lighted." They suspected (probably correctly) that they were going to be the targets of the sword. They went to work, barricading the entrances with what means the room afforded" and spent the rest of the night "in sleepless anxiety." At the crack of dawn, they managed to get out of the house and started to run for their lives— and for the ship. Luckily, the vessel was still waiting for them when they ultimately reached the dock.

After a "long and boisterous" voyage, Bard finally reached New York. Reuniting with his "anxious and longing parents...after five years' absence," the happy event was made even more joyous by the presence of an additional person among the welcomers. Bard's cousin Mary, whose parents had died, had moved in with John and Suzanne Bard. Samuel had been attached to Mary for quite some time, and while in London, had written letters to her expressing his feelings. When he saw her, he was again struck by her beauty, and could not take his eyes off her. The encounter was followed by courtship, but Samuel did not propose until he paid off his debt to his father. They were married in 1770. Their marriage produced eight children, five of whom died at a young age, four from scarlet fever. For more than fifty years of marriage, Samuel continued to love Mary and always thought of her as "a steady, judicious, and affectionate friend, and a dear and excellent wife."[269]

Financial Worries

Samuel was well aware of the economic sacrifices his parents had made to make his European journey possible. He expressed his gratitude on many occasions while he was abroad, and always assured his father that he tried to be thrifty. Even before reaching his destination, he expressed concerns about the expenses he was causing his father. While imprisoned at Bayonne Castle, he had purchased a German flute and hired a teacher "in order to pass any time with some little content in the prison." He expressed his regrets for the expenses: "I have during my stay in France, together with my expenses on my voyage and journey from Plymouth, spent nearly forty pounds sterling. I am afraid you will think this is a very extravagant sum; but I do assure you that there was not twenty shillings, (except my flute), which I spent unnecessarily."[270]

While in London, and wishing to attend the Hunter anatomical school, Bard asked his father for advice: "As Dr. Hunter intends to read lectures on anatomy this winter, I should be glad to know, as it makes a difference of sixteen pounds, whether you would have me attend him as a dissecting pupil, or only his lectures."[271]

Bard returned to the same theme in many of the letters to his father: "You may depend upon it I will not abuse your kindness, but I will regulate them by the strictest economy." In another letter, Bard expressed further gratitude to his father, writing, "I do assure you, sir, I never think of the great expense you are at in my education, without sentiments of the warmest gratitude; at the same time, I feel much uneasiness, lest it should fall heavy upon you."

Despite having been frugal during his time in Europe, when Bard returned to New York, he realized the extent of the economic setback for his father. When he joined his father's practice, he agreed to work without salary for the first three years to pay off some of the debt.

Founding of the Second Medical School in America, and Building the First Hospital in New York

Upon his return to New York, Bard finally tried to realize his dream of a medical school in the city. He understood that he could not do it by himself. His young age, only twenty-four at the time, was a factor that could work against him, and he therefore engaged several more senior colleagues in the efforts. John Jones, twelve years older than Bard, was one of the more influential surgeons in New York, and soon became actively involved in the establishment of the medical school.

In 1767, the board of governors at King's College agreed to start a teaching facility. The school, the Medical Department of King's College, graduated its first medical students two years later. As we have seen, after the Revolutionary War, King's College was renamed Columbia College, and the medical school became the Medical School of Columbia College (presently the Columbia University College of Physicians and Surgeons). Bard was appointed Professor of the Practice of Physic among the initial faculty of the medical school and Jones Professor of Surgery.

When the first medical degrees were conferred on May 16, 1767, Bard delivered the commencement address. His speech was titled "Discourse upon the duties of a physician." When the talk was published shortly thereafter, it had been given the subtitle *With some Sentiments on the Usefulness and Necessity of a Public Hospital.* In his address, Bard started out by reminding his audience that because America suffered from ignorant, untrained doctors, there was a great need of "you Gentlemen, who are Candidates for medical Degrees." He wanted to make sure the students understood that graduation was not the end of hard work, but instead "[their] Labours must have no End."[272] He also pointed out they needed to commit themselves to lifelong learning: "Do not therefore imagine, that from this Time your studies are to cease, [but you are] just entering upon them." He warned that if students did not adhere to the commitment of constant learning, "[they would] fall short of [their] Duty." Bard emphasized the value of learning from those who have gone before us, and following Hippocrates's example. He also encouraged the students to learn from contemporary giants in the field of medicine and surgery, such as "Sydenham, Boerhaave, Huxam, Pringle, and Whytt."

The next section of the discourse deals with moral aspects of physicians' duties. Bard advised the graduates not to badmouth and backstab a colleague, "nor ever attempt to raise [their] Fame on the Ruins of another's Reputation." He devoted significant time to the importance of being kind to patients and remembering their families: "Remember always that your Patient is the Object of the tenderest Affection, to some one, or perhaps to many about him," and "let your Carriage be humane and attentive, be interested in his Welfare."[273] In particular, it was important to look out for individuals who were both sick and poor: "Let those who are at once unhappy Victims, both of Poverty and Disease, claim your particular Attention."

The final part of the address was devoted to the need for a hospital in New York City and the money required to pay for it. He thought it was a disgrace that New York did not have a "proper Asylum, for such unhappy and real Objects of Charity," and complained that it "is truly a reproach." He argued for the need of a hospital for "the laboring Poor," but the benefits from a hospital would not be confined to the poor but "would extend to every Rank." Importantly, a hospital would also be important for the training of doctors, and would be "breeding good and able Physicians."

But the question was, who would pay for the hospital? He pleaded for support from the wealthy in the audience (including the governor): "There are Numbers in this Place I am sure" who would have the means; and he begged for someone to step up to make things happen: "It wants but a Prime Mover, whose Authority would give Weight to the Undertaking... would promote it."

Bard was successful and managed to get the governor and other members of the city authorities to contribute money for the hospital. After King George III granted a charter to establish the Society of the New York Hospital in the City of New York in America, the construction of the hospital began in 1773: "With the funds now collected, three acres of lofty ground, in the upper part of the city, were purchased for a location, and a suitable structure erected." Tragically, when it was almost completed, the building was destroyed in a fire in early 1775. Because of exhausted funds and growing political tensions and unrest, the hospital would not be rebuilt and opened until 1791.

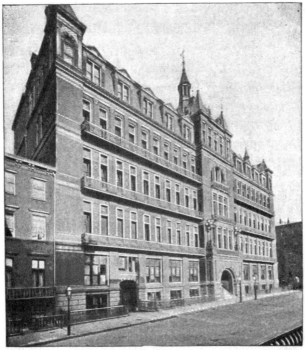

NEW-YORK HOSPITAL, WEST 15TH STREET, NEAR FIFTH AVENUE.

New York Hospital. Samuel Bard, together with John Jones, was a driving force behind New York Hospital. The hospital opened in 1791 after the initial construction was destroyed in a fire, 1775. (BLM Collection)

Building a Medical Practice

When Bard returned to New York, he immediately joined his father's practice, and although he quickly established himself as a successful surgeon and physician, he also encountered challenges. That he did not draw any salary during the initial three years[274] was a drag on his life and, among other things, delayed his marriage to Mary. He also soon realized that New York City was a competitive place for a young surgeon starting out, and he constantly had to compete with older and more established colleagues. He and his father both understood that there was no room for two Doctors Bard in New York. When they discussed different options, Bard's father decided to retire from the practice and move to Hyde Park, something he had thought about earlier. When John Bard retired in 1772, he built a new home at Hyde Park, the "Red House," and settled in for what turned out to be thirty-six happy years of retirement spent with his wife and extended family. He did not miss the hustle and bustle of New York City, or the competitive and sometimes stressful life of a busy surgeon.

After his father's retirement, Samuel continued to expand the practice. His growing practice did not stop him from academic pursuits. In 1771, he had already set the tone when he published, *An Enquiry Into the Nature, Cause and Cure, of the Angina Suffocativa, or, Sore Throat Distemper, as it is Commonly Called by the Inhabitants of This City and Colony.* The work received significant attention and glowing reviews: "Bard's book is wise and accurate. His style is classical and simple, and the description of diphtheria in skin, mucous membrane and larynx is correct and beautiful."

Clouds on the Horizon

Bard was well aware of the political situation and increasing tensions on the continent. He had returned from England only one year after the Parliament imposed the Stamp Act on the colonies, resulting in riots in Albany, Boston, and New York. The Sons of Liberty had been founded, and Samuel Adams was stirring the pot in Massachusetts. Like many fellow colonists, Bard was holding his breath, hoping that political tensions did not escalate into violence and an outright war with the motherland.

In a letter written to his father one week after the battles of Lexington and Concord, Bard expressed his concerns about the situation: "I am most sincerely sorry to confirm the afflicting reports, which, before this, I suppose you have heard." He went on by commenting that "the sword of civil discord is at length unsheathed, and the horrors of that worst of wars begun among us."[275] What he referred to was Lexington and Concord on April 19, and the "body of eight hundred troops" that had "marched suddenly from Boston, in the night, with intention to seize a magazine which had been prepared at Concord, or, perhaps, the delegates, who were there met." Bard wanted to make sure his father had been informed about the events in Massachusetts and described in detail how the British troops had "encountered a company of minute-men exercising, and ordered them to disperse, who refusing to do so, the troops fired twice over their heads, and, as they still stood their ground, a third time, among them, and killed eight."

There is no doubt that Bard was scared. In the letter, he continued, "God, and God alone, knows where these unhappy disputes will end; it can hardly, however, be hoped they will subside we have felt heavily the inconveniences of them." He ended the letter by hoping "that we may again see our former happy days of peace and quiet"—something that would not happen for the next eight years.

Rumors of British troops heading for New York heightened Bard's anxiety, although he commented "this is contrary to the present intention of the ministry." Bard was alarmed by the "gloomy prospect" of seeing Redcoats encamping "upon Harlem commons." This did not seem impossible considering that at the time, Boston was occupied by four thousand British troops.

As the tensions increased, Bard became concerned about the safety of his family. Towards the end of 1775, he moved his wife and two children (Susanne, three, and John, one) to Hyde Park, where they were to stay with the rest of his family.

At this early stage of the Revolution, Bard was not a Patriot, and he was not convinced that there was good in trying to achieve independency. Most of his New York friends were Loyalists. Bard's experiences in England were also fresh in memory, and he felt, as his biographer wrote, that the "long residence in Great Britain, had taught him that there was in it so much of learning and virtue, of science and wisdom, of all that adorns and dignifies humanity, and makes life desirable, that an unwillingness to regard them in light of enemies may be pardoned to him."[276]

This Loyalist leaning made Bard uncomfortable when, after the English were dislodged from Boston, Washington marched the Continental Army down to New York in the spring of 1776. On July 22, Bard wrote in a letter to Mary that "the town is at present little more than a garrison of New-England and New-Jersey troops, who are fortifying it on all sides, so that if any are sent here by government, it will certainly become a scene of blood and slaughter."[277]

Of course, that is exactly what happened. Only a month later, the British arrived with a huge armada of warships and heavily strengthened forces to deal Washington and his army a decisive and humiliating defeat at Long Island.

Independent of his opinion about the Revolution and fight for independence, Bard was mostly concerned about a potential bloodbath when the British showed up in New York. With the family relatively safe at Hyde Park, Bard decided to get out of New York "previous to Sir William Howe taking possession of it," and settled down at Shrewsbury in New Jersey.

Now without an income from his medical practice, Bard looked around for other business opportunities. Somewhat oddly, he "attempted [to] manufacture…salt from sea-water, (an article then much wanted,)"[278] but soon realized this was a failure. The only option he saw to again generate income was to risk moving back to New York and reclaim his home and medical practice. At this point, New York was occupied by the British, and Loyalists were in charge. Bard found his home occupied by "other and no friendly hands," something that happened to most homes that had been deserted when the British took over the city in August 1776.

Finding strangers occupying his home, and realizing many of his old Loyalist friends had turned their backs against him, were hard pills to swallow. The British authorities looked upon Bard with suspicion. In addition to having left the city when the British were approaching, Bard found his situation extremely perilous due to his father residing at Hyde Park within the American lines, and his brother holding a commission in the Continental Army. The military was on the verge of arresting him when the Mayor of New York and old Loyalist friend, David Mathews, came to his rescue. By chance, Bard had run into the mayor a couple of days earlier, and had been asked to attend to a sick member of the mayor's household. A few days later, when a British commandant was just about to issue an arrest order, Mayor Mathews happened to enter the room and hear Dr. Bard's name mentioned. The mayor intervened at once, explaining that Dr. Bard was his family doctor and an honorable friend. Bard was cleared from all suspicions, and was saved from the military arrest. The close call helped Bard to regain both business and friends. He again had a busy practice.

Although Bard had initially not been enthusiastic about the Revolution, and had surrounded himself with Loyalist friends, he was able to mend fences with his previous political opponents. Indeed, after the war, Washington engaged Bard as his personal physician. In 1789, Bard performed surgery on Washington to drain an abscess that the Commander-in-Chief had developed on his left thigh.[279]

1783: A Tragic Year

Although the Peace Treaty of Paris should have made 1783 a celebratory year for most Americans, the year was filled with tragedies for the Bard family. It was the year when Samuel and Mary Bard saw their family decimated by deaths. Four of their six children succumbed to scarlet fever in the fall of 1783. John, nine; Mary, seven; Harriet, four; and Sarah, not yet one year old, all died of the dreaded disease within only a couple of weeks. Seeing four of their six children die shattered Samuel and Mary's lives. Their sorrow and devastation shines through in letters from the period. To support his wife in her grief, Bard took time off from his practice in New York and stayed with his family full time.

In a letter to a younger sister, Bard wrote on September 24, 1783: "How shall I tell you ... of my calamity?"[280] He lamented the death of two of his daughters: "The indisposition of my dear children...has cruelly robbed us not only of...poor little Sarah...but of our most dear and amiable child, my soft-eyed Harriet." He described how "the scarlet fever finished what the meazles [*sic*] had begun; and to add to our distress, our dearest William, and Mary, still continue very weak and feeble."

Two weeks later, Bard wrote: "William, I thank God, ...mends" but "our sweet little prattle Mary is so ill...." Five days later, another letter reported "our sweet little Mary, is out of her misery. She died on Friday morning at one o'clock." He added, "I had the melancholy office of closing her dear eyes." Despite all the love and kindness extended by Bard to his wife, Mary suffered indescribable pain and sorrow. In a letter, she wrote, "My peace of mind is, I fear, gone for ever in this world."[281]

Somehow, the Bards managed to survive the crisis. Dr. Bard returned to his New York practice in the summer of 1784. Samuel and Mary had two more children, but tragedy struck again: a daughter was born in 1786 and was named after her older sister, Harriet, who had died in 1783. The new Harriet died shortly after her birth. Eliza was born in 1789, and was one of only three children who survived to adulthood. The other children who were able to come of age were the firstborn child, Susannah, born in 1772, and William, who had survived the scarlet fever in 1783.

The Doctors' Riot in 1788

In April 1788, the Doctors' Riot ravaged parts of New York City.[282] Surgeons and medical students carried out grave robberies to provide cadavers for anatomical dissections. The riots and violence were directed against physicians and students who, protected by the dark of the night, were digging up newly buried bodies to provide corpses for anatomical dissections. The rampage lasted several days and resulted in at least five deaths (some estimates, however, put the death toll at twenty). Although the protests against body snatching were particularly violent in New York in April 1788, they were certainly nothing new—or even isolated to New York. We have already seen that excavating newly buried bodies caused civil unrest and lawlessness at many places where teaching of anatomy took place. London and Edinburgh were not immune to public uproar against the "resurrectionists." In Philadelphia, Shippen was the target of mobs breaking windows and throwing rocks into the dissecting rooms at his anatomical school. John Warren's Spunkers at Harvard were met by protests among the Bostonians.

The racial aspects of grave robbery made the Doctors' Riot in New York one of the most violent protests of the time. A large number of slaves lived in New York, and when they died, they were required to be buried outside the city limits. Many of the grave robberies took place at the "Negroes Burying Ground." The City Common Council's refusal to take action when a group of freedmen protested against the body snatching increased the sentiments against the medical students and surgeons participating in the activities. This helped the riot spread like wildfire.

Aware that he had not participated in the illegal activities, Bard kept his calm despite the rioting mobs and the possibility that he could become the crowds' next victim. In order to convince the hordes that he had nothing to hide, he did something unusual—and quite courageous. When the screaming and window-smashing crowd approached his house, he ordered the doors and windows to be opened wide and exposed himself in full view inside the opened door. The plan worked. When the protesters saw him, they "gazed a while in silence, and then passed on, with acclamations of his innocence." Yet again, Bard had had a close call.

Bard's Retirement to Hyde Park

Bard continued his practice in New York until he retired at Hyde Park in 1798. Retirement is always a big decision in a person's life, and those times were no different. It influences finances, family life, and social interactions. A physician, in particular, may feel that the identity (serving as someone's doctor) is changed. It is interesting to observe the in-depth thinking Bard gave the decision. He expressed the thought that "some pause of reflection should intervene between the business of life and its close." He resolved to a plan, "which most wise men propose, but few execute—that of retiring voluntarily from the bustle of life."[283]

After Bard had made his decision, he started to inform friends and patients—and received many appeals to reconsider. He felt convinced, however, that it was now time to take the step. Bard felt responsibility towards his patients, and wanted to make sure that their care would be taken over by someone he could trust and "might introduce to his large circle of patients, one to whose medical skill he was content to transfer their safety." Dr. David Hosack fit the bill and was offered a partnership. Bard and Hosack had developed a close friendship and respect for each other, and they continued their relationship for years to come.

Bard followed his father's example and withdrew to Hyde Park when retiring, and "removed to his well known seat, within a short distance from his father's residence." Bard at this point was fifty-six, and ended up enjoying twenty-three years of retirement with his wife, children, and grandchildren. Although Bard, like his father, spent much time on botany and horticulture, he also continued to be actively involved in medical and academic affairs. When the King's College medical school that had become Columbia University merged with the College of Physicians and Surgeons in 1813, Bard was named the first president of the new school.

Bard's kindness became legendary. His personality won him many friends, both among his patients and social acquaintances. He was a soft-spoken and gentle person, something that can also be seen from his free time interests. His biographer commented, "nothing calmed and soothed [Bard's] mind like a walk among his plants and flowers; and he used it as a specific against the petty cares and anxieties of life."[284] In this context, his biographer talked about "his kindness, his patience, and cheering words of consolation, addressed even to the poorest and meanest, ...the value of moral...instruction."

Bard's determination to think good of everyone sometimes led to naïve and risky decisions. On one occasion, he entrusted his wife's and his life savings with an old family friend, who, on his voyage back to London, planned to invest the money in British funds. Before the investments were made, the money was deposited with a banker, who ended up embezzling the riches. When reading about the unfortunate event in a letter from London, Bard cried out, "We are ruined, that is all." Mary tried to comfort her husband, "If that be all, never mind the loss, we will soon make it up again." This, they gradually managed to do.

During his retirement, Bard remained devoted to teaching and scientific writing. He made certain that medical students got proper clinical training at New York Hospital, and published *A Discourse on Medical Education* in 1819. He also continued to serve on the boards of several groups in New York associated with science, medicine, and culture.

Obstetrics and midwifery was a field of surgery and medicine particularly close to Bard's heart. This interest resulted in an 1819 textbook, *A Compendium of the Theory and Practice of Midwifery*, which was the first of its type by an American. For many years, it remained the standard text on the subject.

On one occasion during his retirement, Bard went back to New York to help treat the victims of a yellow fever epidemic that had erupted in the city. During his fearless and unselfish work, he contracted the infection himself. Thanks to the devoted care of his wife, Bard survived the ordeal.

Samuel Bard died in 1821, at the age of seventy-nine, from pleurisy. His wife had succumbed to the same illness only one day earlier. They were buried together in the same grave at Hyde Park.

It took seven years after his death for his family to decide what to do with their beloved Hyde Park. In 1828, they sold the property to Dr. David Hosack. Although not related, Hosack was considered part of the Bard family. He had been close to them for many years and had been a frequent guest at Hyde Park.

Like John and Samuel Bard, Hosack had been touched by the American Revolution. At one time, he had taken care of Alexander Hamilton's son, who had contracted typhoid fever. After the infamous Weehawken, New Jersey duel on July 11, 1804, Hosack also provided care for Hamilton himself during Hamilton's last hours, before he succumbed to the bullet fired by Thomas Jefferson's vice president, Aaron Burr.

Hosack was fifty-nine when he purchased Hyde Park, and would be able to enjoy the beauty of the previous Bard property for another seven years before he died.

CHAPTER 8

JOHN JONES—Father of American Surgery

W hen a medical historian summarized the main characteristics of John Jones, he wrote: "He was small and nonobtrusive. His dress was plain, he wore no wig. He bore the common name of Jones, John Jones, M.D. But this was no common man, rather he was the greatest surgeon in the American colonies and America's first professor of surgery."[285] James Thacher described Jones as being "about the middle size; his chest was moderate.... He was free and easy of access."[286]

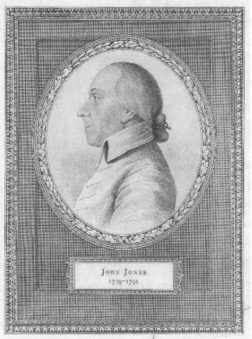

John Jones (1729-1791), professor of surgery,
King's College Medical School, 1787-1776.

John Jones (1729–1791), "Father of American Surgery."
Author of the first surgical textbook written by an
American, *Plain Concise Practical Remarks on the Treatment*
***of Wounds and Fractures* (1775). (Public domain)**

Although other prominent surgeons have been referred to as "the Father of American Surgery," few would dispute that John Jones may be the person most worthy of the epithet: "As a surgeon, Dr. Jones stood at the head of the profession in this country."[287] He was the cofounder of the second medical school in the colonies. He was the first full Professor of Surgery on the American continent. He, more than anybody else, championed the opinion that surgeons should be well educated in internal medicine (physics), in addition to surgery, and should not be regarded as mere technicians, a common sentiment of the medical establishment at the time in both Europe and America.

Family Background and Early Years

Jones' pedigree was that of physicians and surgeons. Born in Long Island into a Quaker family in 1729, he carried on a tradition started by his grandfather, Edward, who, with his wife, Mary, had come to America in 1682 and established a medical practice in the newly founded city of Philadelphia. Edward's son Evan had removed to New York to open his own medical practice after an apprenticeship with his father. With both his grandfather and father being doctors, it is not surprising that John chose a medical career as well.

At the age of eighteen, John entered an apprenticeship with his cousin, Thomas Cadwalader of Philadelphia. Interestingly, Cadwalader had been trained by John's father before traveling to London to study with the anatomist and lithotomist William Cheselden. Subsequently, Cadwalader obtained his MD degree at the University of Rheims in France.

After three years of apprenticeship under Cadwalader, Jones followed in the footsteps of his cousin and teacher and sailed to Europe for studies. In London, he met with an aging Cheselden. He learned anatomy and obstetrics from the renowned scholars and physicians, William Hunter and Colin MacKenzie. These were encounters that came to influence Jones' future clinical interests in midwifery and stone-cutting.

The person in London who had the greatest influence on Jones, however, was Percivall Pott. At the time, Pott was a senior surgeon at St. Bartholomew's Hospital, and was a widely admired and skillful surgeon. He was also an educator of great reputation who had authored important textbooks in surgery. Jones quickly became one of Pott's favorite students. Their interactions resulted in a close and long-lasting friendship.[288]

Understanding the importance of an MD degree, Jones again followed his cousin's example and traveled to the University of Rheims in France. His doctoral thesis, entitled "Observations on Wounds," later became the foundation of the first surgical textbook published in America.

After obtaining his MD degree in 1751 at the young age of twenty-two, it was time for Jones to make the "grand tour." The travels took him to Rouen, Paris, Leyden, and Edinburgh. He had engaging experiences at all of these places. In Rouen, he met with Claude Nicolas Le Cat (1700–1768), famous for lithotomies and cataract surgeries. In Paris, he visited with

Henri François Le Dran (1685–1770), famous for his insights into cancer, hernia surgery, lithotomy, and military surgery. While in Paris, Jones also had an opportunity to "walk the wards" at Hôtel Dieu, an experience that shocked and upset him, and would later influence his plans for the New York Hospital two decades later. Remembering the nightmarish rounds at Hôtel Dieu, Jones wrote, "It is impossible for a man of any humanity to walk through the long wards of this crowded hospital, without a mixture of horror and commiseration, at the sad spectacle of misery which presents itself: the beds are placed in triple rows, with four and six patients in each bed; and I have more than once in the morning rounds found the dead lying with the living...."[289]

In Leyden, the influence of Dutch physician Herman Boerhaaven could still be felt. The idea of a balance between fluids in the body for maintaining health was still prevalent. After Leyden, Jones spent a couple of months in Edinburgh, where Alexander Monro primus, the famous Scottish surgeon and anatomist, was lecturing. His teaching was immensely popular among the students, one reason being that they were delivered in English rather than Latin. In addition, his dissections of human bodies helped put the University of Edinburgh on the map as a place for learning anatomy in the early and mid–1700s. When Jones visited Edinburgh, the anatomical demonstrations had been moved from Surgeons Hall to the safety of the University. This protected Monro from angry mobs protesting against grave robberies.

Returning to New York

Upon returning to New York, Jones was one of the lucky few that had been given the opportunity to obtain medical and surgical training abroad. Around the time of the American Revolution, approximately thirty-five hundred physicians provided care for the about 2.5 million people living in the thirteen colonies. Although several of the surgeons described in this book had studied abroad, this was still rare. The majority of the colonial doctors had learned their crafts through apprenticeships—if they had received any formal education at all. Only about 350 had been fortunate enough to study abroad, and even fewer could put an "MD" after their names. When Jones returned from Europe, well educated and with an MD degree, it was not difficult for him to land a good job.

Jones joined Dr. John Bard, whom we already met in the preceding chapter. Jones was allowed to focus on the surgical cases in Bard's practice, and quickly earned a reputation for being a skillful obstetrician and a courageous and fast lithotomist. Jones's biographer, friend, and apprentice James Mease, reported that Jones was the first to perform "the operation of lithotomy" in New York City. Jones "succeeded so well in several cases…that his fame as an operator became…known," not only locally, but "throughout the middle and eastern states of America."[290] Others in the colonies had tried the operation, but "the want of success attending it, was generally so great, as to prevent it from being performed in future."[291]

Mease described how he "had an opportunity of seeing [Jones] operate, and the honor of being one of his assistants, during the period of my surgical pursuits under his directions."[292] Mease was impressed by Jones's "calm, and firm manner," even in "the most difficult cases." Describing Jones's skills as a lithotomist, Mease commented that "I have seldom known him longer than three minutes in lithotomy, and he sometimes finished the whole procedure in one minute and a half!"[293] The safety of the operation, however, was more important to Jones than the speed: "like his great master POTT, he reprobated the practice frequently pursued of counting the motions of a surgeons [*sic*] hand by a stop watch." Jones "was not so anxious about the shortness of the time in which it was performed as to the certainty of its success," and he "rather wished to accomplish that well, in a little longer time."[294]

The other area in which Jones showed a special interest was obstetrics, and he developed a great reputation as a skillful *accoucheur*. His principal trait was that of a conservative man-midwifery, arguing for natural deliveries with the use of forceps only when absolutely needed; "he seldom had recourse to these artificial aids." This approach provided increased safety for both mother and baby and helped make him a popular male midwife and lecturer of obstetrics.

Jones's surgical skills made him a famous man, with name recognition in the colonies: "his fame became diffused throughout the continent of America." He was often asked for advice by colleagues and "his attendance was frequently desired in the different states."

Despite his stature, Jones remained humble. At the time, other less humble physicians had formed an association that required its members to stand out in society by wearing a wig or having their hair cut in a special way. Others were strutting around using a cane with a golden head, an additional demonstration of their importance. Jones wanted none of "the full bottomed wig, the gold headed cane, and brilliant on the finger."[295] When Jones did not comply, his fellow physicians stopped referring patients to him—but the public sided with Jones. The colleagues had to back down to see "the object of the association…entirely defeated; and the members were under the necessity of wearing their hair like the rest of their fellow citizens."

Military Surgeon During the French and Indian War

The French and Indian War interrupted Jones's practice in New York. In 1755, Jones volunteered to join the British and colonial forces fighting French soldiers who, together with warriors from several Indian tribes, tried to wrestle North America's control from England.

One famous incidence during the war was that of the engagement at Lake George, defending Fort Edward, and the bullet wounds suffered by the French Commander General d'Escaux.[296] The French lost the clash and d'Escaux was taken prisoner. When he realized that Dr. Jones was on site, he requested that his bullet wounds be taken care of by the famous New York surgeon. The request was granted. Jones successfully treated several of the wounds, but a through-and-through wound of the general's urinary bladder did not heal, and instead resulted in a fistula with urine leaking onto the abdominal wall. After the war, d'Escaux was released from prison and sailed back to France, probably with urine still leaking from his bladder.

Re-Establishing the Surgical Practice in New York and Founding the Medical School at King's College

At the conclusion of the French and Indian War in 1763, Jones moved back to New York City and again joined John Bard in his practice. Three years later, Samuel Bard returned from his training in Europe and joined the group. It was a joy for Bard Sr. to see the return of his son, who was well educated and carrying an MD degree. Jones must have also found pleasure in seeing Samuel return from an educational experience similar to his own, and he was probably full of enthusiasm and optimism about the future of American surgery, especially considering Samuel's plans to elevate the medical education in New York. It did not take long for Samuel to talk Jones into the idea of a medical school in New York.

Jones, along with a group of other prominent physicians (Samuel Clossy, Peter Middleton, and James Smith), joined Samuel Bard in petitioning the board of governors of King's College for the establishing of a medical school.[297] The second medical school in the colonies opened in November 1767, only two years behind the College of Philadelphia Medical School.

The faculty of the newly founded medical school consisted mainly of its founders. Jones was appointed Professor of Surgery ("Professor of The Theory of Chirugery with a Course of Operations upon the Human Body"). Although Jones has often been labeled "the first" Professor of Surgery in America, some historians like to point out that he was the first "full" Professor of Surgery, in contrast to William Shippen Jr., who had been appointed Professor of Anatomy and Surgery two years earlier in Philadelphia. This meant that Jones was actually the *second* Professor of Surgery in the colonies. Two hundred and fifty years later, however, this may seem like splitting hairs. Both were pioneers in the field of surgery, and as we have seen from the chapter on Shippen Jr., both made important marks in the annals of medical and surgical history. The other members of the King's College medical faculty were Samuel Bard, Professor of the Theory and Practice of Physick; Samuel Clossy, Professor of Anatomy; Peter Middleton, Professor of Physiology and Pathology; James Smith, Professor of Chemistry and Materia Medica; and John Tennant, Professor of Midwifery.

Jones delivered his inaugural lecture on surgery on November 4, 1767, and continued to give annual lectures until 1775, when the outbreak of the Revolution forced the closure of the college. Part of his teaching was focused on what it takes to become good surgeons and "give the highest degree of perfection to their art." A surgeon, he explained, "ought to have steady hands, & be able to use both alike…strong clear sight…& above all, a mind calm and intrepid…amidst the most severe operations."[298]

Another, perhaps more important part of the lecture was devoted to a discussion of whether surgeons should be mere technicians, or also have good understandings of the diseases that their surgeries would cure: "how necessary it is for the student in surgery to make himself acquainted with all those branches of medicine, which are requisite to form the most accomplished Physician; to which must be super added some peculiar qualifications, to constitute the surgeon, of real merit & abilities." The opinion that surgeons should only keep to the manual work was still prevailing among the medical establishment in Europe, where physicians often looked down on the surgeons, who had been considered mere barbers not long before. In contrast, doctors in America often practiced both physic (internal medicine) and surgery, and Jones wanted to build on that tradition. He was upset by colleagues who continued to consider surgeons the representatives of "a low and mechanical art."

The longer he got into his lecture, the more agitated he seemed to become, and the stronger words he used: "What must we think of the insolence and malevolence of those who represent…[the science of surgery]…as a low mechanical art, which may be taught by a butchers boy in a fortnight—yet such false and absurd representations have been made of it." With a rising voice, trembling full of anger, he told the students that there are medical men who think of themselves as gentlemen, but are "ignorant and weak enough to credit such absurdities."

During the remainder of his career, Jones kept up the fight for the necessity of a surgeon "to make himself truly intelligent in his profession," and continued to detest those "who estimate surgery by operation alone, and believe that nothing but long habit and practice is necessary to form the great surgeon." He stated that, "those surgeons…degrade themselves and their profession" and are "practitioners, whose experience is little more than heaping one blunder upon another." This was indeed the voice of someone who deserved the epithet "Father of American Surgery."

The Medical School at King's College graduated its first (two!) medical students after two years. We have already seen how Samuel Bard used his commencement address in May of 1769 to muster support for a hospital in New York City. Bard also enlisted the collaboration of Jones for this endeavor.

Founding the New York Hospital

In 1770, Jones and Bard, along with Peter Middleton, petitioned King George III for a charter to build a hospital in New York. The petition was approved, and the charter was presented in July 1771. Remembering the horrific rounds at Hôtel Dieu in Paris two decades prior, Jones wanted to make sure the same misery would not be repeated in New York. In particular, he wanted ample space and fresh air, and gave detailed advice to the builders. He was pleased to see what was already accomplished during the construction phase: "The principle wards, which are to contain not more than eight beds, are thirty-six feet in length, twenty-four feet wide and eighteen high. They are all well ventilated, not only from the opposite disposition of the windows, but proper openings in the side walls, and the doors open into a long passage or gallery, thoroughly ventilated from north to south."[299]

In addition to his involvement in the construction of the new hospital, Jones sailed back to London for fundraising and to find equipment for the building. Although these were important enough missions for his second visit to England in 1772–1774, Jones also had two additional plans. First, he wanted to reconnect with his old mentors. He was able to meet with the Hunter brothers and Percivall Pott again. His meeting with Pott was warm and confirmed the respect and friendship the two surgeons held for each other. When the two colleagues said goodbye, Pott presented Jones with a complete copy of his lecture series, which was the basis for a three-volume work on surgery that Pott had just published.[300]

Second, Jones was hoping to see his asthma improve by breathing the London air. Although this seemed to be completely unrealistic, considering the congestion and poor air quality in the British capital, Jones's airways miraculously cleared, and his breathing problems improved. As his biographer Dr. Mease reported, "In the thick smoke, and an atmosphere impregnated with every species of animal putrefaction and effluvia, where so many asthmatics have found such remarkable benefit, he also experienced a considerable alleviation of his complaint."[301] Indeed, the "health-giving air of London" was hard to explain.

When he returned to New York, Jones found the construction of the hospital to be in full swing. In the fall of 1774, the board of governors was ready to appoint the first "Physicians of Ordinary" to the hospital staff. Not surprisingly, both John Jones and Samuel Bard were among the four doctors who were scheduled to admit and treat patients at the New York Hospital. But then tragedy struck.

In February 1775, the almost completed building was destroyed in a fire. The event was reported by the *New York Gazette and Weekly Mercury* on March 6, 1775: "On Tuesday last, between twelve and one o'clock, the new hospital at Ranelagh, a large pile of buildings lately erected and nearly finished, was discovered to be on fire, the workmen being all gone to dinner, and the whole wooden part of the building was, in about an hour, reduced to ashes." Although the rebuilding of the hospital was started immediately, the Revolutionary War—and lack of money—postponed its official opening until January 1791.

Plain Concise Practical Remarks on the Treatment of Wounds and Fractures

In late 1775, Jones published *Plain Concise Practical Remarks on the Treatment of Wounds and Fractures; to which is Added, a Short Appendix on Camp and Military Hospitals; Principally Designed for the Use of young Military Surgeons in North-America*. The volume is remarkable for several reasons. It has gone down in history as the first medical text authored by an American and published on the continent; and it was the first surgical text and the first work on military surgery published in the colonies. Even though the book built on Jones's doctoral thesis written almost twenty-five years earlier, and has been described by some medical historians as "little more than a condensation of the teachings of Henri Le Dran, Percivall Pott, and other European surgeons,"[302] all of whom had mentored Jones in the 1750s, the volume's enormous influence for both the surgical care during the American Revolution, and American surgery in general, cannot be overstated. Because of its significance, the description of the book is given generous space in this chapter.

Although the title was long, the book itself was relatively short and is often referred to as a manual. The publication turned out to be timely, and the book was used by most, if not all military surgeons during the Revolutionary War. A second edition was published after only a year.

The book had four sections. Jones began by dedicating the work to his cousin and mentor, Thomas Cadwalader. The war between the colonists and the motherland had just erupted, and the unrest on the continent colored the words to Cadwalader: "The present calamitous situation of this once happy country...demands the aid and assistance of every virtuous citizen."[303] Jones understood it was too late for a peaceful solution to the conflict between the colonies and England and was pleading to everybody to do what they could: "If he cannot cure the fatal diseases of this unfortunate country; it will, at least, afford him some consolation, to have poured a little balm into her bleeding wounds."

Jones hoped the manual would be particularly useful when fighting started and surgeons needed to treat injuries sustained on the battlefields. He explained that he had selected "the sentiments of the best modern surgeons upon the treatment of those accidents, which are most likely to attend our present unnatural contest." Jones signed his dedication to Cadwalader on October 12, 1775—a time when Boston, occupied by the British, was under siege by Washington and his Continental Army.

The initial pages that paid tribute to Cadwalader were followed by an introduction addressed "To the STUDENTS and young Practitioners in SURGERY, through all America." In this section, Jones repeated many of the points he had made during his inaugural lecture in surgery at the King's College in November 1767. He again elaborated his desire to have surgeons well educated, not only in the manual aspects of their profession but in physics (medicine) as well. This was a theme to which Jones kept coming back. He again expressed his disagreement with those (particularly in Europe) who favored a separation of surgeons (doing the manual work only) from the physicians (understanding the underlying causes of disease and considered intellectually superior to the surgeons).

Jones was especially critical of Dr. Gregory, a celebrated Professor of Physic at Edinburgh, and warned against "the fatal consequences of a total separation of physic and surgery" advocated by many of the European physicians who "arrogated" themselves "an exclusive knowledge of science," which meant that the surgeon should just be an "operator, to whom the mere manual part was committed." Jones scorned this philosophy and claimed that if surgeons only performed manual work without an understanding of the "physics" behind the conditions they treated, they would be like "comedians."[304]

As a professor, Jones also used the introduction to again outline important aspects of the education and character of a good surgeon. Surgeons should be "thoroughly acquainted with most of the branches of medicine, which are requisite to form an accomplished physician." They should have an "accurate knowledge of the structure of the human body,"[305] and they "ought to have firm steady hands." Jones also pointed out other subjects of learning that were important for a successful surgeon, including languages, mathematics, chemistry, and *materia medica*. In addition, he emphasized the importance of continued education and recommended "a diligent, attentive, and repeated perusal of the best English practical writers," among whom Jones considered Pott one of the very best. Finally, Jones ended the introduction by giving harsh words to those "who will neither read nor reason, but practice at a venture, and sport with the lives and limbs of their fellow-creatures" and suggested they should make themselves acquainted with "the sixth commandment, which is *Thou shalt not kill.*"[306]

Having set the agenda, Jones then delved into the eleven chapters that were the meat of the book. It is of interest even for today's surgeons to review some of the points discussed by Jones. There are several examples of treatments that have stood the test of time.

The eleven chapters published in the second 1776 edition were:

Chapter I: Of wounds in general
Chapter II: Of inflammation
Chapter III: Of the division of wounds
Chapter IV: Of wounds penetrating the thorax and abdomen
Chapter V: Of simple fractures of the limbs
Chapter VI: Of compound fractures
Chapter VII: Of amputation
Chapter VIII: Of blows on the head
Chapter IX: Of injuries arising from the commotion of concussion
Chapter X: Of injuries arising from a fracture of the skull
Chapter XI: Of gun-shot wounds

In the first chapter, Jones gave a detailed description of different types of wounds and how they heal. He also mentioned that some wounds are universally fatal, such as injuries to the aorta: "every wound of the aorta must be attended with certain death." Wounds to the arteries of the limbs, however, were survivable if managed correctly; he recommended that a "tourniquet may be applied till the bleeding vessel can be taken up by a ligature."[307] Almost 250 years after Jones's recommendation, modern military surgeons have revived the use of a tourniquet to stop life-threatening hemorrhages.

When Jones described the stages of wound healing, he recounted that the infection and formation of pus commonly seen in those days was actually praiseworthy. The suppuration was "laudable" because it "produces very happy effects, by separating the lacerated vessels and extravasated fluids from the sound parts which then grow up a-fresh." This was the rationale why "laudable pus [was] esteemed by surgeons one of the best signs."

When contemplating how beautifully nature heals wounds, Jones criticized attempts to improve the process by using "balsams, and…nostrums," as often done by "not only quacks and empirics," but also by poorly educated physicians and surgeons. He recommended "nothing but dry, soft lint, to recent wounds, which is usually the best application through the whole course of the cure."

In the second chapter, Jones underscored the importance of understanding inflammation, "a subject of which every person, who intends to practice surgery, should endeavor to acquire just and accurate ideas." Whatever the cause of the inflammation, Jones recommended "anodynes… bleeding, gentle laxatives, warm baths," and soft dressings to "the parts affected." He recommended surgeons' involvement in "the first stage of the disease, where prevention may be happily substituted for a cure." To reduce inflammation, Jones stated that "all stimulating foreign bodies must also be removed," (a recommendation that was somewhat controversial at the time), and "abscesses should be opened."

It is fascinating that inflammation, which is nowadays considered to be involved in many diseases (including cancer, heart disease, and obesity, to mention just a few), was given such a prominent position by Jones, and that he understood the importance of the condition.

Discussing different types of wounds (the division of wounds), Jones elaborated on divergent methods of wound care. A superficial incision, particularly when made in a longitudinal direction of an extremity, could be treated with a "uniting bandage." When deeper or oblique, sutures would be needed. The suture (sometimes called "ligature" here) should be placed with a needle dipped in oil, and the wound edges should be brought together by "making a double knot" of the suture "without wrinkling or puckering the parts." The writing suggests that Jones understood the importance of closing the wound without tension, something that today's students are also still learning.

Jones recommended removal of the sutures a surprisingly short time after closure of the incision: "either [on] the second, or third day, often in twenty-four hours."[308] The use of "a piece of adhesive plaster, embracing a large portion of the external integuments on each side" may explain why early suture removal was possible without dehiscence of the skin. Puncture wounds "which do not penetrate into either cavity of the body" (abdomen or thorax) did not require any particular mode of treatment.

Surgeons differed in their opinions about the treatment of lacerations. Whereas some practitioners favored "removal of the lips" (skin edges), basically converting a slashing into an incisional would, other surgeons, including Jones, favored a more conservative approach, which preserved as much of the skin edges as "the nature of the case will admit." In some cases, however, even Jones recommended a more aggressive approach: "If the torn lips are very unequal" they should be removed "to the state of a simple incisional wound."

An interesting section in this chapter discusses injuries to tendons. Jones explained that if the ends of a cut tendon are "brought into contact, and [preserved] by the means of a proper bandage in that situation; no suture is ever made use of."

In particular, Jones considered rupture of the Achilles tendon. He recommended a conservative approach utilized by the French surgeon Le Dran. In order to approximate the ends of the torn Achilles tendon, the knee was bent, and the foot was extended (positioned with the toes pointing downwards). The extremity was kept in this position by using a "leather knee piece" placed behind the joint. A "piece of thin wood...[was] fixed to the sole of an old slipper, and one end of it projecting near three inches beyond the heel." A strap was used to connect the lower part of the leather knee piece with the end of the protruding piece of wood, and the strap was shortened "to bring the extremities of the divided tendon into perfect contact."[309] The leg and foot were then kept in this position with "absolute rest" for several weeks. The nonsurgical approach described here still remains an option today.

When Jones summarized the treatment of different types of wounds, he added the following statement, reflecting the teaching of the time: "I scarcely need observe, that moderate evacuation, by bleeding, and gentle purging, together with a low diet, are, in these cases absolutely necessary."

"Wounds penetrating the thorax and abdomen" (Chapter IV) were a reality during the Revolutionary War. Whereas wounds to the chest resulting in injury to the aorta or heart were considered nonsurvivable, "because those parts are immediately subservient to life," injuries to the lung and most intra-abdominal organs, including "liver, intestine, kidneys, pancreas, gallbladder, large vessels, spleen, mesentery, bladder and stomach," sometimes saw survivors. It is amazing to read about some of the war injuries and Jones's treatment recommendations, which called for courageous surgeons and heroic patients who suffered through major surgical procedures without the benefit of anesthesia. For example, when Jones recounted abdominal wounds resulting in evisceration of abdominal contents, he wrote, "Should any portion of the intestines or omentum, the usual parts protruded, be forced out, they ought as early as possible to be reduced [pushed back into the abdomen], by placing the patient on his back, with his hips a little elevated, and then with the fore finger of each hand, gently and alternately pressing the protruded part into its proper position."[310]

In the absence of X-rays and other diagnostic tools, the surgeons had to rely on signs, symptoms, and physical examinations. The consequences of penetrating wounds of the thorax, which resulted in injuries to the lungs, had been well known to military surgeons for generations: "The most remarkable of these, are the passage of air through the wound in respiration, and the expectoration of frothy blood from the lungs when they are wounded." If the wound caused bleeding in the chest (hemothorax), Jones understood the importance of removing the blood to allow the victim to breath: "If the wound be made with a bayonet or small sword, the external orfice must be immediately enlarged, in order to give a free discharge of the blood lodged in the cavity."

The management of fractures followed the same basic principles that are adhered to today. In the absence of X-rays, the diagnosis of a fracture was purely clinical. First, the fracture needed to be reduced (set) and the bone fragments aligned as much as possible. The alignment of the fracture was guided by what the surgeon saw and felt when setting the bone. Second, the extremity needed to be retained in the correct position using splints made of wood or leather-covered pasteboards.

If the fracture was associated with a wound of the skin overlying the bone, or protrusion of a bone fragment through the skin, the injury was a compound (open) fracture. A compound fracture was (and still is) a more serious situation, mainly because of the risk of infection and the development of life-threatening sepsis and gangrene.

Because of the risks associated with compound fractures, some surgeons (including Pott in London before his own open fracture) recommended immediate amputation, and others argued for a conservative management and saving the extremity if at all possible. They claimed that the majority of the upfront amputations were done unnecessarily.

Jones made the interesting observation that surgeons who recommended immediate amputation were often big city practitioners, caring for their patients in crowded and dirty hospitals. Surgeons who reported successes when compound fractures were treated conservatively, however, were often private practitioners working in the countryside or small towns, caring for their patients in smaller hospitals or the patients' homes. Jones suspected that the high rates of life-threatening infections and gangrene seen among the patients in the big city hospitals reflected the lack of hygiene with crowded wards filled with patients suffering from putrid wounds and ulcers. Pott and others claimed that the "ill effects of hospital air" was the cause of infections. The surgeons in smaller and cleaner facilities, on the other hand, did not have to contend with such conditions.

In the concluding paragraphs of the chapter on compound fractures, Jones gave the following advice to the young practitioners: "If placed in a large or crowded hospital, speedy amputation should take place, but in private practice, and in pure and healthy air, every effort should be exerted to save the limb."[311]

When amputation (for a compound fracture or for other reasons) was inevitable, the patient was facing not only the horrible pain from the surgery, but also the loss of a leg or an arm. Jones advised "young surgeons" to make certain that patients who were to undergo an amputation were reassured as much as possible. He emphasized that it was important "to support the patient's spirit with a chearful [*sic*] assurance of success." The surgeon should show confidence without arrogance: "the appearance of such a degree of modest confidence as may serve to inspire…[the patient]."

In the chapter on amputations, Jones went on to discuss preparations for the procedure. He recommended that instruments and other equipment be assembled not in front of the patient but (mercifully!) "in a different room." Having the patient watch the amputating knife, saw, tenaculum, needles, and sharp scissors being gathered in full sight would obviously add to the torture.

Jones described in detail the technical aspects of different types of amputations (leg, arm, hand, finger, and toe). Ligatures were to be used to stop bleedings from big blood vessels. Various techniques to cover the end of the bone and to close the wound at the stump were also discussed. Needless to say, in the absence of anesthesia, the pain was horrific. Even if alcohol, typically in the form of wine, and laudanum were used in generous quantities, speed was of essence to shorten the suffering. Jones, however, cautioned against risking severe complications if the amputation was too rushed: "Never affect great expedition, by which very capital and even fatal errors have been committed."

Towards the end of the volume, Jones devoted three chapters to the management of head injuries. In the first of those chapters, he discussed wound injuries of the scalp and pointed out that although many of the injuries could be treated like other wounds, some scalp injuries required special considerations. The closeness to the underlying brain and its membranes, Jones pointed out, posed a risk of infections and abscesses with "symptoms of an oppressed brain." In general, Jones argued for a conservative approach when treating wound injuries of the scalp. This involved keeping as much tissue as possible and refraining from removing too generous pieces of lacerated skin edges: "When a large portion of the scalp has been separated and detached from the pericranium, either by a lacerated or incised wound; the part so separated, after being cleaned from dirt and coagulated blood; ought to be brought as nearly as possible into contact; and then secured by the interrupted suture, with proper compress and bandage."

If the patient developed "a smart fever, severe pain in the head, great anxiety and restlessness, frequent shiverings, a nausea, delirium and convulsions" several days after a "blow on the head" and wound injury of the scalp, Jones warned that "there will be great reason to suspect that the parts within the skull are affected, either by some extravasated fluid, pressing upon the brain, or from an inflammation and suppuration of the dura and pia mater."[312] Under these circumstances, the surgeon should act immediately and perforate the skull bone to make certain that blood or infected material is "speedily removed by proper evacuations."

When describing concussions, Jones provided a list of symptoms that are still the basis for the clinical diagnosis of concussion: "There is generally an immediate suspension of the common functions of the brain, to a certain degree; the patient has a vertigo or giddiness, an inclination to vomit, upon swallowing any liquid, has a wildness in his looks, talks incoherently, is restless and sleepless, with little or no fever." Jones's treatment of patients consisted of "gentle evacuations by bleeding, lenient purgatives and sudorific anodynes." This regiment "frequently removes most of the complaints occasioned by concussion, in twenty-four hours, or two or three days at the farthest."

If the symptoms were to return, "the surgeon ought immediately...be upon his guard, as further mischief, than a mere shock or derangement of the brain is to be suspected." He recommended that "the evacuations already mentioned, in particular bleeding, are to be repeated." If things did not improve, or even worsened, trepanation may be needed. When there was suspicion of an epidural or subdural hematoma or abscess, taking out a circular piece of skull bone using a trephine (a surgical instrument with a cylindrical blade used to cut a hole in the skull bone) was not foreign to the surgeons of the day.

The third chapter devoted to head injuries (Chapter X) dealt with "injuries arising from a fracture of the skull." Jones made the important distinction between "undepressed" and "depressed" fractures (the latter having a bone fragment pushed inwards into the skull). He argued that many patients with undepressed fractures did not need any specific treatment and that "the application of the trephine" would only be necessary for the evacuation of blood or "matter formed in consequence of an inflammation of the dura mater."

When a depressed fracture was encountered, trepanation should always be performed to allow for the insertion of an instrument (elevator) under the depressed bone fragment to lift it up. If blood accumulated between the dura mater and the skull bone, the blood would be evacuated at the same time. If there was suspicion of blood under the durra mater, the dura should be opened "with the point of a lancet, in order to discharge whatever collection may be formed beneath."

Although burring a hole in the skull may seem like a scary proposition (for both patient and surgeon), Jones remarkably seemed to dismiss the anxiety: "As to the operation itself, and particularly the part of it which consists in perforating the bone, there is neither pain, difficulty, nor danger in it." A little further into the chapter, however, Jones pointed out that the surgeon "might fatally plunge the crown of the trephine into the patient's brain; an accident that has happened to some incautious operators."

Gunshot Wounds

The final chapter of *Plain Concise Practical Remarks* elaborated on gunshot wounds, of course highly relevant for surgeons in the Revolutionary War. The management of wounds caused "by a musket of pistol ball" had two purposes: first, the ball should be extracted, and second, the bleeding should be controlled.

Controversy surrounded the first objective. Some surgeons advocated aggressive attempts to remove the bullet, whereas others, including the French surgeon Le Dran, advised "as little search with the probe or forceps as possible" since the irritation caused by aggressive probing of the wound "increases the consequent pain and inflammation." Jones subscribed to the opinion "that we ought not to the attempt the extraction of any thing which lies beyond the reach of the finger." If the surgeon tried to extract the ball, Jones emphasized that the entrance "should be considerably dilated," in order to make it easier to find the bullet.

Cannonballs, of course, caused more severe injures than musket balls, and loss of extremities were not uncommon: "A leg or an arm is frequently carried off by a cannon ball," rendering amputation necessary. Jones pointed out that in such injuries, "the operation should always be performed high enough to leave no fractured bones above the amputated part."

When Jones discussed the consequences of a gunshot wound to the thorax, he described how to manage a pneumothorax (accumulation of air in the chest compressing the lungs and making breathing difficult and ultimately impossible). This could happen if the sharp edge of a fractured rib injured the lung: "The only remedy, capable of affording effectual relief in so distressing a situation, is, to perform the operation of the *paracentesis thoracis,* or opening into the cavity of the chest, through which the confined air may be discharged" (thereby removing the pressure on the lung). He described for the young surgeon in detail how this lifesaving procedure should be performed.

In some cases, the air could escape the chest cavity and enter the subcutaneous space (the space under the skin). Jones described how the subcutaneous air "sometimes distends it [the subcutaneous space] to a monstrous size, extending over great part of the body, face and limbs." If it became too extensive, Jones recommended that multiple small skin cuts be made "with the knife or lancet"—the skin could then be compressed "to force out the confined air."

The Appendix

The last section of *Plain Concise Practical Remarks* was an appendix, added to provide "some short hints on the structure and oeconomy of hospitals." In it, Jones spared no words to express his appall with the conditions of big city hospitals, particularly in London and Paris. He quoted statistics that were staggering: "In the two great hospitals of St. Thomas and St. Bartholomew, in London," he claimed that, "about six hundred patients die annually which is about one in thirteen of those who are admitted as in-patients." To see a death rate of almost 8 percent among 7,800 admissions was indeed upsetting.

The statistics in Paris were even grimmer: "The hotel Dieu, a vast building situated in the middle of that great city, receives about twenty-two thousand persons annually, one fifth of which number die every year." The approximately 4,400 patients who died annually at Hôtel Dieu accounted for one third of all the deaths in the city.

Jones was convinced that bad air in the overcrowded hospitals caused the high death rates, and the state of affairs sickened him. He used strong words to condemn "such glaring absurdities," and blamed them on "sources of darkness and ignorance." He likened the hospitals with "lazarettos or pest-houses." He had already used his experiences at Hôtel Dieu when giving advice to the builders of the New York Hospital: "It evidently appears, how essentially necessary pure fresh air is, to the cure of diseases in general, and particularly those, which arise from putrescent causes either internal or external."

Jones was frustrated when simple measures were not taken to provide open spaces such as making certain windows were opened to allow fresh air to enter. Instead, money was spent on other items, as "in one of the last hospitals built in London…there is more expense bestowed upon an elegant chapel in it, than would have finished four wards." He expanded upon this thought by declaring "the physician and architect, have generally two very opposite and incompatible views."

Jones's cries for fresh air and cleanliness echoed demands made by others. In particular, we have already seen how Benjamin Rush championed the same ideas.

The British Take Over New York City and Jones Leaves to Join the Continental Army

After the Battle of Long Island—a disaster for George Washington and his Continental Army—it was not long before the British had full control of New York City. Jones, one of only two non-Loyalist members of the King's College medical faculty, started to get nervous. He realized he would have to leave to avoid persecution by the British military and the rage of Loyalist New Yorkers who had been assaulted by Sons of Liberty and other opponents of the motherland.

Although Jones was against the aggressive actions taken by some anti-government individuals, it is clear he was on the side of the rebels. Despite being assured of safety, Jones left New York City in September 1776, never to return. When fleeing New York, Jones understood that his property was at risk of being either ransacked and destroyed or taken over by British squatters. He was more concerned, however, about a manuscript and some collectables from Europe. When leaving the city, Jones told Mease that he had a manuscript ready to be published. Its content was meteorological observations made over the last ten years in New York, together with descriptions of common diseases during the same period. When leaving New York, Jones put the manuscript "in a place of apparent safety in a neighboring state" together with anatomical preparations that he had collected during his two visits to England. Unfortunately, a dishonest colleague, "a brother professor," had gotten wind of the hidden treasures and stole them in order to convert them "to his own profit." Jones never saw them again.

Jones traveled north to join the Continental Army in Albany.[313] He was enlisted as an assistant surgeon for the Tenth Massachusetts Regiment and was promoted to surgeon of that regiment one year later. When the British evacuated Philadelphia in 1778, Jones was dispatched to the city on official duty—something he was probably not opposed to since his asthma had started to act up again, and he hoped the change of climate would improve his lung problems.

Unfortunately, his asthma did not get better, and in May 1781, he resigned from the army because of his health. He was to remain in the City of Brotherhood until his death ten years later.

The Years in Philadelphia

After his resignation from the army, Jones built a large and prosperous practice in his new hometown. He was still recognized for his skills in cutting for stone and midwifery, but like most surgeons in those days, he also took care of patients with other surgical and medical ailments. Jones was appointed to the staff of the Pennsylvania Hospital, succeeding John Redman, who was retiring. Jones kept the appointment at the hospital till his demise.

In 1786, the Pennsylvania Hospital was no longer able to provide care for the poor; many previous generous donors were no longer around, and the "paper bills of credit" had been depreciated and lost significant value. To continue to help the poor and sick, a dispensary was established, attended to by both younger and more expert physicians. The poor were "furnished with medicine...and attended by eminent physicians." Jones was among the doctors appointed to attend the patients, and was reelected annually until the end of his career. Mease commented in his biography of Jones that the institution "dispensed health, and removed disease from thousands." Benjamin Rush asked, "In what other charitable institution do we perceive so great a quantity of distress relieved by so small an expense?"[314]

Jones did not only become popular among patients, but was also a respected and admired colleague in the medical community of Philadelphia. In 1787, he cofounded the College of Physicians of Philadelphia along with twenty-three other surgeons, including John Redman, Benjamin Rush, John Morgan and William Shippen Jr. It was indeed an impressive group of physicians and surgeons, who all had played important roles in the American Revolution and in their profession, as we have already seen. Redman was elected the first president of the College and Jones its first vice president.

Jones and Benjamin Franklin's Bladder Stone

Since Jones was one of the most prominent physicians in Philadelphia, it is not surprising that some of its most celebrated residents became his patients. Benjamin Franklin and George Washington were among them.

Benjamin Franklin had suffered from bladder stones for many years, both during his extended periods spent in Europe and after coming back and settling in Philadelphia. During his last years, spells of gout expanded his list of ailments.

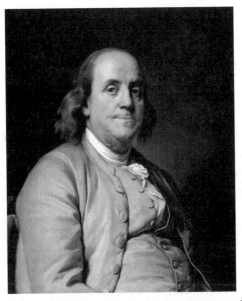

Benjamin Franklin. Portrait painting by Joseph Siffred Duplessis 1778. Franklin suffered from bladder stones for many years. He was a close friend and private patient of Dr. John Jones. (National Portrait Gallery)

Born in Boston in 1706, Franklin had seen the pain and suffering bladder stones caused his own family. Towards the end of his long and otherwise healthy life, his father had had a bladder stone. In 1744, Franklin wrote a letter to his parents, discussing the treatment of his younger brother John's bladder stone. At that time, John was treated with a solvent, primarily based on lye, and Benjamin recommended adding honey and molasses to the mixture in the hope of dissolving the stone—or at least preventing the formation of new stones. The medical treatment was not successful, and the stone continued to agonize John. In particular, he had frequent episodes of inability to pass water and underwent treatment with a stiff silver rod. His physicians passed the rod through the urethra to dislodge the stone when it blocked the outlet from the bladder. Passage of a catheter was also used to empty the bladder when a stone caused stoppage of the urine.

In 1752, Benjamin invented a flexible catheter, a more humane device than the stiff silver rods and catheters used by John's physicians. In a detailed letter to his brother, Franklin explained that the catheter was constructed of flat silver wire wound spirally and was able to pass "any irregularities" of the urethra. He recommended the catheter to be covered with "a small fine gut" or that "tallow be rubbed over it, to smooth it and fill the joints." In addition to the catheter, Franklin provided a wire that could be inserted into the catheter to stiffen it for its passage up the urethra. Before withdrawing the catheter, Franklin emphasized that the wire should be taken out to lessen the diameter of the catheter "whereby it will move more easily." Franklin also continued to recommend different medications to dissolve the bladder stones, although he realized the medication would "probably not dissolve gravel and stone" but "may go a great way toward preventing these disorders."

Franklin himself started to develop symptoms of bladder stones in the mid–1700s. Occasionally, severe manifestations of his stones impacted his involvement in the American Revolution. He was in Paris in 1782 when the peace negotiations between the United States and Britain started (ultimately resulting in the Treaty of Paris in 1783, signaling the end of the American Revolution). Franklin was seventy-six years old and was one of the principle negotiators on the American side. During the fall of 1782, the symptoms from his bladder stones increased both in frequency and severity, and on several occasions, he was unable to attend the negotiations in person.

Franklin remained the United States Ambassador in Paris for two years after the conclusion of the peace negotiations. During this time, his symptoms kept increasing. He described his agony in several letters to friends and colleagues. In December 1783, he wrote to Comte de Vergennes, the French Minister of Foreign Affairs, "Because now being disabled by the Stone, which in the Easiest Carriage gives me Pain, wounds my bladder, and occasions me to make bloody Urine, I find I can no longer pay my Devoirs personally at Versailles, which I hope will be excused."

During this period, Franklin tried medical treatment, including Alexander Blackrie's solvent. He knew that cutting for the stone would be the definitive treatment, but was afraid of the tremendous pain caused by the procedure. There were severe risks for complications and death, particularly at his age: "It is true, as you have heard, that I have the stone, but not that I had thoughts of being cut for it." In an exchange of letters with one of his friends, Franklin wrote, "I thank you much for the Postscript regarding my Disorder the Stone. I have taken heretofore, and am now again taking the Remedy you mention, which is called Blackrie's solvent. It is the soap lie, with lime water, and I believe it may have some effect in diminishing the symptoms, and preventing the growth of the stone, which is all I expect from it." In another letter, penned around the same time and directed to his friend in London, Dr. Benjamin Vaughan, Franklin acknowledged the receipt of "the other Bottle of Blackrie."

Franklin wanted to read and learn more about the solvent, and asked his nephew, Jonathan Williams, to purchase the book by Alexander Blackrie, *A disquisition on medicines that dissolve the stone. In which Dr. Chittick's secret is considered and discovered.*

In July 1785, Franklin wrote to Vaughan, describing his symptoms. He asked Vaughan to send copies of the letter to colleagues requesting their advice, in particular with regards to Franklin's decision not to undergo lithotomy. Vaughan sent the letter to several prominent surgeons in London, including Doctors John Hunter, William Watson, William Heberden, and Adair Crawford.

In the letter to Vaughan, Franklin described his situation in third person, but it was no secret who the patient was. Franklin provided a vivid description of the signs and symptoms caused by his bladder stone. He wrote,

> The patient is now in his 79th year. When a young Man he was sometimes troubled with gravelly Complaints; But they wore off without the use of any Medicine, and he remained more than Fifty Years free from them.

> In the Autumn of 1782, he had a severe Attack.... He daily voided Gravel Stones the Size of small Pease, took now and then some Decoctions of Herbs & Roots that were prescribed him by Friends or Physicians....

Franklin had periods when his symptoms were more tolerable, but then his suffering would reappear:

At length the painful Part of the Disorder left him, and no more large Gravel offer'd; but observing Sand constantly in his Urine…the Malady return'd in the Autumn of 1783, when he first perceived after going in his Carriage on the Pavement, that he felt Pain & made bloody Water. At times when he was making Water in full Stream, something came and stopt the Passage; this he suspected to be small Stone, and he suffered pain by the Stoppage. He found however by Experience that he could be laying down on his Side to cause the Obstruction to remove and continue the Operation. He now thinks the Stone is grown bigger & heavier as he is sensible of its falling from Side to Side, as he turns in his Bed.

Franklin continued the description of the symptoms: "His Inclination to make Water is Sometimes very sudden & very violent, tho' the Quantity small. He feels no Pain, nor is it at all sensible of the Existence of the Stone, except when it obstructs his Making Water, or when he is in his Carriage on a Pavement, or on some sudden Motion or Turn of the Body…." He asked for remedies but made it clear that he did not want surgery: "He would chuse to bear with it rather than have Recourse to dangerous or nauseous Remedies." He also pointed out that if there was no medicine that could dissolve the stone, he would at least be happy if there was something that prevented the stone from growing bigger: "If therefore no safe and sure Dissolvent of the Stone is yet known, he wishes to be informed whether there is a Regimen proper to be observ'd for preventing its Increase…."

As requested, Vaughan made copies of the letter and sent them around for the opinions of several distinguished surgeons. All of them gave interesting suggestions in how the disorder could be managed with different medicines and dietary measures, but they all agreed that cutting for the stone was not an option for the elderly patient. John Hunter wrote, "From the History of the Case, and a distinct account of the patient's feelings, we have no doubt that there is a Stone in the Bladder. Taking into account the Time of Life of the Patient, and that the Symptoms are not so urgent as to render Life uncomfortable, we approve much of his resolution not to risk an operation…." The other consultants gave the same recommendation.

For example, Dr. Heberden wrote that he entirely agreed "in recommending to the gentleman not to think of an operation at such an advanced age" and Dr. Crawford echoed the same sentiment: "An Operation would not be advisable."

So Franklin ended up living with his bladder stone for the rest of his life.

In the summer of 1785, while his case was still being considered and discussed by London doctors, Franklin decided it was finally time to return to America. After a seven-week journey across the Atlantic, he arrived at Philadelphia on September 14. He continued to be plagued by his bladder stone, and the last couple of years of his life turned out to be miserable. Despite that, he tried to be active and involved, both socially and politically. He participated in the Constitutional Convention of 1787. He carried on an extensive correspondence with old friends and colleagues in both America and Europe, and he kept working on his autobiography.

Weakened by the constant pain from his bladder stone (and from recurring episodes of gout), Franklin spent most of his time in bed. He became dependent on opium to get relief from his pain. His optimistic outlook of life failed him, and he lost any belief he might have still had in the medical treatment of bladder stones. In a letter to Vaughan, Franklin wrote, "I am quite discouraged, and have no longer any faith in remedies for the stone. The palliating system is what I am now fixed in. Opium gives me ease when I am attacked by pain, and by the use of it I make life at least tolerable."

Only a couple of weeks before his death, Franklin was visited by his friend Thomas Jefferson, now secretary of state under President Washington and a supporter of the French Revolution. In a letter to the French Revolutionist Louis Le Vieillard, Jefferson gave an account of his visit with Franklin: "I wish I could add to your happiness by giving you a favourable account of the good old Doctor. I found him in bed where he remains almost constantly. He had been clear of pain for some days and was cheerful and in good spirits. He listened with a glow of interest to the details of your revolution and of his friends which I gave him. He is much emaciated. I pressed him to continue the narration of his life and perhaps he will."

Franklin and Jones were intimate personal friends—Franklin had included Jones in his will—but they also had a close patient-doctor relationship. Jones had served as Franklin's physician for several years after Franklin's return to Philadelphia and was well aware of Franklin's bladder stone. During the last couple of weeks before Franklin's death, Jones cared for Franklin almost around the clock.

In an article published both in the *Pennsylvania Gazette* and *Freeman's Journal* four days after Franklin's death, Jones's account of Franklin's last days read in part: "The stone, with which he had been afflicted for several years, had for the last twelve months of his life, confined him chiefly to his bed; and during the extremely painful paroxysms, he was obliged to take large doses of laudanum to mitigate his tortures." Then Franklin's condition deteriorated further, and "about sixteen days before his death he was seized with a feverish indisposition...when he complained of a pain in his left breast, which increased till it became extremely acute...and on the 17th instant, about eleven o'clock at night, he quietly expired, closing a long and useful life of eighty-four years and three months."[315]

President Washington's Pneumonia

The other celebrity whom Jones doctored was Washington. In the summer of 1790, President Washington, who was in the capital, New York City, fell ill from a disease of "inflammatory nature"[316] (probably pneumonia on top of influenza).[317] Mease described the circumstances: "After having been for some days indisposed, [the President] became so ill, that other assistance in addition to that of his attending physician became necessary." The attending physician was Samuel Bard (who had only one year earlier saved Washington's life by cutting open an abscess on the President's leg[318]), and when he saw the condition worsen despite his efforts, he asked his previous partner and mentor, John Jones, for help. Notwithstanding his busy private practice in Philadelphia, Jones dropped everything at hand and hurried up to New York. There, he found that the president's condition "had terminated in an alarming state of debility, and violent spasmodic difficulty of breathing, which threatened the greatest danger." Washington's cabinet members feared for his life, and after the ordeal, Thomas Jefferson wrote, "We have been very near losing the President."

One has to assume that Jones's and Bard's treatment included bleeding and purging, some of the cornerstones in the management of fevers and inflammation during the period. Despite, rather than because of, these therapies, Washington improved and ultimately survived (he was to be less lucky later in life when similar treatments probably contributed to his death). Mease described how "a manifest alteration for the better was perceived, and in a few days the President was out of danger."

When the capital was moved to Philadelphia later that same year, Washington thankfully remembered Jones's efforts during his illness and appointed him his family physician, an honor that Jones kept until his death.

The End

On June 17, 1791, after paying a short visit to the President, Jones returned home feeling frozen and exhausted.[319] The day had started out "very sultry" but had turned cold and chilly in the evening. He was not dressed for the colder temperature, and despite not feeling well, he made a couple of house calls before finally reaching his house. The morning after, Jones woke up feeling miserable with high fever and diarrhea, and "a great prostration of strength." His asthma was again acting up, and over the next several days, Jones became increasingly weaker. After six days of agony, Jones expired in his sleep at the age of sixty-three.

On June 23, 1791, Benjamin Rush wrote in his diary, "This day died Dr. John Jones.... He was much lamented by his friends and patients, as was he by his brother physicians...his manners were gentle and amiable, and his conduct truly liberal in his profession. He was without a rival in surgery in the United States."[320]

Jones was put to rest in the Quaker burial ground at Archer Street in a manner consistent with his character. The humble surgeon, who had once refused to conform to the request from his fellow physicians to mark his importance with a wig and a golden head cane, had repeatedly expressed a desire to have a funeral "without the ridiculous pomp of ceremonious interment, but in a plain manner." His wish was granted.

CHAPTER 9

JAMES THACHER—
Military Journal During the
American Revolutionary War

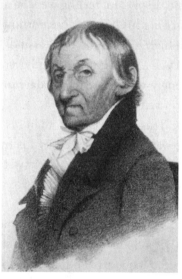

James Thacher (1754–1844). His detailed and voluminous
Military Journal During the American Revolutionary War has
taught us much about what it was like to be a surgeon during
the American War of Independence. (The History Collection)

J ames Thacher (1754–1844) was born at Barnstable on the south coast of Cape Cod. He saw daylight for the first time on February 14, 1754. Two major sources contribute insight into Thacher's life: the annual address on the 110th anniversary of the Massachusetts Medical Society, delivered by Dr. James B. Brewster, that was devoted to the life of Thacher and published the same year in the *Boston Medical and Surgical Journal*; and Thacher's own *Medical Journal During the American Revolutionary War, From 1775 to 1783*, published in 1823.

Medical Training

Thacher decided early in life to go into medicine. He was apprenticed to a local physician, Dr. Abner Hersey, at the young age of sixteen. Although Thacher's proctor was a celebrated Barnstable doctor with the entire Cape Cod as his catchment area, he was also quite a character, described by Brewster as "eccentric in the extreme."[321]

Abner had started his own medical training under his brother James, who was a reputable physician at Barnstable. When James died, only about a year into Abner's training, he left him a thriving practice. Dr. Abner Hersey soon gained the trust of his brother's patients and served many of the seven to eight thousand people living on Cape Cod at the time.

Hersey was probably a little nutty, not only when it came to the ways he dressed and ate, but also with regards to his social skills (or lack thereof). Hersey could be seen traveling around Cape Cod in large and baggy clothes that were lined with green baize. When the weather was bad (not too unusual in this part of New England), he wore a greatcoat made of tanned leather. His diet consisted mainly of vegetables and milk; he did not consume alcoholic drinks.

Reportedly, Hersey did not like company and did not seem to be a happy person in general: "Domestic happiness and social intercourse were strangers in his family." He was known for being rude and abrupt in his behavior. An oft-quoted example of Hersey's unwillingness to engage in social activities is the occasion when his sister-in-law wanted to pay him and his family a visit. When he learned about her plans, he promptly sent her a letter refusing to have her as a guest: "Madam, I cannot have you. I have neither hay nor corn for your horses, I have no servants in my family, and I had rather be chained to a galley oar than wait upon you myself."[322] He sister-in-law got the message and did not come to visit.

Despite Hersey's oddities, he gave Thacher a solid five-year apprenticeship that instilled in Thacher the conviction to focus on surgery in his future career.

Military Surgeon

When Thacher finished his training with Hersey in 1775 at the age of twenty-one, the tensions in the colonies had just erupted into violence. The Battles of Lexington and Concord had ignited the military conflict between the British and the colonists in April of that year, and the Redcoats had slaughtered hundreds of rebels at Bunker Hill in June. Thacher felt compelled to join the fight for independence and realized his training made him qualified to participate in the war. Not only would it help the cause, but it would also offer great opportunities to improve his surgical skills: "Participating in the glorious spirit of the times, and contemplating improvement in my professional pursuits, motives of patriotism and private interest prompted me to hazard my future in the conflict for independence."[323]

Thacher applied for a position in the Medical Department of the Continental Army shortly after finishing his apprenticeship. After a tough examination testing his knowledge in anatomy, physiology, surgery, and medicine, he was accepted as a surgeon's mate in the provincial hospital at Cambridge. The "hospital" was actually a collection of spacious apartments in which soldiers who had been wounded at Bunker Hill were treated under the direction of Dr. John Warren.

In February of the following year, John Morgan appointed Thacher as a mate to surgeon David Townsend, and Thacher joined the forces that had Boston under siege. After the British evacuated the city on March 17, 1776, Thacher spent about five months in Boston, providing experiences that he described in detail in his military journal. In 1777, Thacher was at the scene of the Battles of Saratoga and saw the Northern Army defeating Burgoyne's forces. He was appointed to the Albany general hospital, where both revolutionaries and Redcoats were treated. He was able to observe both British and German surgeons in action, and commented that "the English surgeons performed with skill and dexterity, but the Germans, with few exceptions, do no credit to their profession."[324]

The opportunities to practice and learn war surgeries were abundant. Thacher reported that "amputating limbs, trepanning fractured skulls, and dressing the most formidable wounds, have familiarized my mind to scenes of woe." Curiously, Thacher became involved in the care of a leg injury suffered by General Benedict Arnold, "whom the doctor found an exacting and unreasonable patient."[325]

After about a year with the First Virginia Regiment, Thacher returned to his native state and joined the First Massachusetts Regiment under Colonel Henry Jackson in 1779. With troops from New England, Thacher participated in the siege of Yorktown and witnessed the surrender of Lord Cornwallis and his forces on October 19, 1781. The victory at Yorktown basically ended the military hostilities between England and her colonies. With peace on the horizon, the Continental Congress decided to reduce the army, and Thacher retired from the military in 1783. In March of the following year, Thacher settled in Plymouth, Massachusetts, to build a surgical practice.

Settling in Plymouth, Massachusetts

Already famous and highly regarded from his engagement in the Revolutionary War, Thacher was well received in Plymouth and had no problems establishing himself as a practitioner. He quickly grew a busy practice focused on surgery. He became a highly sought-after consultant both in Plymouth and the surrounding towns. He would remain a busy local surgeon for the next thirty-three years.

Like many successful physicians at the time, Thacher also took on apprentices. During periods, he had between six and eight students living in his household, receiving medical and surgical training. Thacher lectured on anatomy and surgery, and performed human dissections in his teaching. As was the case with other surgeons, the procurement of corpses remained a problem. On one occasion, Thacher had to temporarily suspend his teaching as mobs of angry citizens threatened his home, accusing him of grave robbery.

Authorship

In addition to teaching and running a busy surgical practice, Thacher became a proliferative author, although it would be a while before his pen started to fly. After twenty-six years in Plymouth, he published his first book, *The New Dispensatory, Compiled From the Most Approved Authors, Both European and American.* The book was dedicated to his previous teacher (and chief), John Warren. Thacher submitted his work for review to members of the Massachusetts Medical Society, who approved and recommended the book for publication because "it appears to have been a principal object of Dr. Thacher to adapt the work to American practice, and as he has adopted for the basis of his work the American Pharmacopæia of Massachusetts…it will be for the interest of medical science in this country to encourage the work."[326] The volume was a success and was printed in four editions.

In 1814, Thacher published his next volume, *Observations upon Hydrophobia.* Although rare in this country nowadays, hydrophobia (rabies) was a real threat in the 1700s. Many remedies, which look odd today, were on the market. One of the strangest treatments, highly publicized, was the "Crouse's remedy," named after its inventor, John M. Crouse:

> First. Take an ounce of the jaw-bone of a dog burned and pulverized, or powdered to a fine dust. Second. Take the false tongue of a newly foaled colt, let that also be dried and powdered. Third. Take one scruple of the verdigris which is raised on the surface of old copper by lying in moist earth. The coppers of George I or II are the purest and best. Mix these ingredients together, and if the patient be an adult let him take the common teaspoonful a day, and so in proportion for a child, according to its age. If these should fail, the patient should immediately apply to a physician, who will administer three drachms

of verdigris and one ounce of calomel at one dose, and he
need not be alarmed on account of the size of the dose.

After reviewing Crouse's remedy and several other cures used to treat
hydrophobia, Thacher concluded that they were all more or less worthless.
He called for "properly conducted experiments in animals in some suitable
institution," and was dreaming of an opportunity to become involved in
the development of a vaccine. He wished he would become "the Jenner of
the proposed institution."

In the preface to his next book, Thacher lamented the lack of good
writing on the theory and practice of medicine: "It is confessedly a matter of regret that a country, in which literature and science have been so
honorably and successfully cultivated, should so long remain destitute of
systemic work on practical medicine." These words set the stage for his
book on American modern practice that was published in 1817. Together,
the title and subtitle could almost fill a full page of text: *American Modern
Practice: or, A simple method of prevention and cure of diseases, according to
the latest improvements and discoveries, comprising a practical system adapted
to the use of medical practitioners of the United States. To which is added an
appendix, containing an account of many domestic remedies recently introduced into practice, and some approved formulæ applicable to the diseases of
our climate.*

In the book, Thacher devoted one of the chapters to the character
and qualifications of a physician, and many of his words are applicable
to today's doctors as well. Among other things, he stressed the need for
the practitioner to "possess the strictest integrity of character."[327] He also
emphasized the importance of modesty and humanity, and encouraged
the physician to extend "the hand of relief to the afflicted, especially
to the widow, to the fatherless and to him that hath none to help him."
Furthermore, the practitioner should "avoid all appearance of vanity and
ostentation." At the same time, however, he should exhibit "a modest confidence in his own merits that may command the confidence of others."

Towards the end of the chapter, Thacher emphasized the value of
continued education and the importance of following the most recent literature. He advised his colleagues "to possess themselves of a well-chosen
library," and if they could not afford it, to create "district associations to

accomplish this purpose." Thacher had harsh word for colleagues who were not willing to continue their professional studies, and concluded that those "who practice only by rote, and drudge in in the same beaten track, although they may boast many years' experience, are but novices in many essential points, and utterly incompetent to discharge their calling with satisfaction to themselves or justice to their patients."

Retirement

Thacher had now reached the age of sixty-three, and although he was well aware of colleagues who had continued their practices to much higher age, he felt it was time to retire. His mental faculties were still intact, but "an imperfection of bearing, which he had had from youth, increasing with advancing years," had started to make it difficult for him to "attend upon his patients." It was time "to find employment for his active mind in other pursuits."

In an annual address to the Massachusetts Medical Society, Thacher contemplated upon the importance of a balanced life that allowed time and space for interests outside one's career. This became particularly important when it was time to retire from an active professional life: "Successful men may have gained much to retire *upon,* but nothing to retire *to,* if literature, social ties and philanthropic interests have been lost sight of during the rush and struggle of their thirty years of active life."[328] During the twenty-seven years of retirement that awaited Thacher, he found "occupation and enjoyment in literature, in agriculture, and especially in horticulture." He became an industrious orchardist, planting and training orchards and introducing many new fruit varieties.

Some of these extracurricular activities resulted in publications, including *The American Orchardist* (1822); *A Practical Treatise on the Management of Bees* (1829); *An Essay on Demonology, Ghosts, and Apparitions, and Popular Superstitions; also, an Account of the Witchcraft Delusion at Salem, in 1692* (1831); and *History of the Town of Plymouth, From its First Settlement in 1620, to the Year 1832* (1832).

In addition to reading and writing, growing orchards, and researching the history of Plymouth, Thacher continued his affiliations with colleagues as an active member of the Massachusetts Medical Society. He was elected a fellow of the American Academy of the Arts and Sciences in 1803. Thacher was also one of the earliest members of the Pilgrim Society and the Society of Cincinnati, which reflect his interest in this country's early history.

In addition, Thatcher was known for his piety. He was a devoted churchgoer and always respected the Sabbath. He despised drunkenness and disliked tobacco; he considered both smoking and chewing tobacco "nauseous and disgusting habits."

At a time when owning slaves was considered an unquestioned right by many in the society, including some of the Founding Fathers, such as Washington, Jefferson, and even Benjamin Rush (who despite his passionate fight against slave trade once bought a child slave whom he owned until he freed him in 1794), Thacher expressed his dislike of owning slaves. In 1781, during his time as a surgeon in the Continental Army, he wrote about his antislavery sentiments: "The labor of the Virginia plantations is performed altogether by a species of the human race, who have been cruelly wrested from their native country and doomed to perpetual bondage, while their masters are manfully contending for freedom and the natural rights of man." He continued by lamenting, "Such is the inconsistency of human nature."

The Military Journal

The most influential work authored by Thacher was the *Military Journal During the American Revolutionary War, from 1775 to 1783*. Like many other books at the time, the title page of the Military Journal had several subtitles: *Describing Interesting Events and Transactions of this Period; with Numerous Historical Facts and Anecdotes, from the Original Manuscript. To which is Added an Appendix, Containing Biographical Sketches of Several General Officers.* The first edition of the work was published 1823 with new editions emerging during the next several decades.

During the war, Thacher had carried a diary with numerous, sometimes daily, entries. The first note was listed as "January" (1775), and the second was "March." At that time, Lexington and Concord were still a month in the future, but Thacher expressed his concern that an open conflict was now inevitable: "In short, the horrors of civil war seem stalking, with rapid strides, towards our devoted country."[329] He had noticed that Britain's grip over the country had already started to crumble: "His majesty's name had lost its power; it can have no charms with the sons of liberty." While Thacher felt good about this development, he was afraid of what would happen when angry mobs would take to the Boston streets: "The people are their own rulers, and never was there less need of penal laws." The next entry in the Journal was dated April 21, two days after the battles of Lexington and Concord. The last note was written 316 pages later on January 1, 1783.

Thacher was not writing his diary with an eye on publication but for his own "temporary amusement." Indeed, it would be forty years after the end of the war before Thacher decided to publish the diary. He dedicated the volume to the Governor of Massachusetts, John Brooks. Thacher also sent a copy to ex-president John Adams for his review. In a letter dated September 11, 1824, Adams wrote to the author, "I have had read to me your valuable Journal of your campaigns in the American revolutionary war, and I have no hesitation in saying that it is the most natural, simple, and faithful narration of facts that I have seen in any history of that period." Adams continued by saying, "Posterity will be under great obligations to you for this labor, and every man of the present age who can afford to purchase it, ought to have it."[330]

1775

In January and March of 1775, Thacher described the situation on the continent and the escalating tensions between the colonies and the motherland. He expressed an increasing anxiety about the risk of an open military conflict. He lamented that this was happening when he had just finished his medical training with Abner Hersey, robbing him of "the commencement of a new career in life." Instead, he found his country "about to be involved in all the horror of a civil war."[331]

Thacher described the bad blood between the Tories, "those disaffected individuals, who still adhere to the royal cause," and the "class of people [who] have assumed the appellation of *Whigs;* but by our enemies are stigmatized by the name *Rebels."*

On April 21, Thacher described what had happened two days earlier: "The British troops marched to Lexington and Concord last Wednesday, the 19th instant, for the purpose of destroying some of our military stores." The events at Lexington and Concord became the crisis that ignited the war. Thacher understood that there was now no way back and commented, "The fearful day has arrived; a civil war has actually commenced in our land."

It would be only two months before the next battle. Thacher wrote in his journal, "We are again shocked by intelligence that a terrible battle has been fought between the British regulars and the American soldiers, on Bunker, or rather Breed's hill, in Charlestown, near Boston, on the 17th instant."[332] The slaughter was horrific with losses in the hundreds on the American side and in the thousands among the British. What Thacher grieved most was the death of his colleague, Joseph Warren, "a loss infinitely to be lamented, and which occasions universal grief and sorrow, is that of Major General Joseph Warren."[333]

By then, Thacher had decided to join the fight for freedom. He wanted to connect with the Medical Department but first needed to be approved. In an examination that was "in a considerable degree close and severe," and tested Thacher's knowledge in anatomy, physiology, surgery, and medicine, he landed a position as a "surgeon's mate in the provincial hospital at Cambridge, Dr. John Warren being the senior surgeon." Thacher started his duty in the hospital on July 15. He described the facilities: "Several private, but commodious houses in Cambridge are occupied for hospitals, and a considerable number of soldiers who were wounded at Breed's hill, and a greater number of sick of various diseases, require all our attention."

In November, sick soldiers had started to outnumber soldiers who had been injured at Bunker Hill; "Our hospitals are considerably crowded with sick soldiers from camp; the prevailing disease are autumnal fevers and dysenteric complaints, which have proved fatal in a number of instances."

The siege of Boston had commenced already in May, a month after Lexington and Concord, and had intensified after Bunker Hill. Thacher described the horrible conditions of the Bostonians who were now in the crosshairs of the British forces and the Continental Army. Despite an initial agreement between the British and the Rebels, civilians could now neither come in, nor leave the city. When the lockdown started, families were divided with husbands, wives, and children sometimes separated on different sides of the city border. Inside the city, both soldiers and Bostonians suffered. Thacher described how "the distress of the inhabitants and troops in Boston exceed the possibility of description. They are almost in a state of starvation, for the want of food and fuel. The inhabitants, totally destitute of vegetables, flour, and fresh provisions, have actually been obliged to feed on horse flesh."[334] Winter approaching, people were freezing, and to keep fireplaces going, "they have taken down a number of houses, removed the pews from the church, and are digging up the timber at the wharves for fuel."

During these difficult times, Thacher took solace in the fact that Washington was there, ready to lead. Thacher admired Washington and described in his journal the first occasion he had a chance to see the Commander-in-Chief. One day in July he was "much gratified" to get a glimpse of the General: "His Excellency was on horseback.... It was not difficult to distinguish him from all others; his personal appearance is truly noble and majestic, being tall and well proportioned." What Thacher did not know was that he would end up working under Washington for the next eight years.

1776

In February 1776, Thacher was subjected to yet another medical examination, this time by John Morgan, who had succeeded Church as Surgeon-General of the Continental Army. Thacher passed this examination as well and was appointed surgeon's mate to Dr. David Townsend. With their regiment, they were stationed on Prospect Hill.

In the middle of the night between March 4 and 5, Washington managed to bring cannon and other equipment up the hill of Dorchester Heights. The operation was done right under the nose of the enemy, but was not discovered by the British until the early morning. Thacher was deployed with his regiment as a relief party to Dorchester Heights. They left their camp at Prospect Hill early in the morning, and upon arriving at Dorchester, Thacher was impressed by "the amount of labor performed during the night, considering the earth is frozen eighteen inches deep." Although the prospect of violence scared Thacher ("These are the preparations for blood and slaughter! Gracious God!"), the following day, when his regiment was called back to their camp at Prospect Hill, he "bade adieu to Dorchester heights, without being called to dress a single wound."

General Howe had a rude awakening the morning of March 5. He realized that overnight Washington had managed to secretly install cannon that were now staring down from Dorchester Heights at Boston and its harbor, which was occupied by multiple British warships. According to Thacher's journal, Howe exclaimed, "I know not what I shall do, the rebels have done more in one night than my whole army would have done in weeks."[335] It was time to get out of the city! March 17 became the day of evacuation.

After the evacuation, only a limited number of American soldiers, who had previously had smallpox or been inoculated, were allowed to enter Boston. Whereas some (including John Warren) found the conditions more favorable than feared, Thacher was appalled by the British's destruction. In his journal, he described how "the streets present a scene, which reflects disgrace on their late occupants, exhibiting a deplorable desolation and wretchedness." In particular, Thacher was outraged by what the British troops had done to the churches in town. The Old South Church, which had been "for more than a century consecrated to the service of religion," was ruined. The pulpit and pews had been removed, and the floor had been covered with sand and used as a riding school. A particularly beautiful pew had been demolished and used as a fence for a pigsty. The North Church, meanwhile, had fared even worse. It had been completely demolished and used for fuel. Thacher lamented, "Thus are our houses, devoted to religious worship, profaned and destroyed by the subjects of his Royal Majesty."

The Stone Chapel had been spared the destruction and could serve as the sight of Joseph Warren's funeral on April 8. Thacher, who attended the event, described in the journal how the remains of Warren had been taken "from the earth at Breed's Hill, placed in an elegant coffin, and brought into the chapel." After the ceremony, Warren's body was entombed in the vault under the chapel.

Smallpox kept "lurking in various parts of the town," and in May, Thacher underwent inoculation by his friend, Dr. John Homans. When orders were given to inoculate "all the soldiers and inhabitants in town" against smallpox, Thacher and Townsend became "constantly engaged in this business."

On a happier note, Thacher also took part in the festivities celebrating the Declaration of Independence. On July 18, "the declaration of American Independence [was] proclaimed in form from the balcony of the State House in this town." There were parades in King Street, and the proclamation was met with great joy: "Three huzzas from the concourse of people were given, after which thirteen pieces of cannon were fired" from several locations.

When Washington took most of his army to New York after the British evacuated Boston, Thacher accompanied his regiment to Ticonderoga on Lake Champlain. Curiously, Thacher's first medical rescue at Ticonderoga had nothing to do with surgery but involved a case of a snake bite: "Soon after my arrival here, a soldier had the impudence to seize a rattlesnake by its tail; the reptile threw its head back and struck its fangs into the man's hand."[336] The soldier experienced a severe reaction to the bite with "his whole arm to his shoulder…swollen to twice its natural size." The event scared both the doctor and the patient: "The poor man was greatly and justly alarmed; his situation was very critical." The patient was immediately given "large and repeated doses of olive oil," and his affected limb was rubbed with "a large quantity of mercurial ointment." Luckily, within about forty-eight hours, the man "was happily restored to health."

During the deployment to Ticonderoga, Thacher saw engagements on Lake Champlain between the British naval forces and ships manned by colonists. The British scored overwhelming victories, and Thacher lamented the fact that "out of sixteen of our vessels, eleven were taken or destroyed."

1777

Winter was now approaching, and although Thacher had not brought a thermometer ("I have no means in my possession of ascertaining the precise degree of cold"), everyone agreed that it was "colder here than in Massachusetts at the same season." In January 1777, Thacher noted in his journal that "Lake Champlain is now frozen over, and the ice is about one foot thick, the earth is covered with snow."

Later in February, the temperature started to rise, and in March Thacher reported that the lake was now "open and free from ice in its whole extent." Although this was good news for freezing soldiers, it also meant enemy forces were able to start moving around, again threatening the Rebels stationed at Lake Champlain. The British were coming down from Canada, where they had camped during the winter months, and brought with them local Natives they had engaged in the fight against the freedom fighters. Thacher commented that "the hostile Indians begin to lurk about our lines, laying wait for their prey."[337] With horror, Thacher recalled one episode when "a party of [Natives] in the British interest… discovered about thirty of our unarmed recruits…they immediately made their attack, killed and tomahawked some, made several prisoners, and escaped towards Canada."

In April 1777, Thacher was appointed surgeon's mate in the general hospital at Mount Independence, located directly across the lake from Ticonderoga. (Mount Independence had been connected to Ticonderoga by a "floating bridge" constructed with sections, fifty feet long and twelve feet wide, anchored together with iron chains and rivets.) Several of the buildings on Mount Independence served as its general hospital.

In early summer, the British government appointed General John Burgoyne commander-in-chief of their army in Canada, which was eight to ten thousand men strong. Plans were schemed for Burgoyne to take Ticonderoga and then march down to Albany, where General Howe would meet with British forces who had sailed up the Hudson River from New York City. Feeling threatened by the approaching British army, General Arthur St. Clair abruptly made the controversial decision to abandon the fortifications at Ticonderoga and Mount Independence. Thacher wrote that "at about 12 o'clock, in the night of the 5th instant (July), I was urgently called from sleep, and informed that our army was in motion, and was instantly to abandon Ticonderoga and Mount Independence." Thacher was put in charge to "immediately…collect the sick and wounded and as much of the hospital stores as possible." The evacuation was frantic and accomplished in only three hours.

After some detours, Thacher and his patients ended up in the hospital at Albany. Thacher described the hospital building, "situated on an eminence overlooking the city. It is two stories high…contains forty wards, capable of accommodating five hundred patients, besides the rooms appropriated to the use of surgeons and other officers, stores, &c."

This was the place where Thacher would spend the last four months of 1777. In September and October, the hospital was crowded by soldiers who had been injured in the battles around Saratoga. By the end of October, "not less than one thousand wounded and sick [were] now in this city." The hospital was overwhelmed, and other buildings had to be used for the care of patients, including the Dutch Church "and several private houses." Thacher was working hard every day "from eight o'clock in the morning to a late hour in the evening, to the care of our patients." He saw a vast amount of suffering and despair, including "mutilated bodies, mangled limbs, and bleeding incurable wounds."[338] Many patients were admitted to the hospital, not for injuries sustained on the battlefield, but for unrelated sicknesses. Thacher described the soldiers as "miserable objects, languishing under afflicting disease of every description."

Seeing so many suffering soldiers and fighting to survive, Thacher became irritated by the demanding behavior of the self-important Benedict Arnold. Although Arnold had suffered an injury to his leg "by a musket ball," Thacher found Arnold "very peevish and impatient under his misfortunes," as Arnold continuously requested his "attention during the night." Thacher grew tired of Arnold's complaints and instead "devoted an hour in writing a letter to a friend in Boston."

Some of the injuries Thacher encountered were horrendous. "A young man, received a musket ball through his cheeks, cutting its way through the teeth on each side and the substance of the tongue."[339] The surgeon continued to describe the patient's condition: "His sufferings have been great, but he now begins to articulate tolerably well." Another soldier "had the whole side of his face torn off by a cannon ball, laying his mouth and throat open to view." Thacher did not let us know how this patient fared.

Some of the most challenging injuries were those caused by Native warriors engaged on the British side. Thacher described in detail how victims were scalped: "The Indian mode of scalping their victims is this—with a knife they make a circular cut from the forehead quite round, just above the ears, then taking hold of the skin with their teeth, they tear off the whole hairy scalp in an instant."

By the end of the year, Thacher was exhausted and needed a break. He was happy to pen in the journal on December 20 that he had "obtained a furlough for forty days, and shall tomorrow commence my journey to visit my friends in New England."

1778

After the well-deserved break, Thacher returned to Albany in early February 1778 (actually two days before the expiration of his furlough). He immediately resumed his "duties in the hospital."

In May, Thacher spent a lot of ink describing reports he had received about the conditions the army was experiencing at the Valley Forge winter camp. Thatcher's friend, Major Minnis, who had been at the encampment, wrote to Thacher about "the particular circumstances of the distress and privations, which our army suffered, while in winter quarters."[340] Minnis reported how the march of the soldiers in December 1777 could be followed by tracking the marks "of the men over ice and frozen ground, by the blood from their naked feet." Thacher was also disturbed by the report of soldiers at Valley Forge complaining about "no pay, no clothing, no provisions, no rum."

In June, the hospital at Albany was relocated to High Lands, further down the Hudson River. The new hospital was established on the eastern side of the river, "about two miles from West Point, which is on the opposite shore." Thacher was pleased with the new location, because it made it possible to communicate with both New York and Albany.

Although still working hard and occupying long days taking care of sick and injured soldiers, Thacher also had opportunities to participate in activities outside the infirmary. Some were fun-filled, and others ended in stressful situations. In July, Thacher described how "a number of sheep [were] running at large in the woods belonging to our hospital" had become a nuisance. He volunteered in the efforts to reduce the sheep population, and used his gun "against these harmless animals." Despite "labor and fatigue" for a whole day, Thacher managed to kill only one sheep. Instead, most of his shots missed the target. On his return, people teased him for being such a poor marksman, and Thatcher reported, "Dr. Prescott challenged me to decide our superiority by firing at a mark." Thacher accepted the dare, and "we placed an object at the end of our garden." The competition ended in a disaster that could have been even worse. One of the horses "grazing in a field directly in our range...received a ball through his body," causing an injury that turned out to be fatal. The situation became even more distressing when Thacher and his colleague realized that the horse was not just any horse but "was the property of Brigadier General Glover, and was by him highly prized." General Glover demanded $150 for the creature, and "justice and honor required that we should promptly comply with his demand."

To add to the scary event, Thacher and Prescott were informed that a soldier who was in charge of the horses had been almost hit by another bullet "that struck the ground within a yard of his feet." The shooters realized that "had the poor fellow been the victim, the catastrophe would have been much more melancholy." Thankfully, they understood it was probably wise not to engage in another shooting competition: "The event is sufficiently unfortunate to deter us from again sporting with our guns at random shot."

In August, the hospital again saw a surge in new patients. On the seventh of that month, Thacher reported that "an unusual number of patients have been brought into our hospital within a few days." The patients were not only victims of injuries in battle, but "in many cases their diseases are putrid fever and dysentery." Some of the patients were critically ill, and Thacher feared some of them would not survive: "Many of the cases appear so malignant, that it is feared they will baffle all the skill of the physician."

A surprise visit to the hospital by Washington in October gave Thacher a chance to express his adulation of the Commander-in-Chief. In loving words, Thacher described the general as "the perfect gentleman and accomplished warrior."[341] When painting a picture of Washington's outer features, Thacher was almost at a loss for words. Washington was "remarkably tall, full six feet, erect, and well proportioned." The general impressed on Thacher as a real he-man: "The strength and proportion of his joints and muscles, appear to be commensurate with the preeminent powers of his mind." Even Washington's face was apparently perfect: "There is a fine symmetry in the features of his face, indicative of a benign and dignified spirit. His nose is straight and his eyes inclined to blue."

Like many official inspections of American hospitals today, Washington's visit was unannounced: "His arrival was scarcely announced, before he presented himself at our doors." Thacher and his colleagues were nervous that, since they had had no time "to make preparation for his reception," Washington would find the hospital in less than perfect condition. Thacher was happy to enter in his journal, however, that "we had the inexpressible satisfaction of receiving his Excellency's approbation of our conduct, as respects the duties of our department."

Passing Washington's hospital inspection test was helpful to Thacher's career. In November, he was appointed surgeon to the first Virginia state regiment. His living quarters were upgraded in his new position. He "received a polite invitation to take my quarters in the marquee with Colonel Gibson, and his Lieutenant Colonel, William Brent."

Although Thacher, at this point, had experienced and seen more injuries and diseases than most, he was still a young man. No wonder, therefore, that he enjoyed jolly times with colleagues and officers whenever there were opportunities. He shared some of those occasions with his journal. Good food, wine, and women were part of his leisure time. While still in Albany, he had, along with "several gentlemen belonging to the hospital," taken part in dance lectures given by a Mr. John Trotter, who "had for many years been in the practice of teaching the art in the city of New York." It was the hope that taking advantage of Master Trotter's teaching skills would help Thacher "in due time...to be able to figure in a ball room."

After settling in at the new hospital at High Lands, friendships developed between officers and colleagues on both sides of the Hudson. On July 27, "Colonel Melcome, with his much admired lady, and several other officers, favored us with their company to dine."[342] The dinner was a success, providing the guests with "all the comforts in our power." There was no lack of good wines: "the cheering glass was not removed till evening." After the festivities, the guests were accompanied to the river side, and before finally saying good night, the party "finished two bottles of port on board their barge." As soon as the next day, the favor was reciprocated, and "the gentlemen of our hospital returned the visit to Colonel Malcome, at West Point, and were entertained in the most genteel manner."

The story about Brigadier General Muhlenburg, told by Thacher on November 3, 1778, was another tale about good times that could be had, despite being a wartime surgeon. Muhlenburg was a minister in Virginia who had decided to join the war of independence and had "exchanged his clerical profession for that of a soldier." On the day of his farewell sermon, "he entered his pulpit with his sword and cockade, …and the next day marched at the head of his regiment to join the army." We find Muhlenburg admitted to the hospital (Thacher did not tell us why), and on November 3, he had arranged for a festive dinner in the hospital. Forty-one "respectable officers" were invited, and food and drink were in abundance; "our tables were furnished with fourteen dishes, arranged in fashionable style…a number of toasts were pronounced, accompanied with humorous and merry songs." An untold number of ladies were also present, and after the dinner and toasts, "we were cheered with military music and dancing, which continued till a late hour in the night."

November saw a lull in military activities, so there was time for more parties. The officers "adopted the practice of giving suppers alternately, with music and dancing through half the night." Thacher felt a touch of bad conscience and commented in the journal that "the favorite amusements" did not "accord precisely with my own view of time well spent." It was difficult to resist the temptations, however, and he admitted that he was "frequently enticed to a participation in their banqueting revels."

As Christmas drew closer, the good times intensified, and Thacher wrote that during the holiday season, not a day passed "without receiving invitations to dine, nor a night without amusement and dancing." The holiday spirit continued into the new year, and on New Year's Day, Thacher described in his journal how he and other officers "were introduced to a number of ladies assembled to unite with the gentlemen in the ball room. " Food and drink were again plentiful, "a very elegant supper was provided, and not one of the company was permitted to retire till three o'clock in the morning." Thus have the gallant Virginians commenced the new year.

There is no doubt that Thacher was an integral part of the Revolutionary War, and had a chance to personally meet with several of its leaders. We have already seen how awestruck the doctor was with Washington. At the end of 1778, Thacher was called on to attend Marquis de Lafayette's sickbed. In a note entered in the Military Journal on December 27, Thacher reported how he was introduced to the "great favorite of General Washington." Thacher described how he was "received by this nobleman in a polite and affable manner."[343] Lafayette, twenty-four at the time, was recovering from a fever "and was in his chair of convalescence." Like many other individuals we meet in the journal, Thacher went into some detail of the person's outer appearance. Lafayette was described as a tall, imposing individual, if not necessarily good-looking: "He is nearly six feet high, large but not corpulent.... He is not very elegant in his form... nor is there a perfect symmetry in his features, his forehead is remarkably high, his nose large and long." Despite the big nose, Thacher approved Lafayette's appearance: "His countenance is interesting and impressive." Anyone talking with the Marquis could tell he was recently arrived in the country: "He converses in broken English." Thacher ended his description by summarizing his impression of Lafayette as being "a French nobleman of distinguished character."

1779

In the spring of 1779, Thacher had a meeting with another portal figure of the revolution. On May 28, "the Baron Steuben reviewed and inspected our brigade."[344] As expected, Baron von Steuben did not leave many stones unturned. Thacher described how "the Baron reviewed the line" of troops and scrutinized "each individual and the muskets and accoutrements of every soldier.... He required that the musket and bayonet should exhibit the brightest polish; not a spot of rust, or defect in any part." If he found satisfactory conditions, von Steuben complimented the soldier; otherwise he was condemning, "censuring every fault." His displeasure was expressed in a loud voice with a heavy German accent. Von Steuben concluded his inspection by turning to Thacher, and "required of me, as a surgeon, a list of the sick with a particular statement of the accommodations and mode of treatment, and even visited some of the sick in their cabins."

True to his habit, Thacher also described von Steuben's exterior mien and wrote, "He appears to be about fifty years of age, and is venerable and dignified in his department." One of von Steuben's characteristic traits was his desire to impress his surroundings by dressing in an imposing manner. Thacher described the Baron as "rich and elegant in dress, having a splendid medal of gold and diamonds designating the order of fidelity, suspended at his breast." Thacher added that von Steuben was "held in universal respect, and considered as a valuable acquisition to our country."

A recurring problem during the Revolutionary War was the frequent abandonments by soldiers who found the conditions in the army unbearable, in particular since they often found themselves without pay for long periods of time. Attempted desertion was typically punished by immediate execution. During the spring of 1779, Thacher became the witness of a tragic event revolving around "five soldiers…conducted to the gallows according to their sentence for the crimes of desertion and robbing the inhabitants."[345] In a gripping entry on April 20, Thacher described the gruesome scene of the public hanging: "A detachment of troops and a concourse of people, formed a circle around the gallows," watching how the "criminals were brought in a cart sitting on their coffins, and halters about their necks." Naturally, the young men were scared, "trembling on the verge of eternity." Washington showed clemency and pardoned three of the condemned, but "the two others were obliged to submit to their fate." One of the soldiers who were just about to be hanged was accompanied by "an affectionate and sympathizing brother, which rendered the scene uncommonly distressing, and forced tears of compassion from the eyes of the numerous spectators." The brothers "repeatedly embraced and kissed each other, with all the fervor of brotherly love" and held on to each other until the very end. When the executioner was finally ready to do his duty, the brothers "with a flood of tears, and mournful lamentations…bade each other an eternal adieu." The spectacle ended with double tragedy; "the criminal trembling under the horrors of an untimely and disgraceful death—and the brother overwhelmed with sorrow and anguish for one he held most dear."

1780

Although Valley Forge may have been the nadir of the soldiers' conditions during the war, with circumstances improving somewhat after that winter camp, the army continued to suffer tough conditions during the rest of Revolutionary War. In 1780, Thacher described the miserable situation on several occasions. On the first day of the year, while in winter camp at Morristown, Thacher lamented about how the "canvas covering affords but a miserable security from storms of rains and snow, and a great scarcity of provisions."

That January was particularly cruel: "we experienced one of the most tremendous snowstorms ever remembered." Everybody, from officers and down, were freezing and shivering, but the ill-protected enlisted did worst: "the sufferings of the poor soldiers can scarcely be described."[346] They continued to be badly clothed, "a single blanket to each man... and some are destitute of shoes." The snow continued to pile on, and was now "from four to six feet deep." Not only did the arctic temperatures and snow make the soldiers freeze (sometimes to death), but the deep snow also obstructed the roads and prevented "our receiving a supply of provisions."

In the middle of January, a secret military expedition was undertaken "to attack the enemy in their works at Staten Island." Thacher described how "about two thousand five hundred men...were sent off in about five hundred sleighs," What a sight it must have been! Few knew the reason behind securing all these sleighs, and most had been told that the expedition had the purpose of going "into the country after provision." During the ride on frozen waterways and deep layers of snow, the soldiers gradually understood that the purpose was a surprise attack on the British forces at Staten Island. The British had received intelligence about the approaching army of horses and sleighs, and were prepared. The frozen colonists stayed on the island "twenty-four hours without covering, and about five hundred were slightly frozen." When they gave up and headed back to Morristown, they were pursued by Redcoats, which resulted in casualties among the American soldiers: "Six were killed by a party of horse, who pursued our rear guard." Thacher, however, did not consider the expedition a complete failure because "a number of tents, arms, and a quantity of baggage, with several casks of wine and spirits, were brought off, with seventeen prisoners." The English were not late taking revenge, and only ten days later performed a tit-for-tat counterattack: "A party of the enemy made an excursion from Staten Island in the night, surprised our picquet guard, and succeeded in taking off a major, and forty men."

The hunger and starvation led some soldiers to criminal activities, sometimes resulting in their executions. Thacher described how "some of the soldiers are in the practice of pilfering and plundering the inhabitants of their poultry, sheep, pigs, and even their cattle, from their farms." If caught, the stealing soldiers would face different punishments, ranging from public whipping to "running the gauntlet" to death. When reading about the whipping, one has to wonder if death was not an easier chastising. When condemned to public whipping, "the culprit...securely tied to a tree or post, receives on his naked back the number of lashes assigned him, by a whip formed of several small knotted cords, which sometimes cut through the skin at every stroke." The soldiers were hardened and used to incredibly tough circumstances, and Thacher was amazed that "however strange it may appear, a soldier will often receive the severest stripes without uttering a groan, or once shrinking from the lash, even while the blood flows freely from his lacerated wounds." One way they managed to be whipped without screaming from pain was to "bite the bullet" (similar to patients having surgery without anesthesia). Thacher explained that the receivers of the lashes put "between the teeth a leaden bullet on which they chew while under the lash, till it is made quite flat and jagged."[347]

The number of lashes was often in the hundreds and was sometimes even repeated several days in a row, "in which case the wounds are in a state of inflammation, and the skin rendered more sensibly tender; and the terror of the punishment is greatly aggravated." It is obvious that it would take significant hunger to risk punishments like these.

Being condemned to death for theft or other crimes meant facing the gallows or being shot. Execution by a bullet was considered more dignified than being hanged, and was an "easier death."

Thacher provided several examples of public hangings in his journal. Quite often, large numbers of people gathered to see the otherwise tough and callous soldiers breaking down, trembling, and crying when being put on the gallows. The executions became popular events of entertainment. Thacher told the story of a girl seeking excitement who walked "seven miles in a torrent of rain to see a man hanged." She was, however, upset by the event and "returned in tears," not because of the prisoner's agony, but "because the criminal was reprieved," robbing the girl of the performance.

In May 1780, Thacher described the hanging of a soldier who had been found guilty of forging a number of discharges from the military, allowing him and more than a hundred soldiers to leave the army. His execution was macabre, with the story told by Thacher in an almost comical way. The convict was "a heavy man." When he examined "the halter" applied around his neck, he told "the hangman the knot was not made right, and that the rope was not strong enough." He corrected the knot "round his own neck, (and) was swung off instantly." Sure enough, the rope broke, and he fell down, "by which he was very much bruised." After this, one would think he would ask to be pardoned, but instead "he calmly reascended the ladder" and told the executioner, "I told you the rope was not strong enough, do get a stronger one." With a stronger rope around his neck, "he was launched into eternity."

Less comical was the hanging of John Andre, the British General who conspired with Benedict Arnold during the treason of West Point in September of 1780. Thacher spent several pages in his journal on the treacherous conspiracy of Arnold, and the pages read like a spy novel. While Arnold managed to flee from West Point as Washington had just arrived for an inspection, Andre was less lucky and was caught and brought to justice. He was sentenced to death by a board of general officers quickly assembled by Washington. Andre pleaded with the Commander-in-Chief in a letter (which went unanswered) to be shot rather than hanged. When Andre was led to the place of execution and saw the gallows, surrounded by large throngs of spectators, he realized his wish had not been granted. He exclaimed, "I am reconciled to my death, but I detest the mode."[348] Thacher, who attended the execution on October 2, 1780, "was so near during [Andre's] solemn march to the fatal spot, as to observe every movement, and participate in every emotion which the melancholy scene was calculated to produce." As he often did when describing executions, Thacher lamented the event and found it tragic. In the evening after Andre's hanging, Thacher summarized the events of the day, "Major Andre is no more among the living. I have just witnessed his exit. It was a tragic scene."

1781

This was the year when the British would lose the Revolutionary War. Before Yorktown happened and Lord Cornwallis had to surrender the Royal Army to General Washington, however, Thacher penned several interesting entries in his military journal. These entries described other important events of the year, and included some soul-searching thoughts on slavery and the unjust treatment of the African bondservants.

Although Thacher could have retired from the army on the first day of the year, he decided to retain his commission as military surgeon. Promises by Congress to finally improve the financial outlook, "entitling all officers who shall continue till the end of the war…to receive half pay during life, and a certain number of acres of land, in proportion to their rank," probably played a role in Thacher's decision. Equally important, however, was a feeling of moral obligation to continue the fight and "persevere to the end." Thacher explained that "besides these pecuniary considerations, we are actuated by the purest principles of patriotism." He wanted to stay the course till the end in "the great interest of our native country."

Other army men may not have been as noble as Thacher in their sense of obligations to the Revolution. Along with desertions, revolts were a great problem that persisted throughout the war. Thacher reported on a revolt by "about two thousand men" of the Pennsylvania line of troops that took place in January during winter camp at Morristown. The insurgents contested the length of their enlistment, and challenged the order to stay on beyond the beginning of the new year. They felt particularly betrayed when they saw new recruits receiving much better pay than the "veteran soldiers [who had] served three years for a mere shadow of compensation!" and who had gone through a "total want of pay for twelve months."

Other soldiers followed the example of the Pennsylvania mutineers. Toward the end of January, between two and three hundred New Jersey troops revolted and abandoned their officers. Washington understood that these insurgencies could not stand unanswered, and ordered a detachment of five hundred men to chase down the rebels and serve them the most severe punishment. Thacher was ordered to accompany the detachment pursuing the revolters.

It took four days of marching through snow, "about two feet deep," to find the fleeing insurrectionists. At one o'clock in the morning of the fifth day, after marching eight miles, the fleeing soldiers were finally spotted. Thacher described how the march had "brought us in view of the huts of the insurgent soldiers by dawn of the day." After halting for an hour, "to make the necessary preparations," two cannons were ordered placed in full sight of the insurgents, and the huts were surrounded on all sides by the detachment. The rebels were brutally awakened by the order "to appear on parade in front of their huts unarmed, within five minutes." They probably thought they just had a bad dream, because it was not until the order had been repeated that the soldiers exited the huts. When they found "themselves closely encircled and unable to resist, they quietly submitted to the fate which awaited them."

Three ringleaders were identified and "tried on the spot" by Colonel Sprout, appointed president of the court martial, "standing on the snow, and they were sentenced to be immediately shot." To make the punishment even harder, "twelve of the most guilty mutineers, were next selected to be their executioners." This, of course, was a "most painful task," and when ordered to load, some of them "shed tears." After the first two had been shot with blood pouring out on the white snow, "the third being less criminal, by the recommendation of his officers, to his unspeakable joy, received a pardon."

Thacher ended the distressing entry in his journal with the laconic statement, "Having completed the object of our expedition, we returned to our cantonments on the 31st instant."

Having received news about "our army of the south, under command of Major General [Nathanael] Greene," Thacher described the Battle of Guilford Court House at Greensboro, North Carolina. The fight, which took place on March 15, 1781, was won by the 2,100-man British force under the command of Lord Cornwallis over the 4,500-man strong American force, led by Greene. Although this was a British triumph, Cornwallis suffered severe losses (about a quarter of his forces died, according to some calculations) and historians have described the outcome as a Pyrrhic victory. After the battle, Cornwallis marched his remaining army towards Virginia, trying to connect with Benedict Arnold's forces that were marching south from New York, but instead ended up in Yorktown at Chesapeake Bay.

An arriving fleet of French warships blockaded the bay and cut off Cornwallis's connections with the British forces in New York. After being besieged for a couple of weeks, Cornwallis had to surrender the Royal Army to Washington and his Revolutionary Army, supported by French forces under General Rochambeau. For all practical purposes, the October 19, 1781 surrender by Cornwallis of his seven- to eight-thousand-man army meant the British had lost the war. No further major military engagements took place. It would be another two years, however, before the formal end of the Revolutionary War with the Peace Treaty of Paris in 1783.

Thacher was part of the American forces besieging Yorktown before the British capitulation. He had marched with the army from West Point under Washington, and although the purpose of the troop movements was initially kept a secret, the ultimate goal (Cornwallis at Yorktown) became increasingly clear as the march progressed. In the beginning of the footslog, speculations and rumors about the object of the campaign were rampant. British-occupied New York was high on the list of suspected goals, but Washington was able to keep the purpose of the troop movement secret till at least the end of August. Thacher described the secrecy around the advance in his journal: "…our destination has been for some time matter of perplexing doubt and uncertainty." He recounted how Washington "resolves and matures his great plans and designs under an impenetrable veil of secrecy."[349] Although Thacher was of the opinion that Yorktown had been Washington's secret goal from the beginning of the march, some historians have suggested that Washington actually initially planned to attack New York, but changed his plans after the advance had started and instead decided to go after Cornwallis.[350]

The surrender of Cornwallis was preceded by a siege that grew increasingly violent. Thacher was engaged in treating soldiers on the American side who were injured by cannonades from Cornwallis's defense lines. He was awestruck by the "accuracy an experienced gunner will make his calculations, that a shell shall fall within a few feet of a given point." Casualties were gruesome on both sides: "I have more than once witnessed fragments of the mangled bodies and limbs of the British soldiers thrown into the air by the bursting of our shells."

The besieging forces also suffered casualties. Thacher described how American and French troops saw wounded and killed soldiers, and he gave several examples of his surgical engagements. For example, on September 29, "a cannonade commenced…from the town, by which a man received a wound, and I assisted in amputating his leg." A couple of days later, he assisted in amputating a man's thigh, and on another occasion, he "attended at the hospital, amputated a man's arm, and assisted in dressing a number of wounds."

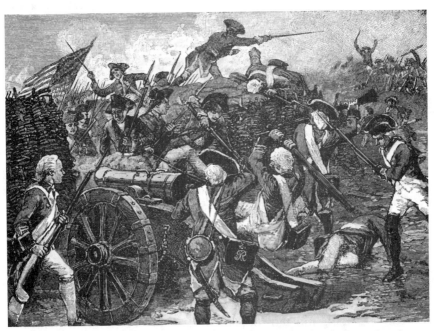

Americans capturing a British redoubt during the Battle of Yorktown 1781. Hand-colored woodcut. James Thacher was with the Continental Army at Yorktown caring for a multitude of injured soldiers. (North Wind Picture Archives)

It was not only direct war-related injuries that were feared, but the enemy was also suspected of what could be called biological warfare. Thacher recounted how "the British have sent from Yorktown a large number of negroes sick with the smallpox, probably for the purpose of communicating the infection to our army."

During the preparations for the siege of Yorktown, Thacher had time to reflect on the situation in Virginia. He provided interesting insight into his thinking about slavery; on September 22, he inked the following entry in his journal: "The population of Virginia is computed at one hundred and fifty thousand whites, and five hundred thousand negro slaves. The labor, therefore, on the Virginia plantations, is performed altogether by a species of the human race, who have been cruelly wrested from their native country and doomed to perpetual bondage, while their masters are manfully contending for freedom, and the natural rights of man. Such is the inconsistency of human nature." Thacher then went on to express hopes that the slaves would be allowed to enjoy the fruits of the American Revolution: "Should Providence ordain that the Americans shall be emancipated from thraldom, it should in gratitude be our prayer, that the African slave may be permitted to participate in the blessings of freedom."

Although Thacher's contemplations clearly showed that he disliked the institution of slavery, he did not expand his commentary due to the fact that several of the Founding Fathers who had signed the Declaration of Independence five years earlier were slave owners. He also did not comment on the fact that Washington busied himself immediately after the victory at Yorktown to chase down slaves who had escaped from Mount Vernon to join the Royal Army (having been promised freedom as a reward).[351]

After Yorktown, Thacher and his regiment marched back to the highlands at Hudson River. They passed through several cities and towns, including Philadelphia, Trenton, and Princeton, where they were celebrated as heroes, and returned at West Point "in triumph." Thacher was hoping that the victorious campaign would have "the most favorable consequences, in bringing this long protracted and distressing war to a happy termination." He realized that he had been allowed to participate in a historical event: "It will be to me a source of inexpressible satisfaction, that I have had an opportunity of participating in the siege and capture of a British army." Thacher concluded by stating, "It is among the blessed privileges and richest incidents of my life."[352]

1782

With major combats out of the way, Thacher could allow himself some relaxation. In April and May, he was given forty-five days of vacation. He used it to visit friends in Massachusetts, and traveled to Boston accompanied by his friend and colleague, Dr. Eustis. Although the visit to Boston was "impeded by foul weather and bad roads," he seemed to have had a good time, reconnecting with family and friends in Boston, Plymouth, and Barnstable. In particular, he enjoyed that "Dr. Eustis kindly introduced me to his father's family, where I received hospitable and polite civilities."

On the 4th of July, Thacher recounted "the anniversary of the declaration of our Independence...celebrated in camp." It was a happy occasion, with "the whole army...formed on the banks of the Hudson on each side of the river." Thacher painted a picture of pomp and circumstance, with "the signal of thirteen cannon being given at West Point, the troops displayed and formed in a line, when a general *feu de joie* took place throughout the whole army."

It is noteworthy that this was only the second time the significance of the 4th of July was mentioned in Thacher's journal. The first time was an entry in July 1776, when Thacher wrote about "the very important intelligence from Philadelphia...now proclaimed, that on the 4th instant, the American Congress declared the thirteen United Colonies, *Free, Sovereign, Independent States.*"

In September, Thacher was sent to Philadelphia "for the purpose of receiving a sum of money at the American Bank, for the payment of our regiment." During his visit, Thacher had the opportunity to meet with Dr. John Jones, "considered at the head of the profession in the United States." Thacher praised Jones for publishing *Plain Remarks on Wounds and Fractures* in 1775 "for the particular benefit of the surgeons of our army, and which has been received with universal approbation."

By now, the Revolutionary War had basically ended. In December, Thacher wrote, "the campaign is now brought to a close...and the prospect of peace is so favorable and encouraging, that our Congress have passed a resolve to discharge a considerable part of the army on the 1st day of January next."

1783

On the first day of 1783, Thacher entered the last note in his military journal: "This day I close my military career, and quit forever the toils and vicissitudes incident to the storms of war."[353] When looking back at his almost eight years in the army, Thacher commented, "While I congratulate my country on the momentous event by which we are about to be elevated to the rank of an Independent Nation, most cordially do I proffer my sympathy for the many lives of inestimable value which have been sacrificed during this ever memorable contest."

Yet Another Impressive Publication

Even after spending much time and energy on the publication of his *Military Journal,* Thacher had enough stamina left for additional research and writing. In 1828, he published two volumes of more than 700 pages of biographies of more than 160 American doctors. The work was titled *The American Medical Biography; or Memoirs of Eminent Physicians who have Flourished in America. To which is Prefixed a Succinct History of Medical Science in the United States From the First Settlement of the Country.* It was dedicated to an old colleague and friend, Dr. Edward Holyoke, who at the time had passed his one-hundredth birthday. We will meet with this remarkable individual in the next chapter of the book.

The End

Looking back, Thacher could certainly be proud of a long and productive life. In his annual address to the Massachusetts Medical Society in 1891 commemorating James Thacher, Dr. Brewster commented that Thacher's life had been "of great activity and industry,—the venerable toiler not resting from his labors even at an age when repose from the cares and toils of life would seem to be imperatively demanded. His usefulness continued even to the end."

Thacher died on May 23, 1844, ninety years old. His wife, Susannah, had gone before him twenty-one years earlier at the age of forty-seven.

CHAPTER 10

EDWARD A. HOLYOKE—
Surgeon and Loyalist Turned Patriot

Perhaps best remembered for reaching the respectable age of one-hundred at a time when getting to fifty was considered old, Dr. Holyoke also left a legacy of a long and successful medical career in the town of Salem, just north of Boston. By the time he died, he had seen thousands of patients in his practice. He also saw a large number of patients by making house calls. To make those visits, he often walked on foot. In 1828, he calculated that he had walked close to 150,000 miles during his lifetime. At the end, he was revered as an old and wise man, and was beloved by the citizens of Salem. Upon his death, "all the church bells of the town tolled, an honor hitherto showed only to presidents of the United States."

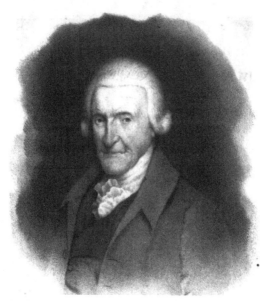

Portrait of Edward Augustus Holyoke (1728–1829). One of the longest living physicians in American history. [Essex Southern District Medical Society - Memoir of Edward A. Holyoke (1829)]

Early Years

Edward Augustus Holyoke was born on August 1, 1728, in Marblehead, Massachusetts.[354] He was the second of eight children of Reverend Edward Holyoke and Margaret (Appleton) Holyoke. The elder Holyoke was a pastor of the second congregational society in Marblehead. In 1737, he was appointed president of Harvard University and moved with his family into the Wadsworth House in Cambridge. He died in 1769 at the age of eighty. At that time, Dr. Holyoke was forty-one years old and a well-established medical practitioner in Salem.

At the age of fourteen, Holyoke was admitted to Harvard University. His written entrance examination was a Latin essay entitled *"Labor Improbus Omnia Vincit"* ("Work Conquers All"), which, considering his future life, was indeed an appropriate topic. He was described as "below the average height, strong, agile, and of lively disposition." Together with his fellow students at Harvard of similar young age, Holyoke participated in activities that created frictions with the faculty at the university. Holyoke and his friends "were fond of the sound of breaking glass, and cutting off the tail of the President's horse was a favorite trick" (notwithstanding the fact that the president at the time was Holyoke's own father!).

Holyoke graduated from Harvard in 1746. After spending about a year teaching at a school in Roxbury, he entered a two-year medical and surgical apprenticeship with Dr. Thomas Berry of Ipswich. In 1749, Holyoke opened a medical practice in Salem.[355] He had to wait until 1783 for his MD degree, which made him the first graduate of Harvard Medical School.[356]

Building a Medical Practice in Salem

The initial years in Salem were difficult. He replaced the beloved Dr. John Cabot, who had passed away at the time Holyoke was finishing his training. Dr. Cabot had been practicing medicine in Salem for a long time and was immensely popular. It was hard for people in Salem to get used to the idea that Dr. Cabot was no longer their doctor and to entrust their care into the hands of a young and inexperienced physician. After two years, Holyoke was so frustrated about the difficulties attracting patients that he seriously thought about giving up. The only thing that stopped him from leaving his practice was the fear of upsetting his father.

Gradually, Holyoke managed to turn things around and was eventually able to build quite a busy practice, seeing patients both locally and from surrounding communities. There were several reasons why Holyoke ultimately was successful. Most importantly, he was a well-trained and well-informed physician. His personality and bedside manner were also helpful. A close friend and previous trainee of Holyoke described several of Holyoke's traits in the *Memoir of Edward A. Holyoke (1829)*, published by Essex South District Medical Society. In that work, Holyoke was described as a lively, cheerful, and humble person: "He possessed much vivacity of disposition, accompanied with great agility of body, and when at college was remarkable for his feats of activity. He was reputed to have been a very good scholar."[357] The memoir emphasized that Holyoke was faithful to his calling and took good care of his patients, regardless of their financial circumstances: "He was very attentive to his professional duties, visiting with equal promptness the poor and the rich. Few physicians in the United States have done so much for the poor. When in the sick chamber his manners were remarkably affable and kind, but preserving a proper dignity of deportment. Such was the success attending his practice, and his great reputation, that it produced to him such a pressure of business, as sometimes scarcely permitted him to take the necessary meals supporting life."[358]

When dealing with colleagues, Holyoke was respectful and willing to share his knowledge. He was a good mentor to the younger colleagues and was not judgmental of their inexperience: "In medical consultations he expressed himself with diffidence and caution, and with junior members of the profession, was free from hauteur, and was communicative, and at the same time candid, and disposed rather to conceal than to expose their errors."

Holyoke also gained respect for his insights into new discoveries in the medical field. He "remained dedicated to the study of medicine and new medical treatments" throughout his career,[359] and was "in the habit of importing, almost every year from England, for some considerable portion of his life, the new medical books of merit." Holyoke's thirst for new knowledge accompanied him throughout his career. He "never neglected to make himself acquainted with the reputed power of new articles…and with the new models of practice which were recommended by others."

In addition to all these acclaims, Holyoke was praised for his positive and happy personality: "Cheerfulness…formed a most conspicuous trait in his character."[360] No wonder he became a beloved figure in Salem and was able to build a thriving practice.

Although in the 1700s, some physicians started to specialize in surgery, many physicians still had a mixed practice, caring for patients with both medical and surgical diseases. Among medical conditions, different epidemics affecting the society were especially feared because of high death rates.

The Great Throat Distemper

A particularly tragic epidemic of "sore throat" was the "Great Throat Distemper" of 1735. Although the epidemic broke out when Holyoke was only eight years old, he must have been influenced by his family and inhabitants of Salem spreading fear, and seeing families horrifyingly affected by the disease. The disease was a reason why Holyoke later in life became a proponent of mercurial medicines in the treatment of inflammatory conditions.

The Throat Distemper mainly affected infants and children and was associated with extremely high mortality rates, making "cruel havoc, sweeping off multitudes of children" and "almost totally destroyed the infant population of the north part of Essex county." The epidemic saw its first victims in Kingston, New Hampshire in 1735 and continued to terrify the population of New England for five years. The disease, which is nowadays recognized as diphtheria, started with symptoms resembling a cold and was associated with an extremely sore throat. The condition then progressed to high fevers and spread to the nose and lungs. We now know that bacteria (*Corynebacterium diphteriae*) caused inflammation of the mucous membranes resulting in a "pseudo membrane" covering the airways. Within a couple of days, the sufferer started having difficulties breathing, and was basically suffocated to death. The disease was called "the strangling angel of children" and killed its victims within a couple of days.

People understood the disease was extremely contagious, but did not understand its cause. One theory, incorrect but popular at the time, was that it was related to the huge increase in caterpillars in 1735. The insects were so numerous that they covered the roads and dwellings and were found in rivers and other waterways.

From its origin in Kingston, New Hampshire, the disease spread north towards Maine and south towards Boston. After reaching Marblehead, it soon also attacked Salem. Later in life, Holyoke addressed the treatment of the epidemic "wherever the baleful influence extended," in a letter published in the first volume of *The New York Medical Repository*. In that essay, he argued for the use of mercurial medicine as a remedy for inflammation and for the beneficial effects it may have had during the "Great Throat Distemper." The use of mercurial medicines in the treatment of inflammatory diseases was not new, but at the time, European physicians had started to express their doubts about the remedy and thought it may even be dangerous, fearing "the most fatal consequences from such a practice." Holyoke, however, remained a strong believer in mercurial medicines and provided an anecdote of a young woman afflicted by the throat distemper:

> A practitioner in a neighboring town, of great repute and extensive practice, being called to attend a young woman dangerously ill of this distemper; having ordered her, among other things, 4 or 5 grs. of calomel, was astonished the next day to find her relieved, greatly beyond his expectation. Upon inquiring of his pupil, to whom he had given his directions, whether his prescription had been followed; he found that his patient had taken 30 grs. of calomel, instead of 4 or 5, to which mistake he attributed the cure. From this time forward in very dangerous cases, he used the medicine in much larger doses than before.

Despite all efforts, the epidemic ravaged New England for several years. Across the region, about five thousand people, mostly infants and children, died between 1735 and 1740. Parents saw their families decimated and often had to bury several of their children in the same grave. In December 1735, Dr. Thomas Berry, Holyoke's future mentor, lost two daughters, Elizabeth, aged five years, and Mary, only eighteen months old. During the month of November 1736, one family lost all their seven children, aged between one and thirteen years.

When the epidemic neared Boston, the *Boston Gazette* offered treatment advice:

> First be sure that a vein be opened under the tongue, and if that can't be done, open a vein in the arm, which must be first done, as all other means will be ineffectual. Then take borax or honey to bathe or annoint the mouth and throat, and lay on the Throat a plaister Vngiuntum Dialthae. To drink a decoction of Devil's bitt or Robbin's

Plantain, with some Sal Prunelle dissolved therein, as often as the patient will drink. If the body be costive use a clyster agreeable to the nature of the Distemper.... But be sure and let blood, and that under the tongue. We have many times made Blisters under the arms, but that has proved sometimes dangerous.[361]

Dysentery and Smallpox

Dysentery was another dreaded disease in the 1700s. Although people understood that it could be spread by unhealthy water, they had no knowledge that bacteria were causing the disease (the discovery of bacteria and what they do was still far in the future). Inflammation of the bowel caused diarrhea that often turned into bloody evacuations. Fever and cramp-like abdominal pain were also part of the clinical picture. Because it became difficult to keep up with the fluid losses, dehydration was a common cause of death. Recurrent epidemics of dysentery plagued the colonies and continued to be a threat well into the 1800s.

Holyoke, like many of his colleagues, became involved in the care of patients with dysentery. His experience with these patients was described in his own words from an outbreak in 1761: "In the beginning of September, of this year, a dysentery began to prevail." He described patients suffering from fever, a "slight chill or rigor," muscle pain, and pronounced weakness. Diarrhea was the main manifestation, with the stools becoming thin and progressing to slime mixed with blood. Nausea, vomiting, and abdominal pain were also part of the picture. Although today, this may seem paradoxical, Holyoke prescribed emetics for the nausea and vomiting, and purging for the diarrhea. To disguise the taste of some of the remedies, he added rhubarb and "a little molasses, or the pulp of a roasted apple."

For the abdominal pain, he prescribed laudanum. He kept purging the sufferers "every day or every other day, as the patient's strength would admit, till the stools began to put on a more healthy appearance." He tried to replenish the fluid losses from the diarrheas with water gruel and large volumes of a decoction of marshmallows and comfrey roots in water or milk and water. In his essay about the 1761 epidemic, he proudly reported that "many dysenteries were cured this season, with the purge and decoction."

With the frequent smallpox epidemics, it is not surprising that Holyoke's practice was touched by this "loathsome pestilence." He also had his personal experience. In 1764, he traveled to Boston to be inoculated by Dr. Nathaniel Perkins, who was in charge of a team of physicians, including Joseph Warren and Benjamin Church, who were appointed to provide the service to the Boston population. Proper preparation was required to "reduce" the subject to be inoculated and to allow him "to receive the disease in the most favorable manner." Adhering to Perkins's instructions, Holyoke prepared himself by taking "a pill at night of five or six grains of Calomel with Antimony" and by "living low."[362] After following this regimen for a couple of days, he was ready for the inoculation. Knowing that the procedure was not without risks, he executed his will before going to Boston on April 6. After the inoculation, he was under observation until April 23, during which time he "had the disease in the most favorable manner" and was then protected from future attacks of the dreaded malady.

In the fall of 1773, Salem was hit by a new outbreak of smallpox. It was a particularly vicious epidemic in which "16 persons died of the first 28 who were attacked with it" (accounting for a death rate of almost 60 percent!). The alarming epidemic prompted inhabitants of Salem to collect money for building a hospital for inoculations. With breakneck speed, a hospital consisting of two buildings was erected in thirty days.[363] The larger of the buildings contained twelve rooms and the smaller had four. In December, the first patients were admitted to the hospital and underwent inoculation.

Holyoke was appointed chief of the hospital in 1777. He inoculated a total of about six hundred individuals, who were divided into groups of two hundred. Holyoke kept detailed records of all the subjects who were inoculated. During the period of illness, Holyoke remained in the hospital and stayed with his patients day and night. Many of his patients testified "to his assiduous and skillful attentions."

Although "only" two patients died from the inoculations, those deaths weighed heavily on Holyoke's mind and caused him so much distress that he almost abandoned the project. When vaccination replaced inoculation, Holyoke was one of the first practitioners to adopt the new method of smallpox prevention. During the first couple of years of the new century, he received vaccine directly from London through a colleague near Salem.

Holyoke and Surgery

Surgery didn't seem to be Holyoke's favorite part of his medical enterprise, and he performed relatively few surgeries with long intervals in between. Still, he was considered a competent surgeon who "had more than a mediocrity of talent and skill."[364] Like other aspects of his practice, he followed the recent literature and "as a matter of necessity held himself qualified for all the normal demands for surgical treatment." Although he had the skills to perform amputations and stone cutting (lithotomy), he performed those procedures infrequently. One reason why amputations were unusual in his practice was that accidents were uncommon among the citizens of Salem, who were "characterized by a greater degree of temperance among laboring people than existed in most large towns."[365] Indeed, people seemed to be well behaved and not much inclined to drinking: "It is believed that there are few seaports in which there is a less number of sots, in proportion to the whole population."

The rareness of bladder stones and need for stone cutting was ascribed to the "perfect purity of the water drank by inhabitants of this town." Despite the fact that bladder stones were uncommon and Holyoke probably did not perform many lithotomies, he remained interested in the subject throughout his career. After his one-hundredth birthday, he was reported to have had a detailed discussion with a colleague about a new method to treat bladder stones, lithotripsy (crushing of the stones followed by removal of the fragments through the urethra).

Although Holyoke was not a very busy surgeon, he was considered skillful and "was occasionally called upon to perform amputations, and other important operations, and in these cases his promptitude and success were such as procured him a high degree of reputation."[366] Holyoke was also considered a skillful orthopedic: "In the management of fractures he particularly excelled. No man handled a broken limb with more tenderness and adroitness."

At the time Holyoke started his practice, midwives delivered most babies in Salem. Physicians were only called to help out in "extraordinary cases." Tragically, Holyoke's first wife, Judith died in childbirth in 1756, after only one year's marriage. This prompted him to learn more about midwifery and to do more obstetric work himself, taking advantage of recent European developments in maternity care. This put him in conflict with the "ignorant midwives" in Salem who were soon outcompeted. Holyoke's obstetric practice became busy, and from 1791, he listed almost one thousand deliveries during the decade.

Marriage and Social Life

After losing his first wife in childbirth, Holyoke found a new love in Mary Viall. They were married in 1759. Mary was a merchant's daughter from Boston. Their "honeymoon" was one week of "sitting up for company." Adhering to the custom of the time, Holyoke and his bride spent a week receiving visitors and congratulations. With the exception of the time spent in Boston in conjunction with his 1764 inoculation against smallpox, this week in Boston turned out to be Holyoke's longest time away from Salem and his practice. Holyoke didn't seem to enjoy the experience too much and described it as "very tedious and irksome."[367]

The marriage with Mary produced twelve children. Most of the children died in infancy, and only two daughters survived into Holyoke's senior years. The eldest daughter, Margaret, became an increasingly important person in Holyoke's life and her father's best friend, particularly after the death of Mary in 1802. When Margaret died in 1825, Holyoke was devastated and felt "an unusual gloom upon his prospects of prolonged life." When reflecting on Margaret's death, Holyoke wrote "*Sit anima mea, tecum, filia carissima.*"

Despite his busy medical practice, Holyoke allowed himself some pleasures in life: "He now and then indulged in a party upon the water in summer." One of his favorite activities in wintertime was skating "in which exercise he was well skilled." He also enjoyed "the sober game of chess." Visiting friends and colleagues in neighboring towns were other activities that provided enjoyment.

A weekly Monday night conversation club was also something Holyoke did not miss. The purpose of these sessions was to improve philosophy and literature skills through reading and conversation. Among the members of the Monday club were some of "the most amiable and distinguished individuals who ever belonged to this town." The Monday club meetings were temporarily interrupted by the outbreak of the Revolution, and were started again in 1779.

Holyoke called himself a religious man. He studied the Bible on a regular basis, including up to his last year, and always tried to arrange his schedule to make it possible to attend church on Sundays. He gave to the poor and needy in society with a "systematic charity proportioned to his means." His gifts were always anonymous and mainly directed to widowed mothers and orphan children. Growing up with a minister father probably in part explains Holyoke's piety in adulthood.

Holyoke and Science

Holyoke kept meticulous notes of the daily events throughout most of his life, and when he died, he left behind a 120-volume diary. He was also known for keeping detailed records related to his medical practice and left behind 122 daybooks at his death.

For almost eighty years, Holyoke recorded the weather conditions on a daily basis hoping to find evidence of a connection between weather patterns and diseases.[368] A thermometer mounted on the doorpost helped him keep track of the temperature, but he also made note of wind and precipitation. Unusual weather events were recorded as well. At the age of eighty-seven, he made a detailed entry about the "September storm of 1815."[369] That year, "the months of August and September were remarkable for storms and violent tempests on the ocean." The winds caused damage a long way inland: "The blast was so violent that it blew the spray of salt water into the country 30 miles or upwards; most likely 90 miles, certainly as far as Worcester, which destroyed the verdure of the leaves upon all the trees—blew all the apples and other fruit to the ground.... We have no record of any storm equal to this, since the settlement of the country."

Holyoke was the author of the first paper of the published "Transactions of the Medical Society of Massachusetts." In that paper, he gave an "account of the state of the weather, diseases, operation of remedies, and deaths, &c. in Salem" for every month of 1786.[370] Although Holyoke was not successful in proving the connection between weather and disease, his meteorological observations illustrate his interest in science, his meticulous mind, and disciplined work habits.

Another interesting scientific endeavor was Holyoke's experiments on the cooling effects of evaporation. In detailed notes from June 1758, he described how he applied "spirit of rosemary" to the foot of a thermometer and observed how the temperature dropped from 68°F to 63°F in about five minutes. After the evaporation had stopped, the temperature started to climb and was back at 68°F in about fifteen minutes. He repeated the experiment using water or saliva instead of the spirit of rosemary and saw the same phenomenon, although this time, it was less pronounced and at a slower pace. In his report, Holyoke concluded that the experiments fully showed "that cold is somehow produced by evaporation."

Holyoke was also interested in astronomy and made observations of planets, comets, and northern lights. He reported the transit of Venus over the sun's disk in 1769, and similar observations when Mercury passed in front of the sun in 1782. In 1827, he wrote a letter to the *American Journal of Science* and described the "beautiful appearance of the heavens in the evening of August 28th, 1827, and of some prior exhibitions of the Aurora Borealis which he had witnessed." True to his passion for astronomy, he donated a twenty-eight-foot telescope to Harvard University in 1769.

The respect for Holyoke as a scientist, both in the medical field and outside, is illustrated by his involvement in some of the most prestigious organizations of the time. He was the founder of the Massachusetts Medical Society and served as its first president 1782–1784 (and was reelected to the post in 1786). Holyoke was a frequent contributor to the published transactions of the Society, the forerunner of the prestigious *New England Journal of Medicine.*

Along with prominent Patriots, such as Samuel Adams, Thomas Jefferson, and John Hancock, Holyoke was an early member of the American Academy of Arts and Sciences. The Academy was founded in

1780 and Holyoke was the third president (1814–1820), succeeding James Bowdoin (president 1780–1790) and John Adams (president 1791–1814).

Holyoke and the American Revolution

When the opposition against "taxation without representation" started to grow strong in the colonies, Holyoke initially sympathized with the sentiments. For example, in 1765, he participated in a local committee that worked for the repeal of the Stamp Act. He could not envision, however, that the protests would ultimately result in a breakaway from England, and he initially opposed the idea of a revolution. He was a good friend of Governor Hutchinson and was considered a Loyalist. This was a reason he lost some of his popularity in Salem. When the Revolution erupted, the local Patriots started to behave in a threatening way against Holyoke and his family. For safety reasons, Holyoke sent his wife and children to Nantucket, where they stayed until 1783.

Holyoke was saddened by the realization that a revolution was coming, and seeing mobs and violence in his beloved Salem. He mentioned to a member of his family "he thought he should have died, with the sense of weight and oppression at his heart."[371] Most of his friends and acquaintances favored the British side at the beginning of the Revolution. Holyoke thought that independency would ultimately be needed, but in 1775, he did not think it was yet the right time. When he saw the violence, he was concerned that the character of the people was declining into manners "which will not be reckoned among its good effects." He was also concerned "there was a falling off in domestic discipline, and a relaxation of wholesome subordination among children."[372]

Several of Holyoke's Loyalist friends decided to leave America when they saw where the winds were blowing, but that option never occurred to Holyoke. With the family tucked away on Nantucket, Holyoke hunkered down in Salem and tried to stay out of trouble as well as he could. During this difficult time, "he kept steadily occupied in his benevolent duties, and such was his prudence, his inoffensive manners, and the universal respect for his virtues, that he did not meet with so much trouble as might have been expected from the unpopularity of his opinions."

Although Holyoke tried to stay away from political involvement during this time, he, along with several other prominent citizens of Salem, signed an address in honor of Governor Hutchinson, who was about to leave the continent. In May 1775, only about a month after the battles of Lexington and Concord, the signers of the address started to get cold feet and realized it might have been a mistake to express warm feelings for Hutchinson, who was hated by the Patriots. Together with eleven other regretful individuals, Holyoke published an apology for their act. In the "Recantation of Toryism" they wrote, "now to our sorrow...[we] find ourselves mistaken."[373] Although the recantation may be considered evidence of opportunism, it also illustrates how fluid the situation was in the colonies at the start of the Revolution. It was not clear which side was going to win, and it could be dangerous to pick a side to support too early. Since Holyoke otherwise tried to stay out of the controversy, it did "not appear that his practice was ever injured."

As the Revolution continued, Holyoke probably had a true change of heart and became a believer in its cause. His 1781 charge by the legislature to organize the Massachusetts Medical Society was evidence that he had gained the trust and respect of the Patriots. His collaboration with several prominent Patriots in founding the American Academy of Arts and Sciences also shows his embrace of the ideas of the American Revolution.

How did Holyoke Manage to get to One Hundred?

Reaching the age of one hundred in the 1700s was indeed remarkable. Although affected by some expected ailments, such as loss of memory and hearing, and declining eyesight (which required reading glasses from the age of forty-five), Holyoke seemed to have retained much of his vigor and stamina up to and even beyond his one-hundredth birthday. Two months after his one-hundredth birthday, Holyoke made hospital rounds with John Warren's son, Edward, who recalled, "in October, 1828...I had the pleasure of going through the wards and offices of the Massachusetts General Hospital with him, then a hale, active man, in full possession of his faculties of mind and body, one hundred years old the 12th of August preceding."[374]

Holyoke's reputation was widespread, and people from far and wide approached him to find out his secrets for a long and productive life. In a detailed letter in response to an individual from North Carolina, written in October 1828, Holyoke described some of the reasons why he thought he had been able to age with grace.[375] The letter provided a fascinating insight into Holyoke's day-to-day living, and discussed topics that are still considered important for a long and healthy life, including exercise, diet, and sleep.

In the letter, Holyoke explained that he had exercised a lot during his life, "having from my 30th to my 80th year walked on foot (in the Practice of my Profession)—probably as many as 5 or 6 miles every day." He calculated that he had probably walked 147,825 miles during ninety-five years of his life. He also confessed that, "In early life, between 20 and 30, I used to ride on Horse back, but being often pestered by my horses slipping their Bridles I found it more convenient to walk."

With regards to eating and drinking habits, he commented that he had always been blessed with a good appetite and tolerated all types of food, the only exception being "fresh roasted Pork." He had, however, found a remedy for this problem "in the Spirit of Sal Ammoniac. Eight or Ten drops of Aqua Ammonia pura in a wine glass of Water, gives me relief after Pork, and indeed after anything else which offends my stomach."

There was one peculiarity in his diet that he thought may have contributed to his good health: "I am fond of Fruit, and have this 30 or more years daily indulged in eating freely of those of the Season, as Strawberries, Currants, Peaches, Plums, Apples, &c. which in summer and winter I eat just before Dinner." With the meal, he drank a mixture of "Good West India Rum...Good Cider" and water. After dinner, he had another glass of the same mixture while smoking his pipe. In the evening he smoked the pipe again and enjoyed another glass of rum and cider.

As an afterthought, Holyoke added a postscript to his letter and described how he had often been called up to see patients "soon after retiring to Rest" and how this had influenced his sleeping habits. In order to not have to be awakened and get out of bed, he "found it most convenient to sit to a late Hour, and thus acquired a Habit of sitting up late, which necessarily occasioned my lying in bed to a late Hour in the Morning—till 7 o'clock in Summer and 8 in Winter." Despite being a night owl, he pointed out that he had "always taken care to have a full proportion of Sleep, which I suppose has contributed to my longevity."

The End

After a long and healthy life, ailments finally started to catch up with Holyoke. When he was between ninety-seven and ninety-eight years old, he reflected on his age and health and reported that, "About 10 or 11 years ago, I found that in walking I was apt to lose my equilibrium, and sometimes to stagger like one intoxicated...this complaint gradually increased."

More recently, Holyoke had also started to experience a strange symptom: "About two months past I perceived an odd and unusual sensation in my head." He had a feeling that fluid was accumulating around his brain and that he could feel the fluctuation of this fluid when he moved his head: "When I turned in my bed, I felt as if it were a fluid flowing from the side I had been laying on, to the other side of my head." He developed a theory to explain this sensation and suggested that as the brain shrinks with age, the resulting empty space fills up with "a serous fluid [to] occupy that void." He consulted several colleagues about the symptoms and his theory, but was not able to convince anybody: "I have stated my case for several physicians, but none of them are disposed to admit of a collection of a fluid between the dura and pia mater"

A couple of months after his one-hundredth birthday, Holyoke started to experience abdominal pain and loss of appetite. The pain "destroyed his usual cheerfulness and spirits, for an hour or more of each day." He grew weaker and became bedridden. About a week before his death, Holyoke suffered a stroke with "the left side paralyzed, the right hand and arm frequently in motion, pulse hardly perceptible." Dr. Holyoke expired "at six o'clock of Tuesday, the 31st of March." He was four months shy of turning 101.

Because of Holyoke's extreme age, there was a great deal of curiosity in the medical community about what his body would look like. After his passing, an autopsy was conducted to which "all the physicians of the town were invited to attend, and most of them were present..."[376] In particular, the physicians were curious about what would be found inside their colleague's skull, considering the unusual symptoms he had reported. The findings at the autopsy were interpreted as supporting Holyoke's symptoms and theory: "Although the utmost care was taken in sawing the cranium, as soon as the saw penetrated the inner table, a transparent fluid began to flow." In addition, "The brain was very firm and dense, and the convolutions very strongly marked; the sulci were wide and deep." These changes were consistent with Holyoke's theory about a shrinking (atrophying) brain that could be expected at his age.

Of even greater interest was what was noticed inside Holyoke's abdomen: "On opening the abdomen, the stomach appeared smaller than common, and contracted about its middle, as if a band was tied round it, and at this part its coats felt solid and much thickened. On opening the stomach, it was found that its middle portion, including about a third of its extent, and making a complete circumference of the viscus, presented the appearance of schirrus, and was contracted so as hardly to admit the passage of a finger." In addition, an ulceration of the gastric mucosa was found: "About the middle of the great curvature was a superficial ulcer of an inch in diameter." Based on these findings, Holyoke most likely had a large gastric cancer (possibly a scirrhous cancer), explaining why he had suffered abdominal pain and loss of appetite towards the end of his life.

When opening the chest, his heart was found to be "of small size and without fat." The other structures of the heart, including the tricuspid and mitral valves, were also in good shape. The big vessels were without evidence of arteriosclerosis: "The descending aorta and the iliac arteries were flexible and free from ossification." His body seemed to have provided evidence for the benefits of exercise, moderate eating, and adding fruit to the menu to prevent cardiovascular disease.

Had Holyoke been able to look down on his own autopsy, he probably would have been smiling at the fact that after a long life devoted to his profession and sharing his knowledge with his fellow physicians, he was able to contribute to the education of his colleagues even after his death.

CONCLUSIONS

This work highlights the important roles played by many surgeons during the American Revolution. The ten surgeons narrated in the book have come at the exclusion of many other medical men in America at the time. The surgeons whose lives were recounted here were chosen because they were arguably the most influential doctors on the continent at the time, from a political, military, and medical standpoint. Their stories have much to teach us about different personalities and characters—some good and some not so good; the role of surgeons in the Continental Army; and the primitive conditions (at least viewed with today's eyes) surrounding the surgeries, which were horrendously painful due to the absence of anesthesia and bloody, dirty, and dangerous.

Different professions were represented among the freedom fighters going to war. In addition to soldiers and military leaders, lawyers and merchants were prominent groups among the supporters of independence. Depending on which side of the conflict they were on, the clergy used their pulpits to indoctrinate their congregants for or against the Revolution. Surgeons, although they were not high in numbers, were crucial for many aspects of the Revolution. As we have seen, some of them participated in laying the foundation for the sentiment of liberty, and worked closely with other essential Patriots during the years leading up to the Revolution. Some were early members of the Sons of Liberty. Others participated in the deliberations of the Continental Congress, and four doctors, including the famous Philadelphia surgeon, Benjamin Rush, risked their lives by signing the Declaration of Independence. Some of the surgeons were involved in economic aspects of the Revolution, and tried to punish the British for different Acts by implementing tariffs and other obstacles that made trade difficult for the Crown.

The narratives told in this book provide evidence for many heroic contributions made by surgeons. The most important example of that side of the story, of course, is the tale of Joseph Warren, who was not only a young and popular surgeon in Boston and strong leader of the political movement, but was also prepared to fight the British on the battlefield and ready to make the ultimate sacrifice. As alluded to in Joseph Warren's chapter, if he had not met a grim and untimely death at Bunker Hill, it is not impossible that today's nation capital could be named Warren DC, rather than Washington DC.

Several of the Revolutionary surgeons were also influential in the field of medical education. John Jones, the Father of American Surgery, wrote the first medical textbook published by an American. The book, *Plain Concise Practical Remarks on the Treatment of Wounds and Fractures*, was the first work on military surgery on the continent. The work would influence surgical care during the Revolution, and for years to come. It is noteworthy that although military injuries gave the surgeons ample opportunities to learn how to manage trauma, more soldiers died from disease than from war injuries during the revolution. It is also remarkable that the first three medical schools in America were founded by Revolutionary surgeons.

Apart from the violence of the war, surgeons were engaged in philanthropy and humanitarianism, reflecting the Enlightenment of the eighteenth century. Dr. Rush was fighting slavery, widespread alcoholism, and the cruel treatment of mentally ill patients. Surgeons were also involved in the fight for the general wellbeing of the population. Smallpox epidemics were regular events during the 1700s, and surgeons were instrumental in protecting the soldiers and the civilian population by performing inoculations, often risking their own lives. Washington's decision to have all soldiers in the army inoculated may have been the most singular factor allowing the revolution to succeed. With the strong support and encouragement of the Commander-in-Chief, the lack of cleanliness and sanitation among the soldiers and in hospitals was aggressively combated by some Revolutionary surgeons.

Although most of the surgeons described in the book come across as noble, there were exceptions. One surgeon, Dr. Benjamin Church, was found guilty of treason only a couple of months into the revolution. Two of the surgeons were at each other's throat for several years and ultimately faced each other at a court martial. The conflict between Doctors Shippen and Morgan involved bitter jealousy and allegations of thefts and other criminal activities, as well as medical malpractice.

Hopefully, this book will help to cast some light on an aspect of the American Revolution that has often been overlooked—the role of surgeons from a political and military standpoint as well as in the advancement of the surgical profession during the trying times of war and conflicts.

ACKNOWLEDGMENTS

To paraphrase, it takes a village to write a book. There are several people I owe a big thank you for making it possible to finish this project. First, I am indebted to my agent, Grace Freedson, who believed in my book proposal and took it on. Grace has provided me with so much valuable insight into the world of book publishing and has also given me many editorial suggestions. Most importantly, Grace found a publisher for the work, Knox Press. The publisher at Knox Press, Roger Williams, has been a delight to work with throughout the project. He has generously given me many hours of his busy life to discuss the book, the process of getting it published, and his passion for the history of the American Revolution. He has also introduced me to several historians writing about the Revolution. Special thanks to Kate Monahan, Managing Editor, who has kept me honest in keeping deadlines for the various parts of the project. I am grateful to my editors, Mara Sandroff and Janice Shay, for their professional and skillful (and detailed!) editing of the manuscript.

I also want to express my gratitude to individuals who took the time to read my manuscript and provide important feedback with critique and constructive suggestions. Some of the reviewers, including Ira Rutkow, Samuel Forman, and Stephen Fried, are proliferative writers in the fields of the American Revolution and Medical History. They gave me many invaluable comments that helped improve my work.

Last, but not least, I want to thank my wife for patiently putting up with piles of books, reprints, and other printed material, covering the floor (and "collecting dust") around my desk throughout the project. I cannot count the number of times you had to take a walk by yourself because I was "working on the book." Thanks for your never wavering love and support!

BIBLIOGRAPHY

Original Sources

Abbe, T. "The Surgery of the Revolutionary War," *Medical Record*, 84 (1913): 277–283.

Bard, John. "A case of an extra-uterine foetus," described by Mr. John Bard, surgeon at New York; in a letter to Dr. John Fothergill, and by him communicated to the society. *Medical Observations and Inquiries by a Society of Physicians in London*, 2 (March 24, 1760): 369–372.

Bard, Samuel. *A Discourse Upon the Duties of a Physician, With Some Sentiments, on the Usefulness and Necessity of a Public Hospital: Delivered Before the President and Governors of King's College, at the Commencement, Held on the 16th of May, 1769*. Carlisle, MA: Applewood Books, first published by A. & J. Robertson, New York, 1769.

Bard, Samuel. *An Enquiry Into the Nature, Cause and Cure, of the Angina Suffocativa, or, Sore Throat Distemper, as it is Commonly Called by the Inhabitants of This City and Colony*. New York: Inslee and Car, 1771.

Butterfield, L. H. (editor). *Letters of Benjamin Rush. Vol II: 1793-1813*. Published for the American Philosophical Society: Princeton University Press, 1951.

Frost, John. *Pictorial Life of George Washington: Embracing a Complete History of the Seven Years' War, the Revolutionary War, the Formation of the Federal Constitution, and the Administration of Washington.* Thomas, Philadelphia: Cowperthwait & Co,1848.

Jones, J. *Plain Concise Practical Remarks, on the Treatment of Wounds and Fractures; To which is Added, An Appendix, on Camp and Military Hospitals; Principally Designed, for the Use of young Military and Naval Surgeons, in North-America.* Philadelphia: Robert Bell, 1776.

Magoon, Elias Lyman. *The Eloquence of the Colonial and Revolutionary Times, With Sketches of Early American Statesmen and Patriots.* Cincinnati: Derby, Bradley & Co. Publishers,1847.

McVickar, John. *The Life of Samuel Bard, M.D.* Carlisle, Massachusetts: Applewood Books, originally published in 1822.

Mease, James. *The Surgical Works of the Late John Jones, M.D. ...To which are added, a Short Account of the Life of the Author. With Occasional Notes and Observations.* Philadelphia: Wrigley and Berriman, 1795.

Morgan, John. *The Journal of Dr. John Morgan of Philadelphia. From the City of Rome to the City of London, 1764; Together With a Fragment of a Journal Written at Rome, 1764, and a Biographical Sketch.* Philadelphia: J.B. Lippincott Company, printed for private circulation, 1907.

Ottley, Drewry. *The Life of John Hunter, F.R.S.* London, England: Longman, Rees, Orme, Brown, Green, and Longman, 1835.

Palmer, James F. *The Works of John Hunter, F.R.S. Volume I.* Cambridge, United Kingdom: Cambridge University Press, 2015. (First edition published by Longman, Rees, Orme, Brown Green, and Longman, London, Great Britain, 1835.)

Rush, Benjamin. *A Memorial Containing Travels Through Life or Sundry Incidents in the Life of Dr. Benjamin Rush. Born Dec. 1745 (old style) Died April 19, 1813. Written by Himself also Extracts from His Commonplace Book as well as A Short History of the Rush Family in Pennsylvania.* Published privately for the benefit of his Descendants by Louis Alexander Biddle. Lanoraie, PA, 1905.

Sparks, Jared. *The Works of Benjamin Franklin; Containing Several Political and Historical Tracts, not Included in Any Former Edition, and Many Letters Official and Private Not Hitherto Published; with Notes and a Life of the Author. Volume V.* Boston: Hilliard, Gray, and Company, 1840.

Swieten, Gerard. *The Diseases Incident to Armies. With the Method of Cure.* Translated from the original of Baron Van Swieten. Philadelphia: R. Bell, 1776.

Thacher, James. *A Military Journal During the American Revolutionary War, From 1775–1783.* Boston: Cottons & Bernard, 1827.

Thacher, James. *American Medical Biography: or Memoirs of Eminent Physicians who have Flourished in America. To which is prefixed a Succinct History of the Medical Science in the United States, from the First Settlement of the Country.* Vol. 1. Boston: Richardson & Lord and Cottons & Bernard, 1828.

Thacher, James. "John Jones, M.D." *American Medical Biography*, Vol. 1, 324–340. Boston: Richardson & Lord and Cottons & Bernard, 1828.

The Committee of the Essex South District Medical Society. *Memoir of Edward A. Holyoke* Boston: Perkins & Marvin, 1829.

Tiffany, Nina Moore. *From Colony to Commonwealth. Stories of the Revolutionary Days in Boston.* Boston: Ginn & Company, 1894.

Toner, Joseph M. *The Military Men of the Revolution.* Philadelphia: Collins Printer, 1876.

Trevelyan, George Otto. *The American Revolution by the Right Hon, Sir George Otto Trevelyan, Bart. (Author of "The Life and Letters of Lord Macaulay" and "The Early History of Charles James Fox.")* New Edition, Volume III. New Impression. London, Bombay, Calcutta, and Madras: Longmans, Green and Co., 1922.

Warren, Edward. *The Life of John Warren, M.D.: Surgeon-General During The War Of The Revolution; First Professor Of Anatomy And Surgery In Harvard College; President Of The Massachusetts Medical Society, Etc.* Boston: Noyes Holmes, and Company, 1874.

Warren, John. "Remarks on angina pectoris." New England Journal of Medicine 1:1–11,1812.

Washington, H.A. (editor). *The Writings of Thomas Jefferson: Being His Autobiography, Correspondence, Reports, Messages, Addresses, and Other Writings, Official and Private.* Vol V. New York: Derby & Jackson, 1859.

Winsor, Justin (editor). *The Memorial History of Boston, Including Suffolk County, Massachusetts. 1630-1880 In Four Volumes. Vol. III The Revolutionary Period. The Last Hundred Years.* Boston: James R. Osgood and Company, 1882.

Wistar, C. *Eulogium on Doctor William Shippen: delivered before the College of Physicians of Philadelphia, March, 1809*. Philadelphia: Thomas Dobson and Son, 1818.

Books

Adelman, J.M. *Revolutionary Networks. The Business and Politics of Printing the News, 1763-1789*. Baltimore: Johns Hopkins University Press, 2019.

Andrlik, Todd. *Reporting The Revolutionary War. Before it was History, it was News*. Naperville, Ill: Sourcebooks Inc., 2012.

Bynum, W.F., and Porter, R. (editors). *William Hunter and the Eighteenth-Century Medical World*. Cambridge, UK: Cambridge University Press, 1985.

Campbell, M, and Flis, N (eds). *William Hunter and the Anatomy of the Modern Museum*. New Haven: Yale Center for British Art,; University of Glasgow: The Huntarian; New Haven and London: Yale University Press, 2018.

Carp, Benjamin L. *Defiance of the Patriots. The Boston Tea Party & The Making of America*. New Haven, CT: Yale University Press, 2011.

Corner, Betsy Copping. *William Shippen, Jr. Pioneer in American Medical Education*. Philadelphia: American Philosophical Society, 1951.

Daughan, George C. *Lexington and Concord. The Battle Heard Round the World*. New York: W.W. Norton & Company, 2018.

Dickey, J.D. *American Demagogue. The Great Awakening and the Rise and Fall of Poplism*. New York: Pegasus Books Ltd., 2019.

Dingwall, Helen M. *A Famous and Flourishing Society. The History of the Royal College of Surgeons of Edinburgh, 1505-2005*. Edinburgh, UK: Edinburgh University Press, 2005.

Di Spigna, Christian. *Founding Martyr. The Life and Death of Dr. Joseph Warren, the American Revolution's Lost Hero*. New York: Crown, 2019.

Drury, Bob, and Clavin, Tom. *Valley Forge*. New York: Simon & Schuster, 2018.

Ellis, Harold. *A History of Surgery*. London: Greenwich Medical Media Limited, 2001.

Ellis, Joseph J. *His Excellency George Washington.* New York: Alfred A. Knopf, 2004.

Fenn, Elizabeth A. *Pox Americana. The Great Smallpox Epidemic of 1775-82.* New York: Hill and Wang, 2001.

Fisher, David. *Bill O'Reilly's Legends & Lies. The Patriots.* New York: Henry Holt and Company, 2016.

Flexner, James T. *Doctors on Horseback: Pioneers of American Medicine.* New York: Collier Books, 1962.

Forman, Samuel. *Dr. Joseph Warren. The Boston Tea Party, Bunker Hill, and the Birth of the American Liberty.* Gretna, LA: Pelican Publishing Co., 2012.

Fried, Stephen. *Rush. Revolution, Madness, and the Visionary Doctor who Became a Founding Father.* New York: Crown, 2018.

Galvin, John R. *The Minute Men. The First Fight: Myths and Realities of the American Revolution.* Washington DC: Potomac Books, 1989.

Gillett, MC. *The Army Medical Department 1775-1818.* Center of Military History, United States Army, Books Express Publishing, 2012.

Gordon, Richard. *The Alarming History of Medicine.* New York: St. Martin's Press, 1994.

Heidler, DS, and Heidler, JT. *Washington's Circle. The Creation of the President.* New York: Random House, 2015.

Ketchum, Richard M. (ed.) *History of the American Revolution.* New York: American Heritage Publishing Company, 1971.

Langguth, A.J. *Patriots – The Men Who Started the American Revolution.* New York: Simon & Schuster, 1988.

Mantel, Hilary. *The Giant, O'Brien. A Novel.* New York: Picador, Henry Holt and Company, 1998.

Moore, Wendy K. *The Knife Man. Blood, Body Snatching, and the Birth of Modern Surgery.* New York: Broadway Books, 2005.

Nagy, John A. *Dr. Benjamin Church, Spy. A Case of Espionage on the Eve of the American Revolution.* Yardley, PA: Westholme Publishing, 2013.

Nelson, Eric. *The Royalist Revolution, Monarchy and the American Founding.* Cambridge, MA: Harvard University Press, 2014.

Olson, James S. *Bathsheba's Breast: Women, Cancer, and History.* Baltimore, MD: The Johns Hopkins University Press, 2002.

O'Reilly, Bill, and Dugard, Martin. *Killing of England. The Brutal Struggle for American Independence.* New York: Henry Holt and Company, 2017.

Philbrick, Nathaniel. *Bunker Hill. A City, a Siege, a Revolution.* New York: Penguin Books, 2013.

Philbrick, Nathaniel. *In the Hurricane's Eye. The Genius of George Washington and the Victory at Yorktown.* New York: Penguin Books, 2018.

Rhodehamel, J. (ed.) *The American Revolution. Writings from the War of Independence 1775-1783.* New York: Literary Classics of the United States, Inc., 2001.

Rutkow, Ira M. *American Surgery. An Illustrated History.* Philadelphia: Lippincott-Raven, 1998.

Rutkow Ira M. *Surgery. An Illustrated History.* Mosby-Year Book, Inc., 1993.

Rutkow Ira M. *The History of Surgery in the United States, 1775-1790, Volume I. Textbooks, Monographs, and Treatises.* San Francisco: Norman Publishing, 1988.

Rutkow, Ira M. *The History of Surgery in the United States, 1775-1900, Volume II. Periodicals & Pamphlets.* San Francisco: Norman Publishing, 1992.

Saunt, Claudio. *West of the Revolution.* New York: W.W. Norton & Company, 2014.

Smithsonian. Jones, J.L. (ed.) *The American Revolution. A Visual History.* New York: Penguin Random House, DK Publishing, 2016.

Standiford, Lee. *Desperate Sons. Samuel Adams, Patrick Henry, John Hancock, and the Secret Bands of Radicals who led the Colonies to War.* New York: Harper Collins Publishers, 2012.

Uhlar, Janet. *Liberty's Martyr. The story of Dr. Joseph Warren.* Indianapolis, IN: Dog Ear Publishing, 2009.

Unger, Harlow Giles. *Dr. Benjamin Rush. The Founding Father who Healed a Wounded Nation.* New york: Da Capo Press, 2018.

Vosburgh, MB. "The disloyalty of Benjamin Church Jr.: A study of the first American Surgeon General." Cambridge, MA: The Cambridge Historical Society, 1944.

Waller, Maureen. *1700: Scenes from London Life. Four Walls Eight Windows,* New York, NY, 2000.

Zabin, Serena R. *The Boston Massacre. A Family History.* New York: Houghton Mifflin Harcourt, 2020.

Peer-reviewed articles

Able, T. "The surgery of the revolutionary war." Medical Record. *A Weekly Journal of Medicine and Surgery.* 4: 1–27, 1913.

Bell, W.J. "The court martial of Dr. William Shippen, Jr., 1780." *Journal of the History of Medicine and Allied Sciences.* 19: 218–238, 1964.

Berman, M. "Salem's physician-meteorologist: Dr. Edward A. Holyoke." *Essex Institute Historical Collections.* 122: 237–245, 1986.

Blake, J.B. "Smallpox inoculation in colonial Boston." *Journal of the History of Medicine and Allied Sciences.* 8: 284–300, 1953.

Bourne, RB. "A history of lithotomy and lithotrity." *Medical Bulletin* (Ann Arbor). 24: 344–351, 1958.

Bowen, E.A. "Shippen and Morgan and Benedict Arnold." *JAMA* 195: 186–187, 1966.

Bradford, C.H. "John Warren." *New England Journal of Medicine.* 292: 1283–1284, 1975.

Brewster, J.B. James "Thacher, M.D., of Plymouth, Mass." *Boston Medical and Surgical Journal.* 124: 571–573, 1891.

Brewster J.B. "James Thacher, M.D., of Plymouth, Mass." *Boston Medical and Surgical Journal.* 124: 595–597, 1891.

Burgdorf, W.H.C., and Hoenig, L.J. "Abigail Adams, smallpox, and the spirit of 1776." *Journal of the American Medical Association (JAMA) Dermatology.* 149: 1067, 2013.

Charles, S.T. "John Jones, American surgeon and conservative patriot." *Bulletin of Historic Medicine.* 39: 435–449, 1965.

Corner, G.W., and Goodwin, W.E. "Benjamin Franklin's bladder stone." *Journal of the History of Medicine and Allied Sciences.* 8:359-377,1953.

Craig, S.C. "John Warren (1753–1815): American surgeon, patriot, and Harvard Medical School founder." *Journal of Medical Biography.* 18: 138–147, 2010.

Dunn, P.M. "Dr. William Hunter (1718–1783) and the gravid uterus." *Archives of Disease in Childhood Fetal Neonatal* 80: F76–F77, 1999.

"John Jones (1729–1791) Physician to Washington and Franklin." *Journal of the American Medical Association* (JAMA). 202: 152–153, 1967.

Editorial. "John Morgan (1735–1789) Founder of American medical education." *Journal of the American Medical Association* (JAMA). 194: 235–236.

Ellis, H. "A history of bladder stone." *Journal of the Royal Society of Medicine.* 72: 248–251, 1979.

Graham, S.D. "Ephraim McDowell (1771–1830) The president's lithotomist." *Invest Urology* 19: 216–217, 1981.

Griesemer, A.D.; Widmann, W.D.; Forde, K.A.; and Hardy, M.A. "John Jones, M.D.: Pioneer, patriot, and founder of American surgery." *World Journal of Surgery.* 34: 605–609, 2010.

Hasselgren, P.O. "The smallpox epidemics in America in the 1700s and the role of the surgeons: Lessons to be learned during the global outbreak of Covid-19." *World Journal of Surgery.* 44: 2837–2841, 2020.

Hume, E.E. "Surgeon John Jones, US Army. Father of American surgery and author of America's first medical book." *Bulletin of the History of Medicine.* 13: 10–32, 1943.

Kimbrough, H.M. "Benjamin Franklin (1706–1790)." *Investigative and Clinical Urology.* 12: 509–510, 1975.

Kirk, N.T. "The development of amputation." *Bulletin of the Medical Library Association.* 32: 132–163, 1944.

Loughlin, K.R. "Benjamin Church: Physician, patriot, and spy." *Journal of the American College of Surgeons.* 192: 215–219, 2001.

Louis, E.D. "William Shippen's unsuccessful attempt to establish the first 'School for Physick' in the American colonies in 1762." *Journal of the History of Medicine and Allied Sciences.* 44: 218–139, 1989.

Mathiasen, H. "Mastectomy without anesthesia: the cases of Abigail Adams Smith and Fanny Burney." *American Journal of Medicine.* 124: 474-480, 2011.

Modlin, M. "A history of urinary stone." *South African Medical Journal.* 58: 652–655, 1980.

North, R.L. "Benjamin Rush, MD: assassin or beloved healer?" *Proceedings of Baylor University Medical Center.* 13: 45–49, 2000.

Peltier, L.F. "John Jones: An extraordinary American." *Surgical History.* 59: 631–635, 1966.

Rogers, B.O. "Surgery in the Revolutionary War. Contributions of John Jones, M.D. (1729–1791)." *Plastic Reconstructive Surgery* 49: 1–13, 1972.

Rutkow, I.M. "James Thacher and his Military Journal During the American Revolution." *Archives of Surgery.* 136, 837, 2001.

Scarlett, E.P. "Fair flower of Harvard (Edward Augustus Holyoke)." *Archives of Internal Medicine.* 116: 611–615, 1965.

Stark, R.B. "John Jones, M.D., 1729–1791 father of American surgery." *NY State Journal of Medicine.* 76: 1333–1338, 1976.

Tefekli, A., and Cezayirli, F. "The history of urinary stones: In parallel with civilization." *Scientific World Journal.* 2013: ID 423964, 2013.

Toledo-Pereyra, L.H. "William Shippen, JR.: Pioneer revolutionary war surgeon and father of American anatomy and midwifery." *Journal of Investigative Surgery.* 15: 183–184, 2002.

Toole, R.M. "Wilderness to Landscape Garden: The early development of Hyde Park." *The Hudson Valley Regional Review* 8: 1–35, 1991.

Wangensteen, O.H.; Smith, J.; and Wangensteen, S.D. "Some highlights in the history of amputation reflecting lessons in wound healing." *Bulletin of the History of Medicine.* 41: 97–131, 1967.

Waserman, M. "Relieving parenteral anxiety: John Warren's 1792 letter to the father of a burned child." *New England Journal of Medicine.* 299:135–136, 1978.

ENDNOTES

1   Di Spigna, C. *Founding Martyr.* 196.
2   *Boston Gazette,* October 27, 1755; *Boston Evening Post,* October 27, 1755. Quoted by Forman, S.A. Dr. Joseph Warren, 26.
3   Di Spigna, C. *Founding Martyr,* 39.
4   ibid. 46.
5   Forman, S.A. *Dr. Joseph Warren,* 35.
6   ibid. 42.
7   ibid. 52.
8   Ellis, H. *A History of Surgery;* Bourne, R.B. *A History of Lithotomy and Lithotrity.*
9   Fann, E.A. *Pox Americana.* 31–43.
10   ibid. 36.
11   ibid. 36.
12   *Boston Gazette,* March 5, 1764,.2, col. 2. Quoted by Nagy, JA. "Dr. Benjamin Church," 12.
13   Forman, S.A. *Dr. Joseph Warren,* 58; Di Spigna, C. *Founding Martyr,* 51.
14   Forman, S.A. *Dr. Joseph Warren,* 92–93.
15   ibid. 100–101.
16   *Boston Gazette,* September 10, 1764; *Boston Post Boy,* September 10, 1764. Quoted by Forman, S.A. *Dr. Joseph Warren,* 180.
17   Forman, S.A. *Dr. Joseph Warren,* 184, 243.
18   ibid. 185.
19   ibid. p185-192; Di Spigna C. *Founding Martyr.* p 139.
20   Forman, S.A. *Dr. Joseph Warren,* 139.
21   Di Spigna, C. *Founding Martyr,* 95.
22   ibid. 96.
23   Forman, S.A. *Dr. Joseph Warren,* 149.

24   Di Spigna C. *Founding Martyr*, 107.

25   ibid. 107.

26   More details about the Boston Massacre are provided in Chapter 3, Benjamin Church.

27   Zabin, S. *The Boston Massacre*, 191–221.

28   Forman, S.A. "Dr. Joseph Warren," 166; Di Spigna, C. *Founding Martyr*, 130.

29   Di Spigna, C. *Founding Martyr*, 133–134; Nagy, J.A. *Dr. Benjamin Church.* 37.

30   Forman, S.A. *Dr. Joseph Warren*, 221.

31   ibid. 224, 262.

32   Di Spigna, C. *Founding Martyr*, 146–147.

33   Forman, S.A. *Dr. Joseph Warren*, 210–212.

34   ibid. 213.

35   Di Spigna, C. *Founding Martyr*, 152.

36   Tiffany, N.M. *From Colony to Commonwealth*, 86.

37   Magoon, E.L. *The Eloquence of the Colonial and Revolutionary Times*, 39.

38   Fisher, D. *Bill O'Reilly's Legend Lies. The Patriots*, 44.

39   Forman, S.A. *Dr. Joseph Warren*, 240–243.

40   ibid. 265.

41   Captain John Parker to his minutemen, April 19, 1775. Quoted in Smithsonian. *The American Revolution*, 55.

42   Galvin, J.R. *The Minute Men*, 206.

43   Forman, S.A. *Dr. Joseph Warren*, 270.

44   Di Spigna, C. *Founding Martyr*, 179.

45   Forman, S.A. *Dr. Joseph Warren*, 291.

46   ibid. 296.

47   ibid. 297.

48   The scene described in a letter by Lt. J. Waller to a friend, June 25, 1775. Quoted by Forman, S.A. *Dr. Joseph Warren*, 301; and by Di Spigna, C. *Founding Martyr*, 186.

49   Forman, S.A. *Dr. Joseph Warren*, 306.

50   O'Reilly, B. Dugard M. *Killing England*, 22.

51   Forman, S.A. *Dr. Joseph Warren*, 307.

52   ibid. 308.

53   ibid. 309.

54   ibid. 311.

55   Edward Warren, John Warren's youngest son, published a biography of his father in 1874. Edward had published a biography of his older brother, John Collins Warren, in 1860.

56   Warren, E. *The Life of John Warren, M.D.* p 4; quoted by Forman, S.A. *Dr. Joseph Warren*, 27.

57   Warren, E. *The Life of John Warren, M.D.*, 5–6.

58 ibid. 11.
59 Craig, S.C. John Warren (1753–1815): American surgeon, patriot and Harvard Medical School founder. *J Med Biography.* 2010; 18: 138–147. 138.
60 Warren, E. *The Life of John Warren, M.D.*, 13; Craig, S.C. John Warren (1753–1815): American surgeon, patriot and Harvard Medical School founder. *J Med Biography.* 2010; 18: 138–147. 139.
61 Warren, E. *The Life of John Warren, M.D.*, 36–37.
62 ibid. 41.
63 ibid. 65.
64 Craig, S.C. John Warren (1753–1815): American surgeon, patriot and Harvard Medical School founder. *J Med Biography.* 2010; 18: 138–147. 140.
65 Warren, E. *The Life of John Warren, M.D.*, 45.
66 ibid. 46.
67 ibid. 48–49.
68 ibid. 72.
69 ibid. 77; Craig, S.C. John Warren (1753–1815): American surgeon, patriot and Harvard Medical School founder. *J Med Biography.* 2010; 18: 138147. 141.
70 Winsor, J. *The Memorial History of Boston*, 163.
71 Gillett, M.C. *The Army Medical Department 1775–1818*, 5657.
72 Warren, E. *The Life of John Warren, M.D.*, 81.
73 Gillett, M.C. *The Army Medical Department 1775–1818*, 66.
74 Warren, E. *The Life of John Warren, M.D.*, 99; quoted by Abbe T. *The Surgery of the Revolutionary War*, 8.
75 Warren, E. *The Life of John Warren, M.D.*, 103.
76 John Warren to George Washington, February 10, 1776. Quoted by Warren, E. *The Life of John Warren, M.D.*, 141–142.
77 Warren E. *The Life of John Warren, M.D.*, 161–162.
78 ibid. 164.
79 John Warren to Samuel Adams, February 13, 1778. Quoted by Warren E. *The Life of John Warren, M.D.* 196.
80 John Warren to Timothy Pickering, May 8, 1780. Quoted by Warren, E. *The Life of John Warren, M.D.*, 207. Timothy Pickering was a politician from Massachusetts, Secretary of State under George Washington and John Adams.
81 John Warren to his Excellency the Governor and the Honorable the Council of the Commonwealth of Massachusetts. Quoted by Warren, E. *The Life of John Warren, M.D.*, 193–194.
82 Warren E. *The Life of John Warren, M.D.* 236.
83 ibid. 246.
84 John Warren to the Board of Overseers (addressed to the Rev. Simeon Willard, December 3, 1782. Quoted by Warren E. *The Life of John Warren, M.D.*, 254.

85 Craig, S.C. John Warren (1753–1815): American surgeon, patriot and Harvard Medical School founder. *J Med Biography.* 2010; 18: 138–147. 145.

86 Salem Tales. Edward Augustus Holyoke, 1728–1829, Physician and Scientist. www.salemweb.com/tales/holyoke.php.

87 Warren, E. *The Life of John Warren, M.D.*, 290.

88 Rutkow, I.M. *Surgery. An Illustrated History*, 315.

89 Warren, E. *The Life of John Warren, M.D.*, 241.

90 Based on the description of the findings at the laparotomy, the patient most likely had an ovarian cystic teratoma (dermoid cysts of the ovary), a tumor originating from multi-potential cells in the ovary. The tumor commonly forms a saclike structure lined by tissue resembling skin and filled with sebaceous, cheesy material. In the tumor, different types of tissues can be found, including hair, teeth, cartilage, and bone (reflecting the ability of the multipotential tumor cells to differentiate into various tissues—what is called stem cells nowadays).

91 The history of early laparotomies in America is described in greater detail in Chapter 5 of this book.

92 Warren, E. *The Life of John Warren, M.D.*, 303–324.

93 ibid. 304.

94 ibid. 323.

95 ibid. 342–349.

96 Gillett, M.C. *The Army Medical Department 1775–1818*, 193.

97 Warren, E. *The Life of John Warren, M.D.*

98 Warren, J. *Mercurial Practice.* Quoted by Gillett MC. *The Army Medical Department 1775–1818*, 7.

99 Olson, J.S. *Jim Olson's Essay on Abigail Adams.* Sam Houston State University.

100 ibid.

101 Butterfield, L.H. *Letters of Benjamin Rush*, 1104.

102 The gruesome mastectomy performed by John Warren (with the assistance of his son John Collins) was described in vivid language by historian James Olson in Olson JS. *Jim Olson's Essay on Abigail Adams.* Sam Houston State University.

103 ibid.

104 It is remarkable that the first paper published in what would become a world premier journal, *The New England Journal of Medicine*, was authored by John Warren and was about angina pectoris: Warren J. Remarks on angina pectoris. *The New England Journal of Medicine and Surgery.* 1812; 1: 1–11.

105 Nagy, J.A. *Dr. Benjamin Church. Spy.*, xi.

106 ibid. 6.

107 ibid. 9.

108 *Boston Post-Boy,* July 2, 1759, 3. Quoted by Nagy JA. *Dr. Benjamin Church. Spy.*, 10.

109 *Massachusetts Spy,* June 10, 1773, 31. Quoted by Nagy JA. *Dr. Benjamin Church. Spy.*, 13.

[110] *Boston Gazette,* March 5, 1764, 2. Quoted by Nagy JA. *Dr. Benjamin Church. Spy.,* 12.

[111] Benjamin Church to Elbridge Gerry, September 8, 1775. Quoted by Nagy JA. *Dr. Benjamin Church. Spy.,* 13.

[112] Langguth, A.J. *Patriots—The Men Who Started the American Revolution.* Quoted by Loughlin, K.R. "Benjamin Church: Physician, patriot, and spy." *Journal of the American College of Surgery* 2001; 192: 215–219. 215.

[113] Appendix A in Nagy, J.A. *Dr. Benjamin Church. Spy.,* 162–163.

[114] Zabin, S. *The Boston Massacre.,* 191–221.

[115] Nagy, J.A. *Dr. Benjamin Church. Spy.,* 34.

[116] The Benjamin Church papers, Massachusetts Historical Society. Quoted by Loughlin, K.R. "Benjamin Church: Physician, patriot, and spy." *Journal of the American College of Surgery* 2001; 192: 215–219. 216.

[117] General Thomas Gage to Lieutenant Colonel Francis Smith ordering the march of British forces to Concord, April 18, 1775. Quoted by Nagy, J.A. *Dr. Benjamin Church. Spy.,* 64.

[118] ibid. 64.

[119] Forman, S.A. *Dr. Joseph Warren,* 248; Di Spigna, C. *Founding Martyr,* 166.

[120] Goss, E.H. *Life of Colonel Paul Revere.* 7th ed., Vol 1, 1906, 208–209. Quoted by Nagy JA. *Dr. Benjamin Church. Spy.,* 64.

[121] Benjamin Church to Thomas Gage, May 24, 1775. French, A. *General Gage's Informers,* 156–157. Quoted by Nagy, J.A. *Dr. Benjamin Church. Spy.,* 78.

[122] Nagy, J.A. *Dr. Benjamin Church. Spy.,* 53.

[123] ibid. 88.

[124] Sparks, J. *The Works of Benjamin Franklin,* 7.

[125] Nagy, J.A. *Dr. Benjamin Church. Spy.,* 40.

[126] Rachel Revere to Paul Revere, April 1775. Quoted by Nagy, J.A. *Dr. Benjamin Church. Spy.,* 69.

[127] "Major Cane," most likely Edward Cane in Boston. Edward Cane had been promoted from captain to major on July 12, 1775. Nagy, J.A. *Dr. Benjamin Church. Spy.,* 95.

[128] Appendix D in Nagy, J.A. *Dr. Benjamin Church. Spy.,* 171.

[129] Nagy, J.A. *Dr. Benjamin Church. Spy.*

[130] Appendix C in Nagy, J.A. *Dr. Benjamin Church. Spy.,* 166–168.

[131] A copy of the proceedings of the Council of War is in Appendix E in Nagy, J.A. *Dr. Benjamin Church. Spy.,* 172–173.

[132] George Washington to the Continental Congress, October 5, 1775. Quoted by Nagy, J.A. *Dr. Benjamin Church. Spy.,* 116.

[133] John Adams to James Warren, October 18, 1775. Quoted by Nagy, J.A. *Dr. Benjamin Church. Spy.,* 116.

[134] Nagy, J.A. *Dr. Benjamin Church. Spy.,* 118–119.

[135] Massachusetts House of Representatives, October 23, 1775. Quoted by Nagy, J.A. *Dr. Benjamin Church. Spy.*, 125.

[136] Nagy, J.A. *Dr. Benjamin Church. Spy.*, 128.

[137] Quoted from Church's ciphered letter, reprinted in Appendix C in Nagy, J.A. *Dr. Benjamin Church. Spy.*, 168.

[138] Nagy, J.A. *Dr. Benjamin Church. Spy.*, 137.

[139] ibid. 138.

[140] ibid. 139.

[141] ibid. 139.

[142] Duncan, Louis. *Medical Men in the American Revolution 1775–1783,* US Army Medical Department, Office of Medical History, 1931.

[143] From the Resolve of the Massachusetts House of Representatives, January 9, 1778. Quoted by Nagy, J.A. *Dr. Benjamin Church. Spy.*, 152.

[144] Church, J. *Descendents of Richard Church of Plymouth.* 1913. 97–98. Quoted by Nagy, J.A. *Dr. Benjamin Church. Spy.*, 153.

[145] McVickar, J. *The Life of Samuel Bard, M.D.*, 34.

[146] Morgan, J. *The Journal of Dr. John Morgan of Philadelphia*, 61–238.

[147] ibid. 64.

[148] ibid. 72.

[149] ibid. 147.

[150] ibid. 103.

[151] ibid. 104.

[152] ibid. 106.

[153] ibid. 151.

[154] Middleton, W.S. John Morgan, father of medical education in North America. *Annals of Medical History* 1927; 9: 13—26. Quoted by Louis, E.D. William Shippen's unsuccessful attempt to establish the first school of physic in the American colonies in 1762. *Journal of the History of Medicine and Allied Sciences,* 1989; 44: 218–239. 231.

[155] Bell, W.J. The court martial of Dr. William Shippen, Jr., 1780. *Journal of the History of Medicine and Allied Sciences,* 1964; 19: 218–238.

[156] Samuel Bard to John Bard, December 29, 1762. Quoted by McVickar, J. *The Life of Samuel Bard, M.D.*, 37–38.

[157] Morgan, J. *The Journal of Dr. John Morgan of Philadelphia*, 35.

[158] John Adams to Abigail Adams, October 20, 1775. Quoted in Morgan, J. *The Journal of Dr. John Morgan of Philadelphia*, 44–45.

[159] Nagy, J.A. *Dr. Benjamin Church. Spy.*, 118.

[160] Journals of Congress, June 12, 1779. Quoted in Morgan, J. *The Journal of Dr. John Morgan of Philadelphia*, 55-56.

161 Benjamin Rush to John Adams, October 1777. Quoted by Bell, W.J. The court martial of Dr. William Shippen, Jr., 1780. *Journal of the History of Medicine and Allied Sciences* 1964; 218–238. 223.

162 Benjamin Rush. Letters. Butterfield, L.H, (ed), Vol 1. Quoted by Bell, W.J. The court martial of Dr. William Shippen, Jr., 1780. *Journal of the History of Medicine and Allied Sciences,* 1964; 218–238. 22.

163 John Morgan to John Jay, June 15, 1779. Quoted by Bell, W.J. The court martial of Dr. William Shippen, Jr., 1780. *Journal of the History of Medicine and Allied Sciences* 1964; 218–238. 225.

164 Bell, W.J. The court martial of Dr. William Shippen, Jr., 1780. *Journal of the History of Medicine and Allied Sciences,* 1964; 218–238. 229,

165 Corner, B.C. *William Shippen, Jr. Pioneer in American Medical Education.* 1951.

166 ibid. 6.

167 William Shippen, Sr. to his brother Edward Shippen, September 2, 1757. Quoted by Corner, B.C. *William Shippen, Jr. Pioneer in American Medical Education*, 7.

168 William Shippen, Jr. to Edward Shippen, March 10, 1759. Quoted by Corner, B.C. *William Shippen, Jr. Pioneer in American Medical Education*, 8.

169 William Shippen, Jr. to Edward Shippen, March 10, 1759. Quoted by Corner, B.C. *William Shippen, Jr. Pioneer in American Medical Education*, 8.

170 Corner BC. *William Shippen, Jr. Pioneer in American Medical Education*, 11.

171 ibid. 16.

172 ibid. 16.

173 Creighton, C. *The History of Epidemics in Great Britain.* Quoted by Corner, B.C. *William Shippen, Jr. Pioneer in American Medical Education*, 41.

174 Corner, B.C. *William Shippen, Jr. Pioneer in American Medical Education*, 21.

175 Waller, M. *1700. Scenes from London Life*, 125–126.

176 Corner, B.C. *William Shippen, Jr. Pioneer in American Medical Education*, 26.

177 William Shippen, Jr. to Edward Shippen, March 10, 1759. Quoted by Corner, B.C. *William Shippen, Jr. Pioneer in American Medical Education*, 8.

178 Corner, B.C. *William Shippen, Jr. Pioneer in American Medical Education*, 15.

179 Waller, M. *1700. Scenes from London Life.* Chapter 9, Coffee-houses, Clubs, Alehouses and Taverns, 195–216.

180 Dickey, J.D. *American Demagogue*, 233; Corner, B.C. *William Shippen, Jr. Pioneer in American Medical Education*, 58.

181 Corner, B.C. *William Shippen, Jr. Pioneer in American Medical Education*, 60.

182 ibid. 59.

183 ibid. 25.

184 Horace Walpole in a letter to the Ambassador to Italy, Sir Horace Mann, August 8, 1759. Quoted by Corner, B.C. *William Shippen, Jr. Pioneer in American Medical Education*, 61.

[185] *London Gazette,* October 17, 1759. Quoted by Corner, B.C. *William Shippen, Jr. Pioneer in American Medical Education*, 63.

[186] Dingwall, H.M. *A Famous and Flourishing Society*, 54.

[187] *Caledonian Mercury,* November 20, 1725. Quoted by Dingwall, H.M. *A Famous and Flourishing Society*, 56.

[188] ibid. 112.

[189] Shippen's doctoral thesis is described in detail in Appendix I of Corner, B.C. *William Shippen, Jr. Pioneer in American Medical Education*, 127–146.

[190] Corner, B.C. *William Shippen, Jr. Pioneer in American Medical Education*, 129.

[191] ibid. 132.

[192] John Morgan to Joseph Shippen. Quoted by Corner, B.C. *William Shippen, Jr. Pioneer in American Medical Education*, 92.

[193] Corner, B.C. *William Shippen, Jr. Pioneer in American Medical Education*, 98.

[194] ibid. 99.

[195] *Pennsylvania Gazette,* November 11, 1762. Quoted by Corner, B.C. *William Shippen, Jr. Pioneer in American Medical Education*, 100.

[196] Sharf and Westcott. *History of Philadelphia.* 1884. Quoted by Corner, B.C. *William Shippen, Jr. Pioneer in American Medical Education*, 102.

[197] *Pennsylvania Gazette,* January 31, 1765. Quoted by Corner, B.C. *William Shippen, Jr. Pioneer in American Medical Education*, 104.

[198] Corner, B.C. *William Shippen, Jr. Pioneer in American Medical Education*, 105.

[199] Fried, S. *Rush*, 42; Corner, B.C. *William Shippen, Jr. Pioneer in American Medical Education*, 99.

[200] The creation of the School of Medicine at Philadelphia and the involvement of Shippen and Morgan have been described in University of Pennsylvania, Archives & Records Center (School of Medicine: Historical development, 1765–1800, www.archives.upenn.edu/histy/features/1700s/medsch.html and School of Medicine. A Brief History, www.archives.upenn.edu/histy/features/schools/med.html) and by Louis ED. William Shippen's unsuccessful attempt to establish the first "School for Physick" in the American colonies in 1762. *Journal of the History of Medicine and Allied Sciences,* 1989. 44: 218–239.

[201] Corner, B.C. *William Shippen, Jr. Pioneer in American Medical Education*, 107.

[202] William Shippen, Jr., to the Trustees of the College, September 17, 1765. Quoted by Corner, B.C. *William Shippen, Jr. Pioneer in American Medical Education*, 109–110.

[203] Bell, W.J. The court martial of Dr. William Shippen, Jr., 1780. *Journal of the History of Medicine and Allied Sciences,* 1964. 19: 218–238. 220.

[204] John Morgan to John Jay, June 15, 1779. Quoted by Bell, W.J. The court martial of Dr. William Shippen, Jr., 1780. *Journal of the History of Medicine and Allied Sciences,* 1964. 19: 218-238. 225.

205 Although the court did not find enough evidence to convict Shippen on the second charge (that he had speculated in goods required by the hospitals and bought and sold wine and sugar on his private account), the court expressed that they considered Shippen's conduct "highly improper, and justly reprehensible." Bell, W.J. The court martial of Dr. William Shippen, Jr., 1780. *Journal of the History of Medicine and Allied Sciences,* 1964. 19:218–238. 232–233.

206 A footling delivery is a delivery when one or both of the baby's feet point downward and will deliver before the rest of the body. This presentation is associated with risk of umbilical cord prolapse and impaired oxygen delivery to the baby, often resulting in hypoxic brain injury. Nowadays, a footling presentation is typically managed with caesarean section, but when that procedure is not an option, version of the fetus—rotating the baby by external manipulation or combined external and vaginal manipulation to make the head the leading part during the delivery—can be employed. A footling presentation is a dangerous situation with risks for fetal injuries and even death, and requires the attention of a highly trained and skillful obstetrician.

207 Corner, B.C. *William Shippen, Jr. Pioneer in American Medical Education,* 118–119.

208 ibid. 121.

209 ibid. 123.

210 Rush, B. *Autobiography,* 323. Quoted by Unger HG. *Dr. Benjamin Rush,* 233.

211 December 24, 1745, is the date of Rush's birth "old style," and was cited by Fried, S. *Rush. Revolution, Madness, and the Visionary Doctor Who Became a Founding Father,* 15. An excellent source of information about Benjamin Rush can be found at the University of Pennsylvania Benjamin Rush Portal created by Stephen Fried and Yen Ho at https://guides.library.upenn.edu/benjaminrush

212 January 4, 1746, is the "new style" cited by Unger, H.G. *Dr. Benjamin Rush. The Founding Father Who Healed a Wounded Nation,* xv; the difference of eleven days between the dates cited for Rush's birthday reflects the new calendar introduced by England in 1752.

213 ibid. 23.

214 ibid. 24.

215 ibid. 24.

216 ibid. 29.

217 ibid. 123.

218 ibid. 41.

219 Bengtsson, B. Founding physicks: the lives and times of the physician signers of the Charters of Freedom. *Journal of Medical Biography,* 2011, 19: 95–104.

220 Gillett, M.C. *The Army Medical Department 1775–1818,* 22.

221 Unger, H.G. *Dr. Benjamin Rush. The Founding Father Who Healed a Wounded Nation,* 47.

222 Rush, B. *Autobiography.* Quoted by Unger, H.G. *Dr. Benjamin Rush. The Founding Father Who Healed a Wounded Nation,* 56.

223 Rush, B. *A Memorial Containing Travels Through Life,* 97.

224 Quoted by Unger, H.G. *Dr. Benjamin Rush. The Founding Father Who Healed a Wounded Nation,*60.

225 Gillett, M.C. *The Army Medical Department 1775–1818,* 39.

226 The feud with Shippen and court martial are described in greater detail in *Chapter 4* of this book.

227 Trevelyan, G.O. *The American Revolution,* 180.

228 Unger, H.G. *Dr. Benjamin Rush. The Founding Father Who Healed a Wounded Nation,* 62.

229 ibid. 80.

230 Gillett, M.C. *The Army Medical Department 1775–1818,* 42.

231 Bell, W.J. The court martial of Dr. William Shippen, Jr., 1780. *Journal of the History of Medicine and Allied Sciences,* 1964.19: 218–228. 223.

232 Rush, B. *Letters.* Butterfield LH (ed). Quoted by Bell, W.J. The court martial of Dr. William Shippen, Jr., 1780. *Journal of the History of Medicine and Allied Sciences,* 1964. 19: 218–228. 223.

233 Fried, S. *Rush. Revolution, Madness, and the Visionary Doctor Who Became a Founding Father,* 264.

234 Unger, H.G. *Dr. Benjamin Rush. The Founding Father Who Healed a Wounded Nation,* 81.

235 ibid. 82.

236 See Chapter 2 for more details about Nabby's breast cancer.

237 Washington, H.A. *The Writings of Thomas Jefferson,* 107.

238 ibid. 107.

239 Unger, H.G. *Dr. Benjamin Rush. The Founding Father Who Healed a Wounded Nation,* 133–137.

240 ibid. 137.

241 Thomas Jefferson to James Madison, September 1, 1793. Quoted by Unger, H.G. *Dr. Benjamin Rush. The Founding Father Who Healed a Wounded Nation,* 140.

242 Gillett, M.C. *The Army Medical Department 1775–1818,* 2.

243 Unger, H.G. *Dr. Benjamin Rush. The Founding Father Who Healed a Wounded Nation,* 174.

244 Fried, S. *Rush. Revolution, Madness, and the Visionary Doctor Who Became a Founding Father,* 387.

245 ibid. 404.

246 Unger, H.G. *Dr. Benjamin Rush. The Founding Father Who Healed a Wounded Nation,* 217–218.

247   Unger, H.G. *Dr. Benjamin Rush. The Founding Father Who Healed a Wounded Nation,,* 235-242; Fried, S. *Rush. Revolution, Madness, and the Visionary Doctor Who Became a Founding Father,* 460.

248   McVickar, J. *The Life of Samuel Bard, M.D.,* 6–7.

249   Rutkow, I.M. Surgery. An Illustrated History, 313.

250   Fothergill, J. *Medical Observations and Inquiries of the Society of Physicians in London,* 369–372.

251   Rutkow, I.M. *Surgery. An Illustrated History,* 314. Interestingly, George Washington consulted Dr. Baynham in the fall of 1799 and sent his plowman, Tom, to Baynham because Tom was losing his eyesight due to a tumor. Tom became blind despite the surgery Baynham performed. The consultation cost Washington $10.

252   McDowell's description of the surgery was quoted in Ellis, H. *A History of Surgery,* 71.

253   McVickar, J. *The Life of Samuel Bard, M.D.,* 8.

254   ibid. 8.

255   ibid. 11.

256   ibid. 12.

257   John Bard to Samuel Bard, September 18, 1761. Quoted by McVickar, J. *The Life of Samuel Bard, M.D.,*14–15.

258   Samuel Bard to John Bard, November 28, 1761. Quoted by McVickar J. *The Life of Samuel Bard, M.D.,* 15–16.

259   McVickar, J. *The Life of Samuel Bard, M.D.,* 16.

260   Samuel Bard to his parents, April 27, 1762. Quoted by McVickar, J. *The Life of Samuel Bard, M.D.,* 20–21.

261   McVickar, J. *The Life of Samuel Bard, M.D.,* 28.

262   Samuel Bard to John Bard, July 9, 1762. Quoted by McVickar, J. *The Life of Samuel Bard, M.D.,* 25.

263   Samuel Bard to his parents, December 5, 1762. Quoted by McVickar, J. *The Life of Samuel Bard, M.D.,* 35.

264   Samuel Bard to John Bard, September 26, 1762. Quoted by McVickar, J. *The Life of Samuel Bard, M.D.,* 33–34.

265   Samuel Bard to John Bard December 29, 1762. Quoted by McVickar, J. *The Life of Samuel Bard, M.D.,* 37–38.

266   McVickar, J. *The Life of Samuel Bard, M.D.,* 74–75.

267   John Bard to Samuel Bard, January 13, 1765. Quoted by McVickar, J. *The Life of Samuel Bard, M.D.,* 63.

268   The examinations for the M.D. degree were described in detail in a letter from Samuel Bard to John Bard on May 15, 1765. Quoted by McVickar, J. *The Life of Samuel Bard, M.D.,* 68–69.

269   McVickar, J. *The Life of Samuel Bard, M.D.,* 89.

270 Samuel Bard to his parents, April 27, 1762. Quoted by McVickar, J. *The Life of Samuel Bard, M.D.*, 21.

271 Samuel Bard to John Bard, June 12, 1762. Quoted by McVickar, J. *The Life of Samuel Bard, M.D.*, 22.

272 Bard, S. *A Discourse Upon the Duties of a Physician*, 13.

273 ibid. 20–21.

274 McVickar, J. *The Life of Samuel Bard, M.D.*, 88.

275 Samuel Bard to John Bard, April 26, 1775. Quoted by McVickar, J. *The Life of Samuel Bard, M.D.*, 97–99.

276 McVickar J. *The Life of Samuel Bard, M.D.* pp 101–103.

277 Samuel Bard to Mary Bard, July 22, 1776. Quoted by McVickar. J. *The Life of Samuel Bard, M.D.*, 105.

278 McVickar, J. *The Life of Samuel Bard, M.D.*, 111.

279 McVickar, J. *The Life of Samuel Bard, M.D.*, 136; Frost, J. *Pictorial Life of George Washington*, 509; Heidler, D.S, and Heidler, J.T. *Washington's Circle*, 73; Rutkow, I.M. *Surgery. An Illustrated History*, 314. Descriptions of Washington's abscess and its treatment have appeared in many places in the literature. There are similarities, but also differences, between the various accounts. Based on a comparison of the different reports, it seems to be well established that Washington developed an abscess on his left leg (probably towards the hip region) and that it was treated by Samuel Bard, who performed an "incision and drainage" (i.e., cutting open the abscess and emptying it of pus). Because Washington had started to develop signs and symptoms of sepsis, Bard's treatment may have saved the president's life. The description of the abscess has varied between "anthrax" (referring to "cutaneous anthrax") and "large tumor" (Ellis, J.J. *His Excellency George Washington*, 190). In the strict sense of the word, "tumor" is correct since an abscess presents as a swelling, or "tumor." Some writings suggest that Samuel's father, John, was also present in Washington's sickroom during the procedure. Despite the pain Washington must have experienced, John allegedly commented, "You see how well he [Washington] bears it," and encouraged Samuel to "cut away—deeper, deeper still!"

280 Samuel Bard to Sally Bard, September 24, 1783. Quoted by McVickar, J. *The Life of Samuel Bard, M.D.*, 115.

281 Mary Bard to Mrs. Barton, January 24, 1784. Quoted by McVickar, J. *The Life of Samuel Bard, M.D.*, 121.

282 McVickar, J. *The Life of Samuel Bard, M.D.*, 150–151.

283 ibid. 158.

284 ibid. 155.

285 Stark, R.B. John Jones, M.D., 1729–1791. Father of American surgery. *N Y State Journal of Medicine*. 1976, 76: 1333–1338.

286 Thacher, J. John Jones, M.D. In Thacher J. *American Medical Biography*, 336.

287 ibid. 337.

288 Mease, J. *The Surgical Works of the Late John Jones, M.D.*, 8.

289 Mease, J. *The Surgical Works of the Late John Jones, M.D.* Quoted by Peltier, L.F. John Jones: An extraordinary American. *Surgery* 1966, 59: 631–635; and by Stark, R.B. John Jones, M.D., 1729–1791. Father of American surgery. *N Y State Journal of Medicine*. 1976, 76: 1333–1338.

290 Mease, J. *The Surgical Works of the Late John Jones, M.D.*, 10–11.

291 ibid. 11.

292 ibid. 40.

293 ibid. 40.

294 ibid. 41.

295 ibid. 14.

296 ibid. 11–12.

297 McVickar, J. *The Life of Samuel Bard, M.D.*, 89.

298 Jones, J. *Plain Concise Practical Remarks, on the Treatment of Wounds and Fractures*, 13.

299 Hume, E.H. Surgeon John Jones, US Army. Father of American surgery and author of America's first medical book. *Bulletin of the History of Medicine* 1943,13: 10–32. 18–19.

300 Mease, J. *The Surgical Works of the Late John Jones, M.D.*, 19.

301 ibid. 17.

302 Rutkow, I.M. *Surgery. An Illustrated History.*, 314.

303 Jones, J. *Plain Concise Practical Remarks, on the Treatment of Wounds and Fractures*, 3.

304 ibid. 11.

305 ibid. 12.

306 ibid. 15.

307 ibid. 17.

308 ibid. 30.

309 ibid. 34.

310 ibid. 37.

311 ibid. 78.

312 ibid. 107.

313 Mease, J. *The Surgical Works of the Late John Jones, M.D.*, 22.

314 ibid. 29.

315 Griesemer, A.D, et al. John Jones, M.D. Pioneer, patriot, and founder of American surgery. *World Journal of Surgery* 2010, 34: 605–609.

316 Mease, J. *The Surgical Works of the Late John Jones, M.D.*, 33.

317 Ellis, J.J. *His Excellency George Washington,*190.

318 Frost, J. *Pictorial Life of George Washington,* 509; Heidler, D.S, and Heidler, J.T. *Washington's Circle. The Creation of the President,* 73.

319   Mease, J. *The Surgical Works of the Late John Jones, M.D.*, 34.

320   Benjamin Rush. Diary note dated June 23, 1791. In possession of the Library Company of Philadelphia. Quoted by Charles, ST. John Jones, American surgeon and conservative patriot. *Bulletin of the History of Medicine* 1965, 39: 435–449; and by Peltier, L.F. John Jones: An extraordinary American. *Surgery* 1966, 59: 631–635.

321   Brewster, J.B. James Thacher, M.D., of Plymouth, Mass. *Boston Medical and Surgical Journal.* 1891,124:,571–573; 595–597. 572.

322   ibid. 572.

323   ibid. 572.

324   Cited by Rutkow, IM. James Thacher and his *Military Journal During the American Revolutionary War.* Archives of Surgery, 2001, 136: 837.

325   Brewster, J.B. James Thacher, M.D., of Plymouth, Mass. *Boston Medical and Surgical Journal,* 1891, 124: 571–573; 595–597; 573.

326   ibid. 595.

327   ibid. 595.

328   ibid. 596.

329   Thacher. J. *A Military Journal During the American Revolutionary War, From 1775–1783*, 14.

330   John Adams to James Thacher, September 11, 1824. Cited in Thacher, J. *A Military Journal During the American Revolutionary War, From 1775–1783*, iv.

331   Thacher, J. *A Military Journal During the American Revolutionary War, From 1775–1783*, 11.

332   ibid. 23.

333   ibid. 28.

334   ibid. 36.

335   General Howe, when detecting the cannon on Dorchester Height, directly threatening Boston. Quoted by Thacher in Thacher J. *A Military Journal During the American Revolutionary War, From 1775–1783*, 43.

336   Thacher, J. *A Military Journal During the American Revolutionary War, From 1775–178,* 54.

337   ibid. 78.

338   Thacher, J, in Thacher, J. *A Military Journal During the American Revolutionary War, From 1775–1783.* Quoted by Rutkow IM. James Thacher and his *Military Journal During the American Revolutionary War. Archives of Surgery,* 2001,136: 837.

339   Thacher, J. *A Military Journal During the American Revolutionary War, From 1775–1783*, 113.

340   Major Minnis to James Thacher. Reported in Thacher, J. *A Military Journal During the American Revolutionary War, From 1775–1783*,126.

341 Thacher, J. *A Military Journal During the American Revolutionary War, From 1775–1783*, 150.

342 ibid. 138.

343 ibid. 153.

344 ibid. 160.

345 ibid. 158.

346 ibid. 181.

347 ibid. 182.

348 ibid. 223

349 ibid. 261. Philbrick N. *In the Hurricane's Eye*, 159.

350 Thacher, J. *A Military Journal During the American Revolutionary War, From 1775–1783*, 260; Philbrick N. *In the Hurricane's Eye*, 146.

351 Philbrick, N. *In the Hurricane's Eye*, 235.

352 Thacher, J. *A Military Journal During the American Revolutionary War, From 1775–1783*. 293.

353 ibid. 315.

354 The Committee of the Essex South District Medical Society, 1829. *The Memoir of Edward. A. Holyoke*. This is a comprehensive description of Holyoke's life and career.

355 Craig, S.C. John Warren (1753–1815). American surgeon, patriot and Harvard Medical School founder. *Journal of Medical Biography*, 2010, 18: 138–147. 138.

356 Salem Tales. Edward Augustus Holyoke 1728–1829, Physician and Scientist. www.salemweb.com/tales/holyoke.php.

357 *The Memoir of Edward A. Holyoke*, 11.

358 ibid. 12.

359 Salem Tales. Edward Augustus Holyoke 1728–1829, Physician and Scientist. www.salemweb.com/tales/holyoke.php.

360 *The Memoir of Edward A. Holyoke*, 12.

361 Quoted in *The Memoir of Edward A. Holyoke*.

362 *The Memoir of Edward A. Holyoke*, 22.

363 Appendix I. *Account of the smallpox hospital, erected at Salem, 1773*. In *The Memoir of Edward A. Holyoke*, 72.

364 *The Memoir of Edward A. Holyoke*, 24.

365 ibid. 24.

366 ibid. 25.

367 ibid. 9.

368 ibid. 15; Salem Tales. Edward Augustus Holyoke 1728-1829, Physician and Scientist. www.salemweb.com/tales/holyoke.php.

369 Appendix C. *September Storm of 1815*. In *The Memoir of Edward A. Holyoke*, 61–62.

370 *The Memoir of Edward A. Holyoke*, 17.

371 ibid. 26.

372 ibid. 27.

373 Appendix N. *Recantation of Toryism, May 30, 1775.* In *The Memoir of Edward A. Holyoke,* 77.

374 Warren, E. *The Life of John Warren, M.D.,* 41. The reference to August 12th as Holyoke's birthday reflects the "new style" (after England changed the calendar) whereas August 1st, as quoted in *The Memoir of Edward A. Holyoke.,* 7, reflects the "old style." Also see endnote 212 regarding the "old style" and the "new style."

375 From Edward Holyoke to an unnamed person in Williamsville Person County, North Carolina, October 1828. Cited in *The Memoir of Edward A. Holyoke,* 39–43.

376 *The Memoir of Edward A. Holyoke,* 52–57.

INDEX

ABOUT THE AUTHOR

Dr. Hasselgren is a surgeon at the Beth Israel Deaconess Medical Center in Boston. He is the Distinguished Professor of Surgery at Harvard Medical School. He has a longstanding interest in surgical and American history.